Cancer Immunology

Immunology and Medicine Series

VOLUME 30

Series Editor:

Professor Keith Whaley, *Kuwait University, Safat, Kuwait*

The titles published in this series are listed at the end of this volume.

Cancer Immunology

Edited by

R. Adrian Robins

University of Nottingham,
Nottingham, U.K.

and

Robert C. Rees

The Nottingham Trent University,
Nottingham, U.K.

KLUWER ACADEMIC PUBLISHERS
DORDRECHT / BOSTON / LONDON

Library of Congress Cataloging-in-Publication Data is available.

ISBN 0-7923-7007-4

Published by Kluwer Academic Publishers,
P.O. Box 17, 3300 AA Dordrecht, The Netherlands.

Sold and distributed in North, Central and South America
by Kluwer Academic Publishers,
101 Philip Drive, Norwell, MA 02061, U.S.A.

In all other countries, sold and distributed
by Kluwer Academic Publishers,
P.O. Box 322, 3300 AH Dordrecht, The Netherlands.

Printed on acid-free paper

Printed in the Netherlands.

We dedicate this volume to the memory of Mike Price,
our friend, colleague and contributor to this work,
who died on the 23rd of November, 2000.

CONTENTS

Immunogenicity of tumour associated antigens
    SHAHID MIAN, R. ADRIAN ROBINS, ROBERT C. REES and
        BERNIE FOX

Recognition of human tumours: cancer/testis antigens
    ALEXEI F. KIRKIN, KARINE N. DZHANDZHUGAZYAN and
    JESPER ZEUTHEN

The immune response to oncogenic fusion proteins
    LORENA PASSONI & CARLO GAMBACORTI-PASSERINI

Anti-idiotypic vaccination
    LG DURRANT, I SPENDLOVE AND RA ROBINS

Genetically modified tumour cells for cancer immunization
    STEPHEN TODRYK, SELMAN ALI, ANGUS DALGLEISH and
        ROBERT REES

Antibody targeted therapy

delivery of radionuclides, toxins and drugs
A.   MURRAY, G. DENTON, M.R. PRICE, and A.C. PERKINS

Escape mechanisms in tumour immunity
GRAHAM PAWELEC

CONTRIBUTERS

SELMAN ALI
Department of Life Sciences,
Nottingham Trent University,
Clifton Lane,
Nottingham NG11 8NS

ANGUS DALGLEISH
Division of Oncology,
St George's Hospital Medical School,
Cranmer Terrace,
London SW17 0RE

GRAEME DENTON
Cancer Research Laboratories
School of Pharmaceutical Sciences
University of Nottingham
Nottingham NG7 2RD
UK.

LINDY G DURRANT
Division of Clinical Oncology
School of clinical Laboratory Sciences
Nottingham University Medical School
Nottingham
NG7 2UH
UK

KARINE N. DZHANDZHUGAZYAN
Department of Tumour Cell Biology,
Institute of Cancer Biology,
Danish Cancer Society,
Strandboulevarden 49,
DK-2100 Copenhagen,
Denmark.

O.J FINN
Department of Molecular Genetics
and Biochemistry,
University of Pittsburgh School of
Medicine,
Pittsburgh, PA

BERNIE FOX
Earle Chiles Research Institute
Portland
Oregan,
97213,
USA

CARLO GAMBACORTI-PASSERINI
Section of Haematology
University of Milan Medical School
San Gerardo Hospital,
Monza,
Italy

JOHN W. GREINER
Laboratory of Tumor Immunology and
Biology,
National Cancer Institute,
National Institutes of Health,
Bethesda, MD
USA

JAMES W. HODGE
Laboratory of Tumor Immunology and
Biology,
National Cancer Institute,
National Institutes of Health,
Bethesda, MD, USA

GENG LI
Department of Life Sciences,
Nottingham Trent University,
Clifton Lane,
Nottingham,
NG11 8NS
UK

STEPHEN MAN
Department of Medicine,
University of Wales College of
Medicine,
Tenovus Building,
Heath Park
Cardiff
CF14 4XX
UK

ANTOINE MÉNORET
Center for Immunotherapy of Cancer
and Infectious Diseases,
University of Connecticut School of
Medicine,
Farmington,
CT 06030,
USA.

SHAHID MIAN
Department of Life Sciences
Nottingham Trent University
Nottingham,
UK.

ANDREA MURRAY
Department of Medical Physics
Queen's Medical Centre
Nottingham NG7 2UH
UK.

ALEXEI F. KIRKIN
Department of Tumour Cell Biology,
Institute of Cancer Biology,
Danish Cancer Society,
Strandboulevarden 49,
DK-2100 Copenhagen,
Denmark.

LORENA PASSONI
Division of Experimental Oncology
Istituto Nazionale Tumori,
Milan,
Italy

GRAHAM PAWELEC
Tübingen Ageing
and Tumour Immunology Group
(TATI),
Section for Transplantation
Immunology,
Zentrum für Medizinische Forschung,
Waldhörnlestr. 22.
D-72072 Tübingen,
Germany

ALAN C. PERKINS
Department of Medical Physics
Queen's Medical Centre
Nottingham
NG7 2UH
UK.

MICHAEL PFREUNDSCHUH
Med. Klinik und Poliklinik,
Innere Medizin I,
Saarland University Medical School;
Kirrberger Str. D-6642;
Homburg
F. R. Germany

CONTRIBUTERS

MIKE R. PRICE
Cancer Research Laboratories
School of Pharmaceutical Sciences
University of Nottingham
Nottingham
NG7 2RD
UK.

ROBERT C. REES
Department of Life Sciences
Nottingham Trent University
Nottingham,
UK.

R. ADRIAN ROBINS
Division of Immunology,
Nottingham University
Queen's Medical Centre,
Nottingham,
UK.

UGUR SAHIN
Med. Klinik und Poliklinik,
Innere Medizin I,
Saarland University Medical School;
Kirrberger Str. D-6642;
Homburg
F. R. Germany

JEFFREY SCHLOM,
Laboratory of Tumor Immunology and
Biology,
National Cancer Institute,
National Institutes of Health,
Bethesda, MD
USA

M. SOARES
Department of Molecular Genetics and
Biochemistry,
University of Pittsburgh School of
Medicine, Pittsburgh, PA

IAN SPENDLOVE
Division of Clinical Oncology
School of clinical Laboratory Sciences
Nottingham University Medical School
Nottingham
NG7 2UH
UK

STEPHEN TODRYK
Division of Oncology,
St George's Hospital Medical School,
Cranmer Terrace,
London
SW17 0RE
UK

KWONG Y. TSANG
Laboratory of Tumor Immunology and
Biology,
National Cancer Institute,
National Institutes of Health,
Bethesda, MD
USA

ÖZLEM TÜRECI
Med. Klinik und Poliklinik,
Innere Medizin I,
Saarland University Medical School;
Kirrberger Str. D-6642;
Homburg
F. R. Germany

JESPER ZEUTHEN
Department of Tumour Cell Biology,
Institute of Cancer Biology,
Danish Cancer Society,
Strandboulevarden 49,
DK-2100 Copenhagen,
Denmark

1
Immunogenicity of tumour associated antigens

SHAHID MIAN, R. ADRIAN ROBINS, ROBERT C. REES and BERNIE FOX

INTRODUCTION

The continuing discovery of new tumor-associated/specific antigens, many of which are discussed in succeeding chapters in the first half of this book, document that at least some (most?) types of cancer are antigenic. Within the past five years, the number of molecular and cellular immunological techniques for identifying tumour-associated antigens has increased to such extent that over 100 distinct genes have now been associated with the transformation process. These antigens have been classified into several sub-groups and include for example proteins that are either mutated [1, 2], over-expressed [3, 4], associated with embryo-genesis [5] or differentiation [6]. They also include novel products that arise due to genetic translocations such as BCR-Abl [7, 8]. Melanoma is particularly interesting from an immunological perspective because it contains a wide spectrum of tissue-restricted proteins (e.g., MART-1, MAGE, gp100, tyrosinase, TRP-1, and TRP-2) that serve as targets of effector T cells in vitro [9-13]; see also Chapters 3 and 4. However, in vivo, adequate spontaneous activation of tumor-specific lymphocytes either does not occur or it results in inefficient tumor protection. Why tumors that are clearly antigenic are so clearly nonimmunogenic has puzzled investigators for years. Aspects of this paradox will be considered in this introductory chapter, including tolerance, antigen processing and the role of dendritic cells, and the nature of the response induced in terms of the balance between cellular immunity (Th1 type response) and antibody responses (Th2 type response).

R.A. Robins and R.C. Rees (eds.), Cancer Immunology, 1–26.

TOLERANCE

Burnett and Fenner have defined tolerance rather simply as "non-reactivity against self". If most tumor antigens are indeed self antigens, and if the tumor-bearing host must ensure "non-reactivity against self," then the host seems doomed to succumb to their cancer. This is what happens all too often to cancer patients. A broader appreciation of tolerance in the tumor-bearing host and how it affects the immune response to tumor antigens is essential to the development of therapeutic cancer vaccines. Our understanding of immunological tolerance has changed dramatically over the past decade. We now recognize a number of measures the host uses to induce tolerance and protect itself from the induction of auto-aggressive T cells. High affinity, auto-reactive T cells may be deleted centrally in the thymus while other non-deletional pathways are available for induction of tolerance in the periphery [reviewed in 14]. Functional silencing (or anergy) can occur as a consequence of T-cell stimulation by antigen and MHC in the absence of costimulation [15, 16]. Antigen-specific immune responses occur in models of tolerance, and appear to be responsible for tolerance induction by developing a non-destructive rather than a destructive immune response, a mechanism referred to as immune deviation [reviewed in 16]. These findings are consistent with the definition of tolerance proposed by Schwartz, "a physiologic state in which the immune system does not react destructively against self." Thus, the production of inefficient immune responses that are not capable of reacting destructively against self may be responsible for the poor results associated with many immunotherapies.

ANTIGEN PROCESSING

Introduction

As with all cellular proteins, tumour associated antigens are processed and degraded to 8-10 amino residue peptides via the 26S proteasome complex. The peptides are transported across the ER membrane in association with chaperone proteins and TAP where they are complexed with MHC class I for cell surface presentation [reviewed by17]. By priming the immune system to recognise cells expressing particular epitope/MHC configurations, these complexes have been shown to act as specific molecular targets for CTL mediated killing [6, 18, 19]. A fundamental and requisite component in eliciting this recognition/killing pathway against tumour cells is the activation of professional antigen presenting cells (APCs). Although B-cells and macrophages are members of this group, it is the dendritic cell that has emerged as the most potent stimulator of immune effector functions in relation to cancer immunotherapy [20].

2

Dendritic Cells

Dendritic cells have been divided into three functional classes that are based primarily upon tissue distribution. Langerhan's cells (LC) for example are found either within the skin or organs possessing mucosal linings [e.g. lungs and nasal passages;21]. Interstitial DCs reside within deeper tissues such as the liver, kidney or heart, while activated/"mature" DCs constitute the final group and represent a class of cells that have altered biochemical and physical properties to those of either the Langerhan or interstitial category [20]. "Immature" cells are known to have an excellent ability to take up antigens from the external medium, but are poor at presenting processed antigens to T-cells, whereas the reverse is true for "mature" DCs. In order to understand how DCs stimulate potent anti-tumour responses via CTL, it is necessary to understand firstly how tumour antigens are processed and presented to the immune system and secondly how accessory receptors are needed to obtain maximal T-cell activation. A summary of how DCs have been used in the clinical treatment of cancer to date will then follow.

Antigen Uptake

To fulfil their role within antigen presentation, it is an obligatory requirement for immature DCs to present antigens that have been derived from both endogenous and exogenous sources, however, it is the latter route that is probably the most common form in which a DC will encounter an antigen from a tumour cell. Endogenous and exogenous antigens are normally presented via MHC class I and class II respectively [reviewed by22], however, for externally derived antigens DCs have evolved two major mechanisms for internalising macromolecules. The first involves macro-pinocytosis and serves to endow the DC not only with an ability to sample large volumes of the external milieu and thus increase the change of coming into contact with a foreign/tumour antigen, but also to enable large soluble molecules to be internalised and presented to the immune system [23, 24]. The second mechanism involves receptor-mediated endocytosis and includes for example both the mannose [23] and Fc cell surface receptors. For proteins glycosylated with mannose, presentation of antigens was reported to be 100 fold higher, if internalisation occurred via mannose-receptor mediated endocytosis [24]. It was also suggested that the system might even function to concentrate antigens (present in low concentrations) on the cell surface [25]. This might in part explain why peptides covalently linked to mannose resulted in 100-10,000 fold greater stimulation of T-cells when compared to the same peptide devoid of sugar residues [26]. The mannose receptor is believed to be a prototypic member of a new family of proteins that recognise the "sugar pattern" coating antigens from foreign agents [27]. It is believed that these pattern recognition receptors are linked to signal transduction pathways and promote the release of cytokines when appropriately stimulated. The mannose-receptor system however, is not universally used by all DC lineages as exemplified by LC. In this scenario, it has been suggested that a reduced rate of antigen uptake/presentation may of benefit to the host, by limiting immune responses to antigens that are encountered frequently within the skin [21]. Immuno-histochemisty data would also suggest that MHC class II molecules and mannose-receptors in fact reside within separate sub-cellular compartments and that the direct transfer of antigens from receptor to MHC class II is unlikely [26, 28, 29].

In contrast to the mannose receptor system, Fc receptors are a group of membrane bound proteins that bind the Fc portion of immunoglobulins such as IgE or IgG and consequently internalise antigens indirectly [30, 31]. Although antigen binding to MHC class I and class II molecules occurs through independent routes, "cross-priming" is an apparent mechanism in which exogenous antigens can be directed into the class I loading pathway. This is known to occur for antigens that are taken up via the Fc gamma R receptor and is dependent upon the both the proteolytic activity of the 26S proteasome and ER transportation involving TAP1/TAP2 [31]. The cross-priming phenomenon is not restricted to receptor-mediated mechanisms. For instance MHC class I presentation of antigens has also been reported for proteins taken up by macropinocytosis. In this pathway, antigen presentation was also contingent upon functional 26S proteasome and TAP transporter proteins [32]. Although discrepancies have existed between in-vitro experiments as to whether cross priming does indeed require the presence of the TAP transporters, Huang et al, have reported an absolute requirement for these proteins in-vivo [33].

Recent evidence is emerging about the existence of a third receptor system involved in antigen uptake and presentation upon MHC class I. DCs have been shown to phagocytose vesicles from apoptotic cells and direct antigen processing towards the class I pathway [34]. The ability to phagocytose apoptotic cells is restricted to immature DCs that express a defined set of surface membrane receptors including for example, the alpha v beta5 integrin and CD36. Upon maturation these two receptors are specifically down regulated and the rate of phagocytosis is reduced. Macrophages are equally adept at phagocytosing apoptotic cells however, they are incapable of presenting antigens via cross priming mechanisms and it has been suggested that this unique ability of DCs is contingent upon alpha v beta5 integrin expression [35]. The inability of macrophages to cross prime antigens derived from exogenous sources was also reported by Ronchetti and colleagues [36]. Antigens that are presented via MHC class I due to cross priming have the ability to actively stimulate CD8[+] T-cells [37]. One possible explanation of how cross priming may occur is that some MHC class I molecules have the ability to enter acidic MHC class II containing compartments. Peptides generated from the degradation of exogenously derived proteins would be able to directly load onto MHC class I before trafficking to the cell surface [38].

Sources of Antigen

The need for APCs to evolve multiple types of receptor and non receptor-mediated pathways for antigen uptake and presentation has resulted primarily in response to the heterogeneity of antigens. For example a single protein antigen can be presented in a variety forms ranging from a simple unmodified form to having a complex array of glycosylated residues attached to the protein backbone. It is also possible that proteins could be presented to dendritic cells not in isolation, but as a complex with other proteins e.g. the heat shock protein family of chaperones. We have also seen that macromolecular structures such as apoptotic bodies bind to specific receptors on dendritic cells before they are engulfed and processed for antigen presentation. As a consequence therefore, the ability of a dendritic cell to mount an effective immune response against a given antigen is contingent not only upon mechanisms in place that will process an antigen regardless of the form in which it is presented, but also in having the capacity to "prioritise" or "rank" antigen potency and to use this as a measure of whether an immune response should be elicited or not. For example antigens that are presented in the form of apoptotic bodies and whose immunogeneicity is low can be made immunogenic by presenting the same apoptotic bodies in the presence of over-expressed HSPs. The same pattern has been demonstrated for peptides coated with mannose residues, in which presentation to T-cells leads to greater stimulation than those that are not. This could suggest that host antigens are often presented to DCs using particular receptor pathways and that these pathways are attenuated so as to prevent improper activation of immune responses against host derived antigens.

MATURATION OF DENDRITIC CELLS IN RESPONSE TO ANTIGEN STIMULATION

Although DCs represent the most potent activators of cell mediated immunity they do however constitute a sub-population of APCs that are present in relatively fewer numbers than their macrophage or B-cell counterparts. In addition, they are also known to be widely distributed throughout tissues which makes them difficult to isolate in large enough numbers for scientific study. To circumvent these problems, DCs have been generated in-vitro using one of either two-precursor cell sources. These include both CD34$^+$ bone marrow stem cells and circulating blood monocytes [39]. In the non-activated or "immature" state, DCs have an extreme proficiency for taking in and degrading exogenously derived antigens however, in order to stimulate a specific immune response towards these antigens it is mandatory for the cell to "mature". The process of maturation is tightly regulated and associated with a specific alteration in function that involves the cell down regulating its ability to engulf/process antigens and up regulating its antigen presentation capacity [39]. There is also a concomitant reduction in MHC class II containing intracellular compartments and an increase in expression of a well-defined set of cell surface markers. These include for example CD1, CD83, Ox40L, CD40, CD80 (B7.1), CD86 (B7.2), as well as an up-regulation of MHC class I and MHC class II [39, 40]. In-vitro DC maturation has been achieved through the use of a number of cytokine "cocktails" depending upon the progenitor cell. Although bone marrow derived DCs have been used in experimental systems for studying a diverse range of immunological functions, human gene therapy experiments have initially concentrated upon using monocyte derived DCs due to the ease of isolating large numbers of cells (discussed below). Monocytes incubated in the presence of GM-CSF and IL-13 for several days are known to alter their morphology/cytology and adopt DC like characteristics including the expression of CD1a and increased MHC trafficking to the plasma membrane [41].

5

Maturation Stimuli

To gain further understanding of the maturation process and to obtain maximal CD4$^+$ T-cell stimulation in response to antigen priming Cella and colleagues conducted studies that assessed the expression kinetics of MHC class II in both immature and mature DC. It was observed that in the immature state, DCs were constantly recycling MHC class II from the surface into highly acidic intracellular endosome type compartments. The half-life of membrane bound MHC class II molecules was noted to be approximately 10 hours. However exposure to inflammatory stimuli resulted not only in an increased rate of gene expression for MHC class II but it also led to a half-life extension of 100 hours for surface bound molecules [42]. DCs are extremely proficient at presenting antigens to T-cells from macromolecular structures such as viruses. In a specific example involving the influenza virus, DC maturation was stimulated both as a direct response to viral infection and as a result of the presence of double stranded RNA. Type I interferon and MxA were shown to be directly up regulated in response to infection and it was suggested a combinatorial effect had occurred that enabled the DC not only to resist the cytopathic effect of the virus (and hence prevent its early demise) but also to augment its overall antigen presenting capabilities [43].

DCs can also be activated in response to "normal" physiological stimuli such as the deletion of cells via apoptosis. This form of programmed cell death is considered the usual route in which cells are removed from tissues upon completing their lifespan [44-46]. There is now an accumulation of evidence suggesting that DCs are capable of taking up apoptotic vesicles through a specific set of receptors [34] and presenting antigens derived from them directly to either CD8$^+$ [35] or CD4$^+$ T-cells. A number of studies have been conducted to assess the relative immunogenicity of apoptotic bodies taken up by DCs and current data would suggest that apoptotic bodies are in fact poor immune activators of DCs [36]. Activation of DCs could only be achieved in the presence of large numbers of apoptotic bodies suggesting that the degree of activation was directly proportional to the number of cells undergoing apoptosis [47]. From a physiological point of view therefore, these data lead to the hypothesis that DCs are unable to activate immune responses against tissues undergoing normal cellular turnover as they produce only low numbers of "poorly" immunogenic apoptotic bodies. An accumulation of these apoptotic bodies above a normal physiological threshold would consequently lead to an effective stimulation of DCs and thus alert the immune system to perturbations occurring in cellular turnover. Maturation of DCs in response to an apoptotic stimulus would result in the presentation of host tissue antigens to the immune system in the absence of activating inflammatory stimuli or "danger signals" [47].

"Danger signals"

The idea of "danger signals" was first developed by Matzinger who suggested that the immune system does not actually discriminate between self and non-self antigens but instead responds to inflammatory stimuli as a means of detecting abnormalities (e.g. microbial infections) within the host [48]. This hypothesis has begun to gain a huge momentum in the field of cancer immunology both in terms of the rational design of cancer "vaccines" and in the manner they would be administered clinically to patients. It is now believed that the immune system is not "actively" engaged in looking for abnormal tumour cells as was once thought, but instead is "ignorant" of them until an appropriate stimulus is received [48]. The critical factor therefore as to whether an immune response will be augmented against a particular antigen, is not whether it is "self" or "non-self" but instead whether an appropriate co-stimulatory signal is also expressed at the time of antigen presentation [48]. These appropriate or "danger signals" can arrive in multiple forms and include for example viruses, lipo-polysaccharide (LPS), cytokine release and necrotic cell death [49]. With respect to the latter it has been shown that DCs have the ability to take up necrotic as well as apoptotic bodies, however, only cells dying by necrotic means have the ability to stimulate DC maturation [49]. Perhaps the most notable members of this group, the heat shock family of proteins (HSPs) [50-54]. The HSP family of proteins have received a great deal of attention as key candidate molecules mediating the "danger signal". Heat shock proteins are discussed in greater detail by A. Menoret (Chapter 10) and consequently, only a brief overview of their function will be conducted here.

HSPs are molecular chaperones that have been implicated in a number of physiological processes ranging from protein folding and transport to the binding of intracellular peptides. Moreover, these proteins are considered as excellent candidates for mediating "danger signals" to DCs as they have an intracellular location under normal physiological circumstances and are only released upon cellular damage [50]. An increase in cellular stress is believed to result in the activation of HSP gene expression ultimately leading to an accumulation of protein [55]. HSPs have been shown to confer resistance to inflammatory cytokines such as TNF alpha and consequently they decrease a cell's likelihood of being killed by external agents [51]. In addition to having a direct effect upon cell survival, HSPs are also known to bind peptides that can be directly transferred to MHC class I molecules for antigen presentation [52, 56]. In a series of elegant studies Suto and colleagues were able to show that heat shock proteins complexed to antigenic peptides could be taken up by antigen presenting cells and transfer their peptides directly to MHC class I for T-cell presentation [57]. It was intimated therefore that in conditions of stress tumour cells might also release peptide bound HSPs that could be taken up by surrounding APCs for T-cell presentation. In-vivo tumour models have been extremely informative about the mechanism of HSP-peptide cross presentation to CD8$^+$ T-cells. In one specific example HSPs were isolated from syngeneic tumour cells and used in a prophylactic immunisation regime to protect against a lethal challenge of tumour cells. Protection occurred only when HSPs were peptide bound and that the peptides were derived from the same tumour type as the challenge. No protection was observed if the HSPs were stripped of tumour peptides, or if the peptides were administered in isolation [52]. This would support the contention that it was the peptide component that was providing a specific immune target for T-cell recognition and the HSP was critical for directing the peptide into the appropriate MHC trafficking pathways [52, 58]. In a recent finding by Todryk et al. inducing HSP 70 expression in tumour cells was found to lead to an increased infiltrate of macrophages, T-cells and DCs within the tumour mass and that immature DCs had the ability to directly take up HSP/peptide complexes and present them to T-cells through cross priming mechanisms [51].

Heat Shock Proteins

It is suggested that heat shock proteins might represent one category of immune modulators possessing the requisite components for mediating "danger signals" to DCs possibly through antigen cross priming. This would not seem unreasonable since HSPs are known to bind peptides in a non-sequence dependent manner and are thus capable of providing an antigenic source. In addition it is now known that these proteins are taken into cells via receptor-mediated endocytosis which might suggest that a functional role in immuno-stimulation has evolved. It might also be implied that under normal physiological conditions, cell death via apoptosis would not lead to immune activation as apoptotic bodies are weakly immunogenic. This is clearly a favourable situation for the host organism and serves to attenuate immune activation for processes that are occurring constantly. If however, a cell becomes stressed due to a change in environmental conditions (e.g. anoxia) and induces the expression of HSPs to counteract these effects, apoptotic bodies produced from these cells (hence accumulating HSPs) would consequently be highly immunogenic. Conditions or stimuli producing large-scale apoptosis in the absence of HSP expression/inflammatory stimuli might also be a situation in which DC activation and maturation could occur.

Co-Stimulatory Molecules

The maturation of DCs is not simply confined to processes involved in optimal antigen presentation to T-cells. For effective T-cell stimulation to occur at the time of antigen presentation, it is necessary to have the simultaneous expression of several cell surface receptors or "costimulatory" molecules. In the absence of these co-stimulators, antigen presentation to T-cells is believed to result in either tolerance or clonal deletion [reviewed by 59]. A number of costimulatory molecules have been identified and their role in T/dendritic cell activation has been elucidated. They include for example B7, CD40 and OX40. While B7 has been extensively studied in relation to its ability to stimulate T-cell activity [reviewed by 60], it is the latter two receptor/ligand systems that have begun to generate a great deal of interest. These are discussed below:

CD40

The ability to cross prime antigens derived from exogenous sources is an extremely powerful means by which DC are able to present antigens to both CD8$^+$ and CD4$^+$ T-cells. Although CTL are the main effector cells for antigen recognition and killing, it has been demonstrated that to cross prime and activate CD8$^+$ T-cells, CD4$^+$ T-cell activation is mandatory [32, 37]. The co-operation between CD4$^+$ T-helper cells and CD8$^+$ CTL has now been shown to occur indirectly, via an intermediary activation of dendritic cells. In this model, antigen recognition by both T-cell subsets is believed to occur upon the same DC via activation of the CD40 receptor (a member of the TNFR super-family) thus obviating the need for direct CD8$^+$/CD4$^+$ interaction [61]. CD40L is up regulated on activated T-helper cells and the binding of ligand to its cognate receptor on DCs is believed to be sufficient to "condition" the DC, promoting both maturation and presentation of co-stimulatory/ accessory molecules. In this state the DC is capable of directly priming naïve T-cells without further involvement of antigen specific T-helper cells [62]. Inhibiting CD40L interactions on DCs is sufficient to abolish CTL activation. The need for "specific" T-cell mediated help has been overcome through the use of antibodies that target CD40 receptors directly and it has been suggested that antibodies used in this manner could have significant value in the therapeutic treatment of cancer [63]. Ligation of the CD40 receptor is known to result in the production of several inflammatory cytokines including TNF-alpha, IL1-beta, IFN-gamma and IL-12. Except for IL-12, antibody depletion studies were shown to have little/no effect upon the DC maturation process and it was suggested that IL-12 release following CD40 ligation served to enhance DC maturation processes [64].

OX40

Another co-stimulatory receptor-ligand complex involved in T-cell activation by dendritic cells is OX40L (a member of the TNF family of proteins). OX40L is present on the surface of dendritic cells and binding to its cognate receptor on CD4$^+$ T-cells results in their cellular activation. Increased cytokine production for TNF alpha, IL-12, IL-1 beta and IL-6 have been reported [65]. In addition CD80 (B7.1), CD86 (B7.2), CD54 and CD40 expression were augmented to levels sufficient for T-cell activation [65]. The functional significance of up-regulating CD40 expression on DCs, would be to ensure maximal stimulation via CD40L and thus lead to full DC maturation. To gain a better understanding of OX40-OX40L interactions between T-cells and APCs, Gramaglia and co-workers engineered artificial APCs transfected with OX40L and/or B7.1 co-stimulatory molecules and studied T-cell proliferative responses. CD4$^+$ T-cells stimulated with antigen alone were able to produce OX40 for approximately two to three days post exposure after which a decline in receptor expression was noted. For APCs expressing OX40L in isolation, only a weak stimulation of IL-2 release was noted, however for OX40L$^+$ cells expressing the co-stimulatory molecule B7.1, CD4$^+$ T-cells were induced to proliferate and to secrete large amounts of IL-2. These authors suggested that OX40-OX40L interactions serve to prolong T-cell proliferation, enhance cytokine production and could even have a role in producing long-term memory CD4$^+$ cells [66]. OX40L has been implicated in a number of other roles including T-cell homing and B-cell activation. In a recent publication by Chen et al., [67] OX40L knockout mice were studied to address specific questions in relation to its function as a co-stimulatory molecule. OX40L -/- mice were deficient in contact hypersensitivity responses due an inability to correctly stimulate T-helper cells. These mice did not however, exhibit inappropriate T-cell homing or defective humoral immune responses. In-vitro, dendritic cells obtained from these knockout mice were unable to stimulate T-cell cytokine production and as a result OX40L was implicated as a co-stimulatory molecule necessary for dendritic/T-cell interactions. In parallel studies conducted by Kopf and colleagues [68], OX40 receptor knockout mice were generated and the formation of both extrafollicular plasma cells and antibody responses were measured. No perturbations were detected for either of these processes and consequently were

9

considered to be independent of OX40 involvement. The generation of primary and memory cytotoxic T-cells in response to viral infection were not affected either, however, the number of IFN-gamma producing CD4$^+$ T-cells was greatly reduced as were the number of CD4$^+$ cells infiltrating lung tissue following viral infection. The authors concluded that OX40 had a pivotal role in generating optimal CD4$^+$ responses in-vivo.

Th1 and Th2 cytokine release in response to DC maturation following antigen stimulation

The type of immune response elicited by a DC is of crucial importance in determining whether effective anti-tumour immune cells are mobilised [69, 70]. As outlined previously, DCs have the ability to take in, process and present antigens to both CD4$^+$ and CD8$^+$ T-cells through cross priming mechanisms. Following an up-regulation of requisite co-stimulatory molecules, T-cells become and activated and induced to proliferate in an antigen specific manner. What is becoming evident however, is that helper responses are not generic in nature, but are instead polarised between either Th1 associated cytokines such as IL-2, IL-12, IFN-gamma or Th2 associated e.g. IL-4 and IL-10. Th1 cytokines lead to the activation and proliferation of CTL, NK cells and the production of IgG2a isotype specific antibodies. In contrast, Th2 cytokines elicit B-cell activation and the production of IgG1 associated antibodies in the absence of substantial CD8$^+$ CTL activation. There is mounting evidence to suggest that the cytokine profile associated with a tumour might indeed have a strong bearing on the clinical outcome; this is considered in more detail in the context of experimental models in section 5 below.

In the clinical context, a similar trend has been bserved. For example, it was noted in 10 tumour biopsies taken from patients with SCLC, that high levels of IL-4, IL-6, IL-10 and TGF-beta1 were expressed in tumour infiltrating lymphocytes while IL-2 mRNA expression was low [70]. Th1 (IL-2, IFN-γ) and Th2 associated cytokine release (IL-4, IL-6 and IL-10) was measured from mitogen activated PBMCs derived from patients possessing bladder, prostate or renal cell carcinomas. It was found that the levels of Th1 cytokine secretion were drastically reduced in comparison to age matched controls and the suggestion was made that there is not a concerted shift from Th1 to Th2 but rather that the Th1 cytokine cascade is not functioning correctly [71]. The ratio of Th1:Th2 cytokine expression has also been determined in tumour samples from patients diagnosed with non-SCLC. It was found that a higher Th1 ratio was associated with patients with operable tumours while the converse was true for patients with recurring tumours [69].

Cancer patients often produce antibody responses against the tumour and this has often been looked upon as a favourable sign, but other authors would suggest that an antibody response might actually favour tumour growth [72]. With a deeper understanding of how cytokines polarise immune responses, one might envisage a scenario in which the activation of Th1 associated cytokines is mandatory for the effective eradication of tumours. Shifting the balance towards Th2 and therefore predominantly an antibody response would ultimately result in the attenuation of CTL and NK responses. If Th2 responses favour tumour growth, one might even speculate that the ability to actively subvert the immune system towards a Th2 immune response could indeed provide a distinct survival advantage for a tumour.

Summary of DC properties

To elicit effective ant-tumour responses it is necessary to activate and mobilise T-cells capable of recognising tumour-associated antigens. In order to achieve this goal, co-stimulatory molecules must be present on DCs at the time of antigen presentation as these receptors serve to enhance T-cell function and thus home their ability to recognise and kill target cells. CD40/CD40L and OX40/OX40L interactions serve to enhance the maturation of DCs making them effective antigen-dependent stimulators of CD8$^+$ T-cells. In this context, T-cells are activated and not tolerised to MHC restricted tumour antigens. Another important consideration is not simply whether an immune response is elicited against a tumour antigen but whether the immune response is primarily CTL and not antibody based. For this to occur therefore, it is necessary to favour the development of Th1 cytokine cascades (IL-2, IL-12, IFN-γ) over those stimulating T-helper cells to release Th2 associated cytokines (IL-4, IL-5, IL-10, and IL-13).

Type 1 and Type 2 tumour immune responses

It is now generally accepted that both T helper (Th) cells and T cytotoxic (Tc) cells can be segregated into two general categories based on their cytokine release patterns [73-76]. A type 1 cell (T1) selectively secretes IL-2, IFNγ and TNFβ/LT, whereas type 2 cells (T2) secrete IL-4, 6, 9 and 13. IL-5 and 10, generally thought of as T2 cytokines can be more promiscuous and also found associated with cells of a T1 phenotype. All of these cells appear to share a common precursor that can differentiate along either pathway. The final pathway is determined by the cytokine milieu in which the T cells are activated and undergo differentiation [77]. The presence of T1 or T2 cytokines, will drive uncommitted T cells to develop a cytokine profile similar to that which they are exposed, while at the same time inhibiting the development of cells with the reciprocal phenotype. Thus, IFNγ selectively expands T1 cells and inhibits proliferation of T2 cells, while IL-4 and IL-10, can selectively inhibit cytokine secretion by T1 cells [75, 78, 79]. This ability to inhibit the maturation of cells producing cytokines of the alternate type may account for the tendency to see a predominant cytokine profile. Therefore, the presence of T2 cytokines during the initial interaction between the T cell and tumor antigen presented by APC in the draining lymph node would facilitate the development of a T2 antitumor response. This could be caused by secretion of T2 cytokines by tumor cells, by secretion of IL-4 by NK1.1 T cells, or by IL-6 secreted from APC, [75, 80-84]. The secretion of IFNγ by NK cells or IL-12 by APC acts reciprocally and would be expected to activate T1 and inhibit T2 cells [75, 84-86].

Exposure to antigen in the absence of costimulation also induces T2 responses [87, 88]. This in turn blocks the release of IL-12 by dendritic cells, inhibits production of T1 cells and allows T2 responses to be established. The dose of antigen used to sensitize T cells also affects the type of cytokine response. High concentrations lead to a predominant T1 response in CD4 cells, whereas low doses of antigen promote differentiation of predominantly T2 cells that produce high levels of IL-4 [reviewed in 87, 89]. A T2 profile also may develop as the default response if antigen is presented to T cells in the absence of inflammatory cytokines.

The importance of T1 or T2 responses in the pathogenesis and control of a number of diseases has been reviewed [75]. T1 responses protect or cure animals infected by protozoa, bacteria or fungi and appear to cause the destruction observed in transplant rejection and in the following autoimmune diseases: EAE, multiple sclerosis, psoriasis vulgaris, insulin-dependent diabetes mellitus, and rheumatoid and reactive arthritis. In contrast, T2 responses appear to be important in models where helminths are studied, and causative for allergic reactions, including atopic asthma and Omenn's syndrome.

The differential effects of T1 and T2 responses in tumor-bearing animals has only been appreciated recently. [90, 91]. Aruga et al demonstrated that the efficacy of T cells in an adoptive transfer model could be abrogated by neutralizing Mabs to IFNγ and GM-CSF, and augmented by treatment with anti-IL-10 [91]. Examining the effect of IL-12 administration on cytokine production at the tumor site in the same murine tumor model found that tumors from untreated mice had a rim of CD3+ T cells associated with production of IL-2, 4 and 10 (T2 response), but no IFN-γ [90]. However, tumors from IL-12 treated mice, exhibited high levels of IFN-γ production (T1 response) while IL-2, 4, and 10 production was decreased. This suggests that the balance between the production of T1 and T2 cytokines is a key determinant of whether or not a therapeutic effect is seen.

Using a B-cell lymphoma model, Lee and colleagues have reported that a cytotoxic T-cell immune response could be elicited in animals susceptible to tumour growth and that the response was rapid, being detected as early as 4 days post-challenge. The difference between resistant and susceptible animals was attributed to the type of helper responses being produced in the former group. It was found that Th1 cytokines were preferentially being secreted and that CTL development was stronger and earlier in the resistant group of animals [92]. It is known that antigen presentation can occur through DCs, macrophages or B-cells and the extent to which one particular population of cells might be recruited to present antigen has been speculated to play a role in the process of tumour progression. Qin et al. have reported that animals devoid of B-cells were resistant to tumour challenge and that their re-introduction resulted in sub-optimal helper responses for stimulating CTL activity.

This concept is supported by two further clinical studies in which T1 responses were associated with tumor regression. Kawakami et al, noted higher response rates in patients treated with tumor-infiltrating lymphocytes (TIL) exhibiting gp100-specific IFN-γ production, and Lowes et.al. demonstrated that mRNA levels for T1 cytokines were significantly higher in spontaneously regressing melanomas compared to progressing lesions [13, 93]. These data support the hypothesis that induction of a T1 response is necessary for tumor regression and that type 2 responses are either ineffective or potentially harmful because of their ability to inhibit T1 responses.

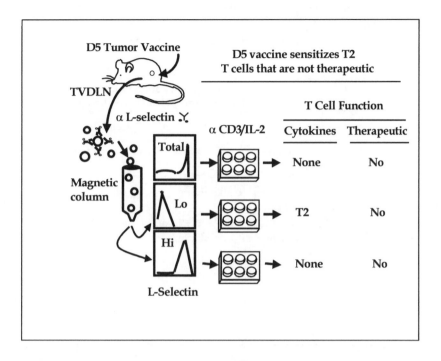

Figure 1.1. Day 7 D5-TVDLN were harvested and T cells isolated and labeled with anti-L-selectin magnetic beads. T cells were separated by passage over a magnetic column, into populations expressing low or high levels of L-selectin. These cells were activated with anti-CD3 for 2 days and expanded in low dose IL-2 for 3 more days. T cells were then assayed for tumor-specific cytokine secretion and adoptively transferred into mice bearing 3 day established pulmonary metastases.

However, it is generally accepted that the failure of vaccination with poorly/non immunogenic tumors to protect the host from a subsequent tumor challenge is because the host fails to generate an antitumor immune response.

Recent data from Hu and colleagues demonstrate that this scenario is not true for the poorly immunogenic B16BL6-D5 tumor. They used a method pioneered by Kagamu et al., to isolate tumor-reactive T cells [94]. This method exploits the observation that T cells responding to antigen in tumor vaccine draining lymph nodes (TVDLN) will down regulate expression of L-selectin (CD62L), a well established marker of recently activated T cells [95-99]. Kagamu isolated T cells with reduced expression of L-selectin (L-selectin^{LO}) from lymph nodes draining an immunogenic sarcoma and documented that all the therapeutic activity was confined to the T cells with the L-selectin^{LO} phenotype [94].

Based on these studies, Hu and colleagues examined lymph nodes draining the poorly immunogenic melanoma, B16BL6-D5 (D5), and observed reduced expression of L-selectin, suggesting that T cells were responding to the tumor vaccine [100]. They then used the same approach used by Kagamu et al., to see if the enriched population of potentially tumor-reactive T cells would mediate tumor regression in an adoptive transfer model (Figure 1.1).

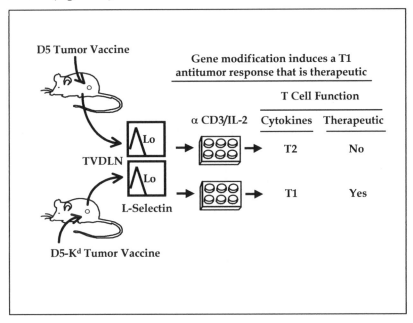

Figure 1.2. Day 7 TVDLN were harvested from mice vaccinated with either D5 or the allo-modified (D5-K^d) vaccine and T cells were separated, by passage over a magnetic column, into populations expressing low levels of L-selectin (L-selectin^{LO}). These cells were activated with anti-CD3, expanded in IL-2, and assayed for antitumor activity as described in figure 1. Effector T cells generated from the D5 vaccine exhibited a tumor-specific T2 cytokine profile and were non therapeutic, while effector cells generated from the D5-K^d vaccine exhibited a tumor-specific T1 cytokine profile and mediated tumor regression.

Although L-selectin$^{Lo/-}$ T cells were not therapeutic in vivo, they exhibited a strong tumor-specific cytokine response to stimulation with D5 tumor in vitro; the dominant cytokines produced were type 2; IL-4 and IL-10. These results demonstrated that T cells in lymph nodes draining the poorly immunogenic tumor were not ignoring the tumor, but were specifically responding to tumor with a T2 cytokine response. The reason that this observation had not been made previously probably relates to the requirement to enrich for tumor-specific (L-selectin^{LO}) T cells in order to identify the low level of tumor-specific IL-4 secretion.

Hu and colleagues, then directly compared the L-selectin^{LO} TVDLN from mice vaccinated with both the non therapeutic (D5) and the therapeutic (D5-K^d) vaccine [100]. T cells from either vaccine were phenotypically identical, but while non therapeutic T cells exhibited a tumor-specific T2 response, therapeutic T cells made a T1 response (Figure 1.2).

While these data support the hypothesis that immune deviation occurs following exposure to D5, they do not offer proof that immune deviation is responsible for the failure of vaccination. To directly test this possibility they next examined whether it was possible to polarize D5 primed TVDLN away from a T2 profile and towards a T1 cytokine profile. Adding neutralizing anti-IL-4 Mab and a source of IL-12 to the culture media during the in vitro activation and expansion of D5 TVDLN T cells they were able to polarize tumor-specific T cells to a T1 cytokine profile (Hu et al., manuscript in preparation). Coincident with this "repolarization" the T1 T cells aquired therapeutic activity while the tumor-specific T2 cells did not (Figure 1.3).

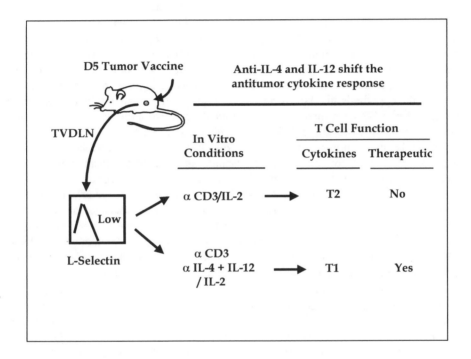

Figure 1.3. L-selectin[LO] T cells were isolated from day 7 D5-TVDLN. Half the cells were cultured as described above and the remainder were cultured similarly, but with the addition of a neutralizing anti-IL-4 and a source of IL-12 during the anti-CD3 activation step. While the standard anti-CD3 and IL-2 culture generated T cells with a tumor-specific T2 cytokine response that were not therapeutic, the T1 promoting culture generated T cells with a dominant tumor-specific T1 cytokine response that mediated significant tumor destruction.

These results beg the question: Do animals that are vaccinated with other poorly/non immunogenic tumors recognize them and make a T2 immune response that is non destructive? Do immunogenic tumors prime a T1 response? Before you can ask this question it is important to have a standard definition and understanding of the term "immunogenicity". In tumor models, immunogenicity is functionally defined by whether vaccination with irradiated unmodified tumor provides protection from a subsequent challenge with a dose of viable tumor cells that will uniformly generate tumors in naïve mice. Since the dose of tumor cells used for vaccination can make a major difference in the efficacy of the vaccine, 10^7 cells given 10,000 rads are routinely used [100]. Since the timing and dose of tumor cells used to challenge can substantially effect vaccine efficacy, mice are generally challenged with two to five times the TD100 (lowest dose of cells that form tumors in 100 % of naïve animals) 14 days following vaccination. Using this method, vaccination with poorly immunogenic or non-immunogenic tumors will not protect any animals from a tumor challenge, while vaccination with weakly immunogenic tumors will protect 20-40 percent of animals from a tumor challenge. In contrast, vaccination with strongly immunogenic tumors will uniformly protect 90 to 100 percent of animals from a tumor challenge.

To determine how generalizable this T1/T2 paradigm might be for predicting immunogenicity, a panel of murine tumors were analyzed to see if a correlation could be drawn between induction of a T1 response to vaccination and protection from a tumor challenge. The data presented in table 1.1 summarizes a series of experiments and supports the hypothesis that poorly/non immunogenic and weakly immunogenic tumors induce either a T2 or a mixed T1-T2 response while strongly immunogenic tumors induce a dominant T1 response (Winter et al., manuscript in preparation).

While these preliminary findings document a strong correlation between induction of a T1 antitumor immune response and vaccine efficacy, others have documented T2 effector mechanisms that can mediate tumor regression [101-103]. Clearly, additional studies will need to evaluate how these tumor-specific T2 cytokine responses, generated in mice with cytokine transduced tumor vaccines or using TCR transgenic T cells, will compare to the correlation we have made between the primary response to tumor vaccination and the ability to induce protective immunity. It is likely that different mechanisms will mediate tumor regression in vaccine challenge experiments and adoptive transfer studies. Our own studies document a reliance on IFN-γ in vaccination challenge experiments with the D5 tumor, but additional T1 cytokines appear to compensate, in the absence of IFN- γ, and mediate tumor regression in adoptive transfer studies using the same tumor (Winter, Hu and Fox manuscript in preparation). These findings should not be viewed as controversial, but as a compliment to the diversity of the immune response, particularly as it relates to tumor immunity.

Unlike the rather straightforward T1/T2 paradigm seen in infectious disease models, the preliminary findings in tumor models infers that a more complicated series of effector mechanisms exist. Even vaccines that normally induce strong T1 responses can not do so in a vacuum: Development of an effective antitumor T1 cytokine response has been shown to require some IL-4 during the initial priming of the immune response [104].

Another potential problem with the hypothesis that T1 cytokine responses are effective at mediating tumor destruction lies in defining the mechanism of tumor destruction. While not ruling out the role for cytokines, conventional wisdom has long held that for most T cell-mediated mechanisms, tumors are destroyed by cytolytic T cells. Since the two principal methods of cytolysis are via perforin or Fas/FasL [105], Winter and colleagues examined whether tumor-specific T1 T cells, from animals deficient in either of these two lytic mechanisms, could mediate tumor regression. Their results clearly show that T cells from perforin knock-out (PKO) or FasL mutant (gld) animals can mediate highly therapeutic antitumor activity (Figure 1.4)[106].

Table 1.1 Tumor-specific T2 cytokine profile of TVDLN effector T cells predicts vaccine failure.

Tumor TVDLN	Strain	Histology	Immuno- genicity	Cytokine profile
B16BL6-D5	C57BL/6	melanoma	non/poor	T2
MPR-5	C57BL/6	prostate	non/poor	T2
4T1	BALB/c	breast	non/poor	T2
MCA-310	C57BL/6	sarcoma	weak	T2=T1
MCA-304	C57BL/6	sarcoma	strong	T1
MCA-309	C57BL/6	sarcoma	strong	T1

While these studies rule out a critical role for either cytolytic effector mechanism in the B16BL6-D5 melanoma model, it is possible that compensatory mechanisms may allow FasL to be more active in PKO mice and vice-versa in gld mice, or that other effector mechanisms exist. To further examine this possibility Yamada has developed multiple gene knock-out animals to further examine this hypothesis (Yamada and Fox unpublished observation).

Considering these findings, Schwartz's definition of tolerance as it relates to patients with cancer might be better stated as follows: "a physiological state in which the immune system does not react destructively against cancer". We have provided evidence that the "non immunogenic" D5 tumor does sensitize tumor-specific T cells in vivo; however, because they produce T2 cytokines, tumor cells are not destroyed. The allo-modified or GM-CSF secreting vaccine induces T1 T cells that can mediate therapeutic activity in adoptive transfer studies.

These observations clearly identify immune deviation, a mechanism of tolerance, as being operational during the initial immune response following vaccination in the D5 tumor model and suggest possible sites to examine in patients with cancer. Recent studies suggest that separation strategies that exploit reduced L-selectin expression are useful in analyzing TVDLN of patients on vaccine trials [107]. Careful examination of a patient's initial immune response to vaccination could be predictive of a vaccines therapeutic potential and may provide a platform for the design and monitoring of a new generation of clinical trials.

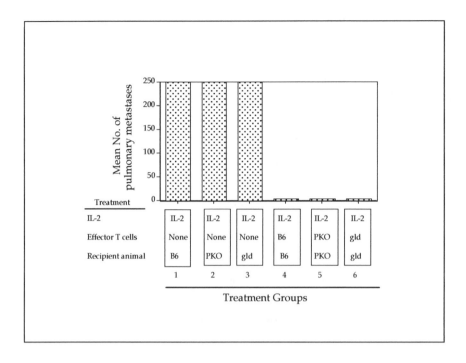

Figure 1.4. C57BL/6 (B6), perforin knock out (PKO) or FasL mutant (gld) mice were vaccinated with a GM-CSF producing D5 tumor (D5-G6) in order to generate effector T cells with a tumor-specific T1 response. B6, PKO and gld mice bearing 3 day established pulmonary metastases were treated with either IL-2 alone (Groups 1-3, 90,000 IU bid x 4 days) or with IL-2 and $7x10^7$ effector T cells, matched for the same genotype (groups 4-6, B6, PKO, gld). Similar results were obtained in two additional experiments.

IMMUNOTHERAPY TREATMENT OF CANCER PATIENTS USING DC BASED VACCINES

There is now a concerted effort to use immunological based vaccines for the treatment of cancer due to the inefficiency and toxicity problems that are associated with conventional treatments. The number of clinical trials involving DCs is increasing steadily and the approaches being used are varied. For example in the treatment of prostate cancer, phase I clinical data has been published regarding the efficacy of dendritic cell based vaccines pulsed with peptides from the prostate specific membrane antigen (PSMA). The patients (who were clinically refractive to hormone ablation therapy) were divided into groups receiving either peptide, DC or DC pulsed with peptide. Clinical responses (as measured by a reduction in the level of prostate specific antigen (PSA)) were detected only in the group receiving DC pulsed with PSMA peptides [108]. In a follow up study, patients responding to treatment were monitored closely for a variety of prostate markers including PSA, free PSA, PSMA and alkaline phosphatase. Many of these patients were still found to be clinically responsive to treatment 200 days post vaccination, suggesting that treatment was long lived and contingent upon the presence of DCs for effective anti-tumour responses [109, 110]. In order to determine whether GM-CSF might increase the immunogenicity of DCs pulsed with PSMA, patients were also given co-administrations of the cytokine; no augmentation in immune response was detected [111]. In a similar study Nestle and co-workers pulsed autologous DCs (obtained from patients diagnosed with melanoma) with peptides from known melanoma associated antigens. Keyhole limpet haemocyanin was added as a CD4$^+$ helper antigen and immunological tracer molecule. Objective responses were detected in 5 out of 16 patients – two showed complete whereas three patients had partial responses and regression of metastasis was noted in the skin, soft tissue, lung and pancreas. One patient was noted as having a minor response during the course of therapeutic treatment. No side effects or autoimmunity was detected from any of the patients [112]. Dendritic cell immunotherapy has not been restricted to solid tumours. DCs from patients diagnosed with follicular B-cell lymphomas were pulsed with a tumour specific idiotype protein. Although the number of patients involved in the study was limited (4), all patients were able to mount detectable anti-tumour immune responses. One patient had complete tumour regression, one with partial and a third resolved all evidence of disease as measured by molecular assays [113].

Future of cancer immunotherapy using dc based vaccines

There is no doubt that the number of clinical trials based upon DC vaccine technology will increase exponentially within the next five years. As more is learned with respect to costimulatory molecules (e.g. B7, CD40, OX40 etc) it is likely that DCs will be "appropriately primed" (e.g. via CD40 ligation) for maximum antigen presenting and T-cell stimulatory capacity. The feasibility of this idea has already been tested in in-vivo animal models as highlighted by the work of Diehl et al. These authors noted that animal immunisations regimes consisting of peptide alone, resulted in T-cell tolerance whereas the addition of activating antibodies against CD40 in combination to a CTL specific antigen was sufficient to change a tolerance signal to a CD8$^+$ T-cell stimulatory signal. It was suggested that this type of approach might be an effective way in which to stimulate an immune response against pre-established tumours [114]. The idea of stimulating an appropriate T-helper response in parallel to providing specific CTL epitopes is gaining such momentum that MHC class II binding epitopes from known tumour antigens are now being actively sought. To date several have been discovered and it is likely that they will be used as part of an immune "adjuvant" for stimulating a maximal CD8$^+$ T-cell response against tumours [115]. An alternative approach for activating T-helper cells was developed by Wu et al., who used DNA targeting constructs to take endogenously synthesized antigens directly into the class II processing pathways for presentation to CD4$^+$ T-cells [116, 117]. DNA based vaccines represent a powerful tool in the fight against cancer since they can be produced and administered to patients relatively easily and once constructed, DNA vaccines are known to have a uniform and consistent quality. DNA "minigene" vaccines have received a great deal of attention because they code only for MHC class I CTL epitopes [118-122]. Several epitopes can be arranged in a linear manner to produce a single protein and this has been shown to be an extremely effective mechanism for inducing anti-tumour immunity. This immunity is likely to work through either direct or indirect transfection (e.g. taking up of apoptotic bodies from transfected cells) of DCs. One might envisage a scenario in which haplotype specific "minigenes" for a given tumour antigen is given in combination with MHC class II encoding DNA vaccines to produce maximal effect. DCs have been shown to release vesicles commonly referred to as "exosomes", that contain MHC class I, MHC class II and co-stimulatory molecules. Antigen specific peptide pulsing of "exosomes" resulted in the formation of CTL clones followed by the suppression or eradication of pre-established tumours [123]. While the ease and reproducibility of "exosome" preparations for tumour immunotherapy is questionable, it has stimulated the idea of creating artificial liposome structures that possess "appropriate" co-stimulatory molecules necessary for maximising T-cell activation. If this could be achieved, it would circumvent problems associated with isolating host specific DCs, quality of preparation, reproducibility and cost since these molecules could be manufactured consistently on a large scale. Another area receiving attention is the development of HSP based immunological vaccines that carry tumour antigens into DCs. As outlined previously heat shock proteins are known to bind peptides in a relatively non-specific manner thus making them superb candidates as immune adjuvants for dendritic cells. There is a lot of supporting evidence that these molecules could have a dual function in not only carrying peptides directly into MHC class I loading pathways but also in acting as an immune adjuvant ("danger signal") boosting CTL responses against tumours.

SUMMARY

If "danger signals" are found to be absolutely necessary for successful immune priming against tumours then it is likely that vaccination strategies must encompass the use of both MHC class I and class II targeted epitopes in conjunction with a potent immune adjuvant. MHC class II binding epitopes would be mandatory for stimulating optimal CD4[+] T-cell activity, concomitantly leading to full CTL maturation. In addition, co-stimulatory molecules are fundamental in the antigen priming process and it is likely therefore, that an appropriate immune adjuvant would have to be employed in order to ensure maximal expression at the time of antigen presentation to T-cells. In the absence of co-stimulation, peptide presentation would almost certainly result in tolerance rather than activation. It is possible therefore that a survival advantage would ensue if tumours had the ability to present antigens to T-cells in the absence of co-stimulatory molecules. This would serve to promote T-cell tolerance and prevent the activation of an effective immune response against the tumour. One might envisage a scenario therefore, in which immunisation regimes would be administered to patients on a regular and consistent basis and thus help to overcome any tolerising activity initiated directly from the tumour.

REFERENCES

1. Hainaut P and Hollstein M, p53 and human cancer: The first ten thousand mutations. Adv Cancer Res, 2000; 77: 81-137.
2. Zweemer RP, Shaw PA, Verheijen RMH, Ryan A, Berchuck A, Ponder BAJ, Risch H, McLaughlin JR, Narod SA, Menko FH, Kenemans P, and Jacobs IJ, Accumulation of p53 protein is frequent in ovarian cancers associated with BRCA1 and BRCA2 germline mutations. J Clin Pathol, 1999; 52: 372-375.
3. Duffour MT, Chaux P, Lurquin C, Cornelis G, Boon T, and vanderBruggen P, A MAGE-A4 peptide presented by HLA-A2 is recognized by cytolytic T lymphocytes. Eur J Immunol, 1999; 29: 3329-3337.
4. Ruschenburg I, Kubitz A, Schlott T, Korabiowska M, and Droese M, MAGE-1, GAGE-1/-2 gene expression in FNAB of classic variant of papillary thyroid carcinoma and papillary hyperplasia in nodular goiter. Int J Mol Med, 1999; 4: 445-448.
5. Fuller GN, Rhee CH, Hess KR, Caskey LS, Wang RP, Bruner JM, Yung WKA, and Zhang W, Reactivation of insulin-like growth factor binding protein 2 expression in glioblastoma multiforme: A revelation by parallel gene expression profiling. Cancer Res, 1999; 59: 4228-4232.
6. Kittlesen DJ, Thompson LW, Gulden PH, Skipper JCA, Colella TA, Shabanowitz JA, Hunt DF, Engelhard VH, and Slingluff CL, Human melanoma patients recognize an HLA-A1-restricted CTL epitope from tyrosinase containing two cysteine residues: Implications for tumor vaccine development. J Immunol, 1998; 160: 2099-2106.
7. Eder M, Battmer K, Kafert S, Stucki A, Ganser A, and Hertenstein B, Monitoring of BCR-ABL expression using real-time RT-PCR in CML after bone marrow or peripheral blood stem cell transplantation. Leukemia, 1999; 13: 1383-1389.
8. Osarogiagbon UR and McGlave PB, Chronic myelogenous leukaemia. Current Opinion in Haematology, 1999; 6: 241-246.
9. Boon T, Cerottini JC, Vandeneynde B, Vanderbruggen P, and Vanpel A, Tumor antigens recognized by T lymphocytes. Annu Rev Immunol, 1994; 12: 337-365.
10. Vanderbruggen P, Traversari C, Chomez P, Lurquin C, Deplaen E, Vandeneynde B, Knuth A, and Boon T, A gene encoding an antigen recognized by cytolytic lymphocytes-t on a human-melanoma. Science, 1991; 254: 1643-1647.
11. Brichard V, Vanpel A, Wolfel T, Wolfel C, Deplaen E, Lethe B, Coulie P, and Boon T, The tyrosinase gene codes for an antigen recognized by autologous cytolytic T lymphocytes on HLA-A2 melanomas. J Exp Med, 1993; 178: 489-495.
12. Kawakami Y, Eliyahu S, Sakaguchi K, Robbins PF, Rivoltini L, Yannelli JR, Appella E, and Rosenberg SA, Identification of the immunodominant peptides of the MART-1 human-melanoma antigen recognized by the majority of HLA-A2-restricted tumor-infiltrating lymphocytes. J Exp Med, 1994; 180: 347-352.
13. Kawakami Y, Eliyahu S, Delgado CH, Robbins PF, Sakaguchi K, Appella E, Yannelli JR, Adema GJ, Miki T, and Rosenberg SA, Identification of a human-melanoma antigen recognized by tumor-infiltrating lymphocytes associated with in-vivo tumor rejection. Proc Natl Acad Sci U S A, 1994; 91: 6458-6462.
14. Schwartz RH, *Immunological Tolerance*, in *Fundamental Immunology*. 1993, Raven Press: New York. p. 677.
15. Linsley PS and Ledbetter JA, The role of the cd28 receptor during t-cell responses to antigen. Annu Rev Immunol, 1993; 11: 191-212.
16. Rocken M and Shevach EM, Immune deviation - The third dimension of nondeletional T cell tolerance. Immunol Rev, 1996; 149: 175-194.
17. Fruh K, Gruhler A, Krishna RM, and Schoenhals GJ, A comparison of viral immune escape strategies targeting the MHC class I assembly pathway. Immunol Rev, 1999; 168: 157-166.
18. Lee PP, Yee C, Savage PA, Fong L, Brockstedt D, Weber JS, Johnson D, Swetter S, Thompson J, Greenberg PD, Roederer M, and Davis MM, Characterization of circulating T cells specific for tumor-associated antigens in melanoma patients. Nat Med, 1999; 5: 677-685.
19. Skipper JCA, Gulden PH, Hendrickson RC, Harthun N, Caldwell JA, Shabanowitz J, Engelhard VH, Hunt DF, and Slingluff CL, Mass-spectrometric evaluation of HLA-A*0201-associated peptides identifies dominant naturally processed forms of CTL epitopes from MART-1 and gp100. Int J Cancer, 1999; 82: 669-677.

CANCER IMMUNOLOGY

20. Takashima A and Morita A, Dendritic cells in genetic immunization. J Leukoc Biol, 1999; 66: 350-356.
21. Mommaas AM, Mulder AA, Jordens R, Out C, Tan MCAA, Cresswell P, Kluin PM, and Koning F, Human epidermal Langerhans cells lack functional mannose receptors and a fully developed endosomal/lysosomal compartment for loading of HLA class II molecules. Eur J Immunol, 1999; 29: 571-580.
22. Rees RC and Mian S, Selective MHC expression in tumours modulates adaptive and innate antitumour responses. Cancer Immunology Immunotherapy, 1999; 48: 374-381.
23. Sallusto F, Cella M, Danieli C, and Lanzavecchia A, Dendritic Cells Use Macropinocytosis and the Mannose Receptor to Concentrate Macromolecules In the Major Histocompatibility Complex Class-Ii Compartment - Down-Regulation By Cytokines and Bacterial Products. J Exp Med, 1995; 182: 389-400.
24. Lutz MB, Rovere P, Kleijmeer MJ, Rescigno M, Assmann CU, Oorschot VMJ, Geuze HJ, Trucy J, Demandolx D, Davoust J, and RicciardiCastagnoli P, Intracellular routes and selective retention of antigens in mildly acidic cathepsin D/lysosome-associated membrane protein-1/MHC class II-positive vesicles in immature dendritic cells. J Immunol, 1997; 159: 3707-3716.
25. Engering AJ, Cella M, Fluitsma D, Brockhaus M, Hoefsmit ECM, Lanzavecchia A, and Pieters J, The mannose receptor functions as a high capacity and broad specificity antigen receptor in human dendritic cells. Eur J Immunol, 1997; 27: 2417-2425.
26. Tan MCAA, Mommaas AM, Drijfhout JW, Jordens R, Onderwater JJM, Verwoerd D, Mulder AA, vanderHeiden AN, Ottenhoff THM, Cella M, Tulp A, Neefjes JJ, and Koning F, Mannose receptor mediated uptake of antigens strongly enhances HLA-class II restricted antigen presentation by cultured dendritic cells. Adv Exp Med Biol, 1997; 417: 171-174.
27. Stahl PD and Ezekowitz RAB, The mannose receptor is a pattern recognition receptor involved in host defense. Curr Opin Immunol, 1998; 10: 50-55.
28. Kleijmeer MJ, Ossevoort MA, Vanveen CJH, Vanhellemond JJ, Neefjes JJ, Kast WM, Melief CJM, and Geuze HJ, MHC class-II compartments and the kinetics of antigen presentation in activated mouse spleen dendritic cells. J Immunol, 1995; 154: 5715-5724.
29. Engering AJ, Cella M, Fluitsma DM, Hoefsmit ECM, Lanzavecchia A, and Pieters J, Mannose receptor mediated antigen uptake and presentation in human dendritic cells. Adv Exp Med Biol, 1997; 417: 183-187.
30. Maurer D, Fiebiger E, Ebner C, Reininger B, Fischer GF, Wichlas S, Jouvin MH, SchmittEgenolf M, Kraft D, Kinet JP, and Stingl G, Peripheral blood dendritic cells express Fc epsilon RI as a complex composed of Fc epsilon RI alpha- and Fc epsilon RI gamma-chains and can use this receptor for IgE-mediated allergen presentation. J Immunol, 1996; 157: 607-616.
31. Regnault A, Lankar D, Lacabanne V, Rodriguez A, Thery C, Rescigno M, Saito T, Verbeek S, Bonnerot C, RicciardiCastagnoli P, and Amigorena S, Fc gamma receptor-mediated induction of dendritic cell maturation and major histocompatibility complex class I-restricted antigen presentation after immune complex internalization. J Exp Med, 1999; 189: 371-380.
32. Brossart P and Bevan MJ, Presentation of exogenous protein antigens on major histocompatability complex class I molecules by dendritic cells: Pathway of presentation and regulation by cytokines. Blood, 1997; 90: 1594-1599.
33. Huang AYC, Bruce AT, Pardoll DM, and Levitsky HI, In-Vivo Cross-Priming Of Mhc Class-I - Restricted Antigens Requires the Tap Transporter. Immunity, 1996; 4: 349-355.
34. Albert ML, Sauter B, and Bhardwaj N, Dendritic cells acquire antigen from apoptotic cells and induce class I restricted CTLs. Nature, 1998; 392: 86-89.
35. Albert ML, Pearce SFA, Francisco LM, Sauter B, Roy P, Silverstein RL, and Bhardwaj N, Immature dendritic cells phagocytose apoptotic cells via alpha(v)beta(5) and CD36, and cross-present antigens to cytotoxic T lymphocytes. J Exp Med, 1998; 188: 1359-1368.
36. Ronchetti A, Rovere P, Iezzi G, Galati G, Heltai S, Protti MP, Garancini MP, Manfredi AA, Rugarli C, and Bellone M, Immunogenicity of apoptotic cells in vivo: Role of antigen load, antigen-presenting cells, and cytokines. J Immunol, 1999; 163: 130-136.
37. Bennett SRM, Carbone FR, Karamalis F, Miller JFAP, and Heath WR, Induction of a CD8(+) cytotoxic T lymphocyte response by cross-priming requires cognate CD4(+) T cell help. J Exp Med, 1997; 186: 65-70.

38. Gromme M, Uytdehaag FGCM, Janssen H, Calafat J, vanBinnendijk RS, Kenter MJH, Tulp A, Verwoerd D, and Neefjes J, Recycling MHC class I molecules and endosomal peptide loading. Proc Natl Acad Sci U S A, 1999; 96: 10326-10331.
39. Herbst B, Kohler G, Mackensen A, Veelken H, Kulmburg P, Rosenthal FM, Schaefer HE, Mertelsmann R, Fisch P, and Lindemann A, In vitro differentiation of CD34(+) hematopoietic progenitor cells toward distinct dendritic cell subsets of the birbeck granule and MIIC-positive Langerhans cell and the interdigitating dendritic cell type. Blood, 1996; 88: 2541-2548.
40. Bernhard H, Disis ML, Heimfeld S, Hand S, Gralow JR, and Cheever MA, Generation Of Immunostimulatory Dendritic Cells From Human CD34+ Hematopoietic Progenitor Cells Of the Bone-Marrow and Peripheral- Blood. Cancer Res, 1995; 55: 1099-1104.
41. Allavena P, Piemonti L, Longoni D, Bernasconi S, Stoppacciaro A, Ruco L, and Mantovani A, IL-10 prevents the differentiation of monocytes to dendritic cells but promotes their maturation to macrophages. Eur J Immunol, 1998; 28: 359-369.
42. Cella M, Engering A, Pinet V, Pieters J, and Lanzavecchia A, Inflammatory stimuli induce accumulation of MHC class II complexes on dendritic cells. Nature, 1997; 388: 782-787.
43. Cella M, Salio M, Sakakibara Y, Langen H, Julkunen I, and Lanzavecchia A, Maturation, activation, and protection of dendritic cells induced by double-stranded RNA. J Exp Med, 1999; 189: 821-829.
44. Watanabe M, Choudhry A, Berlan M, Singal A, Siwik E, Mohr S, and Fisher SA, Developmental remodeling and shortening of the cardiac outflow tract involves myocyte programmed cell death. Development, 1998; 125: 3809-3820.
45. Frade JM and Barde YA, Genetic evidence for cell death mediated by nerve growth factor and the neurotrophin receptor p75 in the developing mouse retina and spinal cord. Development, 1999; 126: 683-690.
46. Gumienny TL, Lambie E, Hartwieg E, Horvitz HR, and Hengartner MO, Genetic control of programmed cell death in the Caenorhabditis elegans hermaphrodite germline. Development, 1999; 126: 1011-1022.
47. Rovere P, Vallinoto C, Bondanza A, Crosti MC, Rescigno M, RicciardiCastagnoli P, Rugarli C, and Manfredi AA, Bystander apoptosis triggers dendritic cell maturation and antigen-presenting function. J Immunol, 1998; 161: 4467-4471.
48. Matzinger P, Tolerance, danger, and the extended family. Annu Rev Immunol, 1994; 12: 991-1045.
49. Gallucci S, Lolkema M, and Matzinger P, Natural adjuvants: endogenous activators of dendritic cells. Nat Med, 1999; 5: 1249-1255.
50. Melcher A, Todryk S, Hardwick N, Ford M, Jacobson M, and Vile RG, Tumor immunogenicity is determined by the mechanism of cell death via induction of heat shock protein expression. Nat Med, 1998; 4: 581-587.
51. Todryk S, Melcher AA, Hardwick N, Linardakis E, Bateman A, Colombo MP, Stoppacciaro A, and Vile RG, Heat shock protein 70 induced during tumor cell killing induces Th1 cytokines and targets immature dendritic cell precursors to enhance antigen uptake. J Immunol, 1999; 163: 1398-1408.
52. Blachere NE, Li ZH, Chandawarkar RY, Suto R, Jaikaria NS, Basu S, Udono H, and Srivastava PK, Heat shock protein-peptide complexes, reconstituted in vitro, elicit peptide-specific cytotoxic T lymphocyte response and tumor immunity. J Exp Med, 1997; 186: 1315-1322.
53. Chandawarkar RY, Wagh MS, and Srivastava PK, The dual nature of specific immunological activity of tumor-derived gp96 preparations. J Exp Med, 1999; 189: 1437-1442.
54. Yedavelli SPK, Guo L, Daou ME, Srivastava PK, Mittelman A, and Tiwari RK, Preventive and therapeutic effect of tumor derived heat shock protein, gp96, in an experimental prostate cancer model. Int J Mol Med, 1999; 4: 243-248.
55. Jaattela M, Escaping cell death: Survival proteins in cancer. Exp Cell Res, 1999; 248: 30-43.
56. Schoenberger SP, vanderVoort EIH, Krietemeijer GM, Offringa R, Melief CJM, and Toes REM, Cross-priming of CTL responses in vivo does not require antigenic peptides in the endoplasmic reticulum of immunizing cells. J Immunol, 1998; 161: 3808-3812.
57. Suto R and Srivastava PK, A Mechanism For the Specific Immunogenicity Of Heat-Shock Protein-Chaperoned Peptides. Science, 1995; 269: 1585-1588.
58. Basu S and Srivastava PK, Calreticulin, a peptide-binding chaperone of the endoplasmic reticulum, elicits tumor- and peptide-specific immunity. J Exp Med, 1999; 189: 797-802.
59. Ganss R, Limmer A, Sacher T, Arnold B, and Hammerling GJ, Autoaggression and tumor rejection: it takes more than self-specific T-cell activation. Immunol Rev, 1999; 169: 263-272.

60. Slavik JM, Hutchcroft JE, and Bierer BE, CD28/CTLA-4 and CD80/CD86 families - Signaling and function. Immunol Res, 1999; 19: 1-24.
61. Bennett SRM, Carbone FR, Karamalis F, Flavell RA, Miller JFAP, and Heath WR, Help for cytotoxic-T-cell responses is mediated by CD40 signalling. Nature, 1998; 393: 478-480.
62. Ridge JP, DiRosa F, and Matzinger P, A conditioned dendritic cell can be a temporal bridge between a CD4(+) T-helper and a T-killer cell. Nature, 1998; 393: 474-478.
63. Schoenberger SP, Toes REM, vanderVoort EIH, Offringa R, and Melief CJM, T-cell help for cytotoxic T lymphocytes is mediated by CD40-CD40L interactions. Nature, 1998; 393: 480-483.
64. Bianchi R, Grohmann U, Vacca C, Belladonna ML, Fioretti MC, and Puccetti P, Autocrine IL-12 is involved in dendritic cell modulation via CD40 ligation. J Immunol, 1999; 163: 2517-2521.
65. Ohshima Y, Tanaka Y, Tozawa H, Takahashi Y, Maliszewski C, and Delespesse G, Expression and function of OX40 ligand on human dendritic cells. J Immunol, 1997; 159: 3838-3848.
66. Gramaglia I, Weinberg AD, Lemon M, and Croft M, Ox-40 ligand: A potent costimulatory molecule for sustaining primary CD4 T cell responses. J Immunol, 1998; 161: 6510-6517.
67. Chen AI, McAdam AJ, Buhlmann JE, Scott S, Lupher MLJ, Greenfield EA, Baum PR, Fanslow WC, Calderhead DM, Freeman GJ, and Sharpe AH, OX40-ligand has a critical co-stimulatory role in dendritic cell:T cell interactions. Immunity, 1999; 11: 689-698.
68. Kopf M, Ruedl C, Schmitz N, Gallimore A, Lefrang K, Ecabert B, Odermatt B, and Bachmann MF, OX40 deficient mice are defective in Th cell proliferation but are competent in generating B cell and CTL responses. Immunity, 1999; 11: 699-708.
69. Ito N, Nakamura H, Tanaka Y, and Ohgi S, Lung carcinoma - Analysis of T helper type 1 and 2 cells and T cytotoxic type 1 and 2 cells by intracellular cytokine detection with flow cytometry. Cancer, 1999; 85: 2359-2367.
70. Asselin-Paturel C, Echchakir H, Carayol G, Gay F, Opolon P, Grunenwald D, Chouaib S, and MamiChouaib F, Quantitative analysis of Th1, Th2 and TGF-beta 1 cytokine expression in tumor, TIL and PBL of non-small cell lung cancer patients. Int J Cancer, 1998; 77: 7-12.
71. Elsasser-Beile U, Kolble N, Grussenmeyer T, SchultzeSeemann W, Wetterauer U, Gallati H, Monting JS, and vonKleist S, Th1 and Th2 cytokine response patterns in leukocyte cultures of patients with urinary bladder, renal cell and prostate carcinomas. Tumor Biology, 1998; 19: 470-476.
72. Qin ZH, Richter G, Schuler T, Ibe S, Cao XT, and Blankenstein T, B cells inhibit induction of T cell-dependent tumor immunity. Nat Med, 1998; 4: 627-630.
73. Salgame P, Abrams JS, Clayberger C, Goldstein H, Convit J, Modlin RL, and Bloom BR, Differing lymphokine profiles of functional subsets of human cd4 and cd8 t-cell clones. Science, 1991; 254: 279-282.
74. Croft M, Carter L, Swain SL, and Dutton RW, Generation of polarized antigen-specific cd8 effector populations - reciprocal action of interleukin (il)-4 and il-12 in promoting type-2 versus type-1 cytokine profiles. J Exp Med, 1994; 180: 1715-1728.
75. Mosmann TR and Sad S, The expanding universe of T-cell subsets: Th1, Th2 and more. Immunol Today, 1996; 17: 138-146.
76. Li L, Sad S, Kagi D, and Mosmann TR, CD8Tc1 and Tc2 cells secrete distinct cytokine patterns in vitro and in vivo but induce similar inflammatory reactions. J Immunol, 1997; 158: 4152-4161.
77. Seder RA and Paul WE, Acquisition of lymphokine-producing phenotype by cd4+ t-cells. Annu Rev Immunol, 1994; 12: 635-673.
78. Nakamura T, Lee RK, Nam SY, Podack ER, Bottomly K, and Flavell RA, Roles of IL-4 and IFN-gamma in stabilizing the T helper cell type 1 and 2 phenotype. J Immunol, 1997; 158: 2648-2653.
79. Gollob JA, Kawasaki H, and Ritz J, Interferon-gamma and interleukin-4 regulate T cell interleukin-12 responsiveness through the differential modulation of high-affinity interleukin-12 receptor expression. Eur J Immunol, 1997; 27: 647-652.
80. Tamada K, Harada M, Abe K, Li TL, Tada H, Onoe Y, and Nomoto K, Immunosuppressive activity of cloned natural killer (NK1.1(+)) T cells established from murine tumor-infiltrating lymphocytes. J Immunol, 1997; 158: 4846-4854.
81. vonderWeid T, Beebe AM, Roopenian DC, and Coffman RL, Early production of IL-4 and induction of Th2 responses in the lymph node originate from an MHC class I-independent CD4(+)NK1.1(-)T cell population. J Immunol, 1996; 157: 4421-4427.
82. Inoue M, Minami M, Fujii Y, Matsuda H, Shirakura R, and Kido T, Granulocyte colony-stimulating factor and interleukin-6-producing lung cancer cell line, LCAM. J Surg Oncol, 1997; 64: 347-350.

83. Rincon M, Anguita J, Nakamura T, Fikrig E, and Flavell RA, Interleukin (IL)-6 directs the differentiation of IL-4-producing CD4(+) T cells. J Exp Med, 1997; 185: 461-469.
84. Bendelac A, Rivera MN, Park SH, and Roark JH, Mouse CD1-specific NK1 T cells: Development, specificity, and function. Annu Rev Immunol, 1997; 15: 535-562.
85. Schartonkersten T, Afonso LCC, Wysocka M, Trinchieri G, and Scott P, IL-12 is required for natural-killer-cell activation and subsequent t-helper-1 cell-development in experimental leishmaniasis. J Immunol, 1995; 154: 5320-5330.
86. Scharton T and Scott PA, Natural killer cells are a source of interferon gamma that drives differentiation of CD4 T cell subsets and induces early resistance to Leishmania major in mice. J Exp Med, 1993; 176: 567.
87. Constant SL and Bottomly K, Induction of TH1 and TH2 CD4+ T cell responses: The alternative approaches. Annu Rev Immunol, 1997; 15: 297-322.
88. McKnight AJ, Perez VL, Shea CM, Gray GS, and Abbas AK, Costimulator dependence of lymphokine secretion by naive and activated cd4(+) t-lymphocytes from tcr transgenic mice. J Immunol, 1994; 152: 5220-5225.
89. Hosken NA, Shibuya K, Heath AW, Murphy KM, and Ogarra A, The effect of antigen dose on cd4(+) t-helper cell phenotype development in a t-cell receptor-alpha-beta-transgenic model. J Exp Med, 1995; 182: 1579-1584.
90. Tsung K, Meko JB, Peplinski GR, Tsung YL, and Norton JA, IL-12 induces T helper 1-directed antitumor response. J Immunol, 1997; 158: 3359-3365.
91. Aruga A, Aruga E, Tanigawa K, Bishop DK, Sondak VK, and Chang AE, Type 1 versus type 2 cytokine release by V beta T cell subpopulations determines in vivo antitumor reactivity - IL-10 mediates a suppressive role. J Immunol, 1997; 159: 664-673.
92. Lee PP, Zeng DF, McCaulay AE, Chen YF, Geiler C, Umetsu DT, and Chao NJ, T helper 2-dominant antilymphoma immune response is associated with fatal outcome. Blood, 1997; 90: 1611-1617.
93. Lowes MA, Bishop GA, Crotty K, Barnetson RS, and Halliday GM, T helper 1 cytokine mRNA is increased in spontaneously regressing primary melanomas. J Invest Dermatol, 1997; 108: 914-919.
94. Kagamu H and Shu SY, Purification of L-selectin(low) cells promotes the generation of highly potent CD4 antitumor effector T lymphocytes. J Immunol, 1998; 160: 3444-3452.
95. Mobley JL and Dailey MO, Regulation of adhesion molecule expression by cd8 t-cells invivo .1. Differential regulation of gp90mel-14 (lecam-1), pgp-1, lfa-1, and vla-4-alpha during the differentiation of cytotoxic lymphocytes-t induced by allografts. J Immunol, 1992; 148: 2348-2356.
96. Mobley JL, Rigby SM, and Dailey MO, Regulation of adhesion molecule expression by CD8 t-cells in-vivo .2. Expression of l-selectin (CD62L) by memory cytolytic T-cells responding to minor histocompatibility antigens. J Immunol, 1994; 153: 5443-5452.
97. Hou S and Doherty PC, Partitioning of responder CD8(+) t-cells in lymph-node and lung of mice with sendai virus pneumonia by lecam-1 and CD45rb phenotype. J Immunol, 1993; 150: 5494-5500.
98. Andersson EC, Christensen JP, Marker O, and Thomsen AR, Changes in cell-adhesion molecule expression on T-cells associated with systemic virus-infection. J Immunol, 1994; 152: 1237-1245.
99. Bradley LM, Duncan DD, Tonkonogy S, and Swain SL, Characterization of antigen-specific CD4+ effector T-cells invivo - immunization results in a transient population of mel-14-, CD45rb- helper-cells that secretes interleukin-2 (il-2), il-3, il-4, and interferon-gamma. J Exp Med, 1991; 174: 547-559.
100. Hu HM, Urba WJ, and Fox BA, Gene-modified tumor vaccine with therapeutic potential shifts tumor-specific T cell response from a type 2 to a type 1 cytokine profile. J Immunol, 1998; 161: 3033-3041.
101. Dobrzanski MJ, Reome JB, and Dutton RW, Type 1 and type 2 CD8(+) effector T cell subpopulations promote long-term tumor immunity and protection to progressively growing tumor. J Immunol, 2000; 164: 916-925.
102. Rodolfo M, Zilocchi C, Accornero P, Cappetti B, Arioli I, and Colombo MP, IL-4-transduced tumor cell vaccine induces immunoregulatory type 2 CD8 T lymphocytes that cure lung metastases upon adoptive transfer. J Immunol, 1999; 163: 1923-1928.
103. Hung K, Hayashi R, LafondWalker A, Lowenstein C, Pardoll D, and Levitsky H, The central role of CD4(+) T cells in the antitumor immune response. J Exp Med, 1998; 188: 2357-2368.
104. Schuler T, Qin ZH, Ibe S, NobenTrauth N, and Blankenstein T, T helper cell type 1-associated and cytotoxic T lymphocyte-mediated tumor immunity is impaired in interleukin 4-deficient mice. J Exp Med, 1999; 189: 803-810.

25

105. Henkart P, *Cytotoxic T lymphocytes*, in *Fundamental Immunology*. 1999, Raven Press: New York. p. 1021.
106. Winter H, Hu HM, Urba WJ, and Fox BA, Tumor regression after adoptive transfer of effector T cells is independent of perforin or Fas ligand (APO-1L/CD95L). J Immunol, 1999; 163: 4462-4472.
107. Chu Y, Hu HM, Winter H, Wood WJ, Doran T, Lashley D, Bashey J, Schuster J, Wood J, Lowe BA, Vetto JT, Weinberg AD, Puri R, Smith JW, Urba WJ, and Fox BA, Examining the immune response in sentinel lymph nodes of mice and men. Eur J Nucl Med, 1999; 26: S50-S53.
108. Murphy G, Tjoa B, Ragde H, Kenny G, and Boynton A, Phase I clinical trial: T-cell therapy for prostate cancer using autologous dendritic cells pulsed with HLA-A0201-specific peptides from prostate-specific membrane antigen. Prostate, 1996; 29: 371-380.
109. Tjoa BA, Erickson SJ, Bowes VA, Ragde H, Kenny GM, Cobb OE, Ireton RC, Troychak MJ, Boynton AL, and Murphy GP, Follow-up evaluation of prostate cancer patients infused with autologous dendritic cells pulsed with PSMA peptides. Prostate, 1997; 32: 272-278.
110. Salgaller ML, Lodge PA, McLean JG, Tjoa BA, Loftus DJ, Ragde H, Kenny GM, Rogers M, Boynton AL, and Murphy GP, Report of immune monitoring of prostate cancer patients undergoing T-cell therapy using dendritic cells pulsed with HLA-A2-specific peptides from prostate-specific membrane antigen (PSMA). Prostate, 1998; 35: 144-151.
111. Simmons SJ, Tjoa BA, Rogers M, Elgamal A, Kenny GM, Ragde H, Troychak MJ, Boynton AL, and Murphy GP, GM-CSF as a systemic adjuvant in a phase II prostate cancer vaccine trial. Prostate, 1999; 39: 291-297.
112. Nestle FO, Alijagic S, Gilliet M, Sun YS, Grabbe S, Dummer R, Burg G, and Schadendorf D, Vaccination of melanoma patients with peptide- or tumor lysate-pulsed dendritic cells. Nat Med, 1998; 4: 328-332.
113. Hsu FJ, Benike C, Fagnoni F, Liles TM, Czerwinski D, Taidi B, Engleman EG, and Levy R, Vaccination of patients with B-cell lymphoma using autologous antigen-pulsed dendritic cells. Nat Med, 1996; 2: 52-58.
114. Diehl L, denBoer AT, Schoenberger SP, vanderVoort EIH, Schumacher TNM, Melief CJM, Offringa R, and Toes REM, CD40 activation in vivo overcomes peptide-induced peripheral cytotoxic T-lymphocyte tolerance and augments anti-tumor vaccine efficacy. Nat Med, 1999; 5: 774-779.
115. Chaux P, Vantomme V, Stroobant V, Thielemans K, Corthals J, Luiten R, Eggermont AMM, Boon T, and vanderBruggen P, Identification of MAGE-3 epitopes presented by HLA-DR molecules to CD4(+) T lymphocytes. J Exp Med, 1999; 189: 767-777.
116. Wu TC, Guarnieri FG, Staveleyocarroll KF, Viscidi RP, Levitsky HI, Hedrick L, Cho KR, August JT, and Pardoll DM, Engineering an intracellular pathway for major histocompatibility complex class-ii presentation of antigens. Proc Natl Acad Sci U S A, 1995; 92: 11671-11675.
117. Lin KY, Guarnieri FG, Staveleyocarroll KF, Levitsky HI, August JT, Pardoll DM, and Wu TC, Treatment Of Established Tumors With a Novel Vaccine That Enhances Major Histocompatibility Class-Ii Presentation Of Tumor-Antigen. Cancer Res, 1996; 56: 21-26.
118. Rodriguez F, An LL, Harkins S, Zhang J, Yokoyama M, Widera G, Fuller JT, Kincaid C, Campbell IL, and Whitton JL, DNA immunization with minigenes: Low frequency of memory cytotoxic T lymphocytes and inefficient antiviral protection are rectified by ubiquitination. J Virol, 1998; 72: 5174-5181.
119. Yu ZY, Karem KL, Kanangat S, Manickan E, and Rouse BT, Protection by minigenes: a novel approach of DNA vaccines. Vaccine, 1998; 16: 1660-1667.
120. Ishioka GY, Fikes J, Hermanson G, Livingston B, Crimi C, Qin MS, delGuercio MF, Oseroff C, Dahlberg C, Alexander J, Chesnut RW, and Sette A, Utilization of MHC class I transgenic mice for development of minigene DNA vaccines encoding multiple HLA-restricted CTL epitopes. J Immunol, 1999; 162: 3915-3925.
121. Iwasaki A, DelaCruz CS, Young AR, and Barber BH, Epitope-specific cytotoxic T lymphocyte induction by minigene DNA immunization. Vaccine, 1999; 17: 2081-2088.
122. Petersen TR, Bregenholta S, Pedersen LO, Nissen MH, and Claesson MH, Human p53(264-272) HLA-A2 binding peptide is an immunodominant epitope in DNA-immunized HLA-A2 transgenic mice. Cancer Lett, 1999; 137: 183-191.
123. Zitvogel L, Regnault A, Lozier A, Wolfers J, Flament C, Tenza D, RicciardiCastagnoli P, Raposo G, and Amigorena S, Eradication of established murine tumors using a novel cell-free vaccine: dendritic cell-derived exosomes. Nat Med, 1998; 4: 594-600.

2
Recognition of human tumours: cancer/testis antigens

ALEXEI F. KIRKIN, KARINE N. DZHANDZHUGAZYAN and JESPER ZEUTHEN

INTRODUCTION

During the last few years, significant progress has been achieved in the identification of human tumour-associated antigens recognised by T cells [1,2]. The largest group is the group of cancer/testis (CT) antigens. Originally discovered in melanomas [3], they have been found in many human malignancies. Among normal tissues they are expressed in testes (therefore they have been designated cancer/testis antigens [4]) and in some cases in placenta, both structures in which they are not accessible for the recognition by cells of immune system. The majority of cancer/testis genes have been mapped to the X chromosome. Many CT antigens can be grouped into subfamilies that include several members. They are MAGE-A, MAGE-B, MAGE-C, GAGE, PRAME (MAPE), LAGE and SSX subfamilies (Table 2.1). For the other antigens only one individual member has been discovered so far. These are BAGE, SCP-1, SART-1, SART-3, TSP50, CT9 and CTp11 antigens. SART-1 and SART-3 antigens are different from the other CT antigens in that they are expressed in some normal non-testes cells on mRNA levels, but the protein product has been detected only in tumour cells and in testes. In this they resemble another tumour antigen, p15, which is expressed at the RNA level in all investigated tissues, but only tumour cells are recognised by a TIL culture isolated from a melanoma patient [5]. Despite the fact that only for some of the CT antigens recognition by T cells has been described and corresponding peptide epitopes have been found (Table 2.2), all CT antigens should be considered as potential targets for immunotherapy. In this review we will give the detailed description of their properties.

R.A. Robins and R.C. Rees (eds.), Cancer Immunology, 27–43.

PROPERTIES OF CANCER/TESTIS ANTIGENS

One of the largest groups of CT antigens is the group of MAGE proteins. The *MAGE* genes comprise three families, *MAGE-A, MAGE-B* and *MAGE-C*. *MAGE-A* genes represent a family of 12 closely related genes located on the long arm of chromosome X (region Xq28) [6], including the first identified gene coding for the CT antigen MAGE-A1 (previously designated MAGE-1) [3]. In the majority of the investigated tumours only the expression of *MAGE-A1, -A2, -A3, -A4, -A6* and *–A12* genes has been demonstrated. Recently the expression of *MAGE-A11* [7] and *MAGE-A10* [8] has also been detected in several tumours. The ability to present peptide epitopes recognised by cytotoxic T lymphocytes (CTL) has been shown for MAGE-A1 [3], MAGE-A2 [9], MAGE-A3 [10], MAGE-A4 [11], MAGE-A6 [12] and MAGE-A10 [8]. Eight antigenic epitopes of MAGE-A1 have been identified: two recognised by melanoma-specific CTL clones isolated from patient PBLs and restricted by HLA-A1 (epitope EADPTGHSY [13]) and HLA-Cw16 (epitope SAYGEPRKL [14]; one based on the ability of a predicted peptide to induce tumour-specific CTLs (the HLA-A24-restricted epitope NYKHCFPEI [15]); one epitope present in several MAGE-A molecules and restricted by HLA-B*37 [12]; and four epitopes identified after *in vitro* immunisation with dendritic cells transfected with the *MAGE-A1* gene [16]. These are HLA-A3-restricted epitope 96-104 (SLFRAVITK), HLA-A28-restricted epitope 222-231 (EVYDGREHSA), HLA-B53-restricted epitope 258-266 (DPARYEFLW) and HLA-Cw2-restricted epitope 62-70 (SAFPTTINF)). For the MAGE-A2 protein, four peptides have been identified: two HLA-A2-binding peptides (KWVELVHFL and YLQLVFGIEV) have been shown to induce the formation of CTL in transgenic mice able to kill MAGE-A2-expressing cells [9]; one HLA-A24-binding peptide (156-163, EYLQLVFGI) was shown to induce melanoma-specific CTLs [17]; and one HLA-B37-restricted epitope (134-143, REPVTKAEML), shared with MAGE-A1 [12]. For the MAGE-A3 protein, nine epitopes recognised by CTLs have been identified, one recognised by HLA-A1-restricted CTL clones from the patient MZ2 (EVDPIGHLY [10]), four based on the ability of peptides predicted by known HLA class I binding motifs to stimulate the formation of CTL recognising melanoma cells, namely the HLA-A2-restricted epitope FLWGPRALV [18], two HLA-A24-restricted epitopes, IMPKAGLLI [19] and 97-105 (TFPDLESEF), and the HLA-B44-restricted epitope MEVDPIGHLY [20], one shared with MAGE-A1 HLA-B37-restricted epitope 134-143 (REPVTKAEML) [12], two HLA-A2-restricted epitopes identified after vaccination of patients with a polyvalent melanoma vaccine (159-169, QLVFGIELMEV and 188-198, IMPKAGLLIIV) [21], and one HLA-A*52-restricted epitope (143-151, WQYFFPVIF) identified after immunisation with dendritic cells loaded with apoptotic bodies [22]. Other MAGE-A antigens that are able to create epitopes recognised by CTLs are MAGE-A4 [11], MAGE-A6, which has three epitopes shared with MAGE-A3 and one epitope shared with several other MAGE-A proteins, MAGE-A10 [8], and MAGE-A12, the expression of which has been detected in various tumours and which has epitopes present in MAGE-A2 and MAGE-A3 antigens. T-helper cells also recognise MAGE-A3, and some corresponding epitopes have been identified. They are the DR11-restricted peptide TSYVKVLHHMVKISG (281-295) [23], and two DR13-restricted peptides AELVHFLLLKYRAR (114-127) and FLLLKYRAREPVTKAE (121-134) [24].

The expression of MAGE-A antigens has been further investigated in a number of different studies. These antigens are generally highly expressed in cutaneous melanomas (up to 65% for MAGE-A3 [6]), but not in ocular melanomas [25]. To a lesser extent they are expressed in other types of tumours such as mammary carcinomas, head and neck tumours, lung carcinomas, sarcomas and bladder carcinomas (for review see [26]). A high expression of MAGE-A1 (80%) was found in hepatocarcinomas [27]. In contrast, myelomonocytic leukemias have been consistently negative [28,29], and colon or renal carcinomas are rarely positive. A correlation of the expression of MAGE-A antigens with tumour progression has been found in a number of malignancies [30-33]. Peptides from MAGE-A1 and MAGE-A3 have been tested for their ability to induce anti-melanoma immune responses *in vivo*, and limited anti-tumour activity has been shown only for the MAGE-A3 peptide EVDPIGHLY [34,35].

TABLE 2.1. Human cancer/testis antigens.

Family	Members	Chromosome Localisation	References
MAGE-A	MAGE-A1 – MAGE-A6, MAGE-A8 – MAGE-A12	Xq28	[6]
MAGE-B	MAGE-B1 – MAGE-B4	Xp21.3	[36]
MAGE-C	MAGE-C1/CT7	Xq26	[40,41]
	CT10	Xq27	[42]
GAGE	GAGE-1 - GAGE-8	Xp11.2- p11.4	[48-50]
	PAGE-1 - PAGE-4	Xp11.23	[49,51]
	XAGE-1 - XAGE-3		[52]
LAGE	LAGE-1a (1S), -1b (1L)	Xq28	[61]
	NY-ESO-1	Xq28	[57]
SSX	SSX-1 – SSX-5	Xp11.2	[4,62]
Separate CT antigens			
	BAGE	ND	[47]
	SCP-1 (HOM-TES-14)	1p13	[64,65]
	PRAME (MAPE)	22q11.2-q12	[53]
	SART-1		[70]
	SART-3		[72]
	CTp11	Xq26.3-Xq27.1	[67]
	TSP50	3p14-p12	[68]
	CT9/BRDT	1p22-p21	[69]

The *MAGE-B* genes represent a family of 4 genes located in the region p21.3 of X chromosome [36]. *MAGE-B1* has previously been also described as *MAGE-Xp* [37] or *DAM-10* [38], and *MAGE-B2* as *DAM-6* [38]. The coding regions for these genes share 66-

81% nucleotide identity and show 45-63% identity with those of the *MAGE* genes located in Xp28. Only two genes, *MAGE-B1* and *MAGE-B2*, are expressed in a significant fraction of tumours of various histological types. A potential HLA-A2-restricted CTL epitope for MAGE-B1 and MAGE-B2 has recently been identified as the peptide FLWGPRAYA [39]. The *MAGE-C1* gene, a member of the *MAGE-C* family located in Xq26, has been recently identified by analysis of the selective gene expression in testis and melanomas [40]. Its expression pattern strongly resembles the expression pattern of *MAGE-A* genes. The protein MAGE-C1 carries a unique feature when compared to the other MAGE proteins since in addition to a 275-amino acid MAGE-homologous segment on its COOH terminus, it has in its NH_2 part an 867-amino acid region composed of tandem repeats of three types. 53 % of all amino acid residues of this large repetitive region are serine, proline, or glutamine residues. This region may be of interest as a target for immunotherapy, as it contains several potential HLA class I-restricted peptides, which, due to their repetitive appearance in the protein sequence, may reach a high density on the cell surface.

TABLE 2.2. Peptide epitopes of cancer/testis antigens recognised by T cells

Antigen	HLA restriction	Epitope	Sequence	References
MAGE-A1				
	A1	161-169	EADPTGHSY	[13]
	A3	96-104	SLFRAVITK	[16]
	A24	135-143[a]	NYKHCFPEI	[15]
	A28	222-231	EVYDGREHSA	[16]
	B37	127-136	REPVTKAEML	[12]
	B53	258-266	DPARYEFLW	[16]
	Cw2	62-70	SAFPTTINF	[16]
	Cw3,Cw16	230-238	SAYGEPRKL	[14,16]
MAGE-A2				
	A2	112-120[a]	KMVELVHFL	[9]
	A2	157-166[a]	YLQLVFGIEV	[9]
	A24	156-163[a]	EYLQLVFGI	[17]
	B37	134-143	REPVTKAEML	[12]
MAGE-A3				
	A1	168-176	EVDPIGHLY	[10]
	A2	159-169[b]	QLVFGIELMEV	[21]
	A2	188-198[b]	IMPKAGLLIIV	[21]
	A2	271-279[a]	FLWGPRALV	[18]
	A24	195-203[a]	IMPKAGLLI	[19]
	A24	97-105[a]	TFPDLESEF	[92]
	A52	143-151	WQYFFPVIF	[22]
	B37	134-143	REPVTKAEML	[12]
	B44	167-176[a]	MEVDPIGHLY	[20]
	DR11	281-295	TSYVKVLHHMVKISG	[23]
	DR13	114-127	AELVHFLLLKYRAR	[24]
	DR13	121-134	FLLLKYRAREPVTKAE	[24]

TABLE 2.2 (continued)

Antigen	HLA restriction	Epitope	Sequence	References
MAGE-A4				
	A2	230-239	GVYDGREHTV	[11]
MAGE-A6				
	A2	159-169[c]	QLVFGIELMEV	
	A24	97-105[c]	TFPDLESEF	
	A52	143-151[c]	WQYFFPVIF	
	B37	134-143	REPVTKAEML	[12]
MAGE-A10				
	A2	254-262	GLYDGMEHL	[8]
	B53	290-298[d]	DPARYEFLW	
MAGE-A12				
	A2	157-166[e]	YLQLVFGIEV	
	A2	271-179[c]	FLWGPRALV	
	A24	156-194[e]	EYLQLVFGI	
MAGE-B1/B2				
	A2	271-279	FLWGPRAYA	[39]
BAGE				
	Cw16	2-10	AARAVFLAL	[47]
GAGE-1,(-2,-8)				
	Cw6	9-16	YRPRPRRY	[48,50]
GAGE-3,(-4,-5,-6,-7B)				
	A29	10-18	YYWPRPRRY	[50]
PRAME				
	A24	301-309	LYVDSLFFL	[53]
NY-ESO-1				
	A2	157-165	SLLMWITQC	[93]
	A2	157-167	SLLMWITQCFL	[93]
	A2	155-163	QLSLLMWIT	[93]
	A31	53-62	ASGPGGGAPR	[59]
	DRB4*0101-0103	115-132	PLPVPGVLLKEFTVSGNI	[60]
	DRB4*0101-0103	131-138	VLLKEFTVSGNILTIRLT	[60]
	DRB4*0101-0103	139-156	AADHRQLQLSISSCLQQL	[60]
LAGE (CAMEL)				
	A2	1-11	MLMAQEALAFL	[94]
SART-1				
	A24	690-698	EYRGFTQDF	[71]
	A26	736-744	KGSGKMKTE	[70]
		749-757	KLDEEALLK	[70]
		785-793	VLSGSGKSM	[70]
SART-3				
	A24	109-118	VYDYNCHVDL	[72]
		315-323	AYIDFEMKI	[72]

[a] Predicted epitopes, to which induced CTL can kill tumour cells
[b] Epitopes identified after vaccination with polyvalent melanoma vaccine.
[c] Epitope identified for MAGE-A3.
[d] Epitope identified for MAGE-A1.
[e] Epitope identified for MAGE-A2.

Using the SEREX method, Chen and co-workers identified a similar gene, which they named *CT7* [41] and the *CT7* sequences differed from *MAGE-C1* in having additional nucleotides in the 5′ untranslated region, and also in a 14 single nucleotide differences in the coding region, resulting in 11 corresponding amino acid differences. *CT7* and *MAGE-C1* probably represent different alleles of the same gene. Another protein with a strong homology in the C-terminal part to MAGE-C1 is CT10 [42], which also was discovered by selective gene expression analysis. The gene is localised in the Xq27 region. In contrast to MAGE-C1, the protein has no repetitive part.

Several proteins with homology to MAGE proteins have been identified which exhibit a different distribution from the classical CT antigen distribution in the organism. Two of these proteins are localised at locus 15q11-q12 and both are thought to associate with the Prader-Willi syndrome. These are the MAGEL2 protein, expressed in foetal and adult brain and placenta [43], and necdin, or neuronal growth suppressor, expressed in many tissues and in neurons [44]. Two other genes are coded in the p11 region of the X chromosome and expressed practically in all tissues and organs. These are the *MAGE-D1* [45], and the *MAGE-D* [46] genes. The gene structure of *MAGE-D* is significantly different from the gene structure of *MAGE-A*, *-B*, and *-C* genes in that it is composed of 14 exons with 11 of them coding for protein. Other *MAGE* genes have only three – four exons, with the entire MAGE coding sequence contained in the last exon. Lucas and co-authors [46] suggest that *MAGE-D* has maintained the structure of the ancestor of all the *MAGE* genes, whereas the other *MAGE* genes would have originated by retrotransposition of mRNA of this ancestral gene.

BAGE codes for a putative protein of 43 amino acids [47]. Its pattern of expression in tumour samples is extremely similar to the pattern of the expression of MAGE antigens with an overall lower frequency of expression (22% in melanomas, 15% in bladder carcinomas, 10% in mammary carcinomas and 8% in head and neck squamous cell carcinomas). As for the MAGE antigens, the expression of BAGE correlates with the stage of tumour progression. The antigenic peptide epitope was identified as AARAVFLAL (residues 2-10). Experiments demonstrating the immunogenic properties and the protective effect of this antigen have not yet been performed.

An additional antigen present in melanoma cells of patient MZ2 (these melanoma cells and this patient's PBLs have been used for the identification of several CT antigens) was identified as a HLA-Cw6-restricted epitope (YRPRPRRY) encoded by the *GAGE-1* gene [48]. This gene belongs to a large family of genes, including the *GAGE-1 – GAGE-8* genes [48-50], *PAGE-1 – PAGE-4* genes [49,51], and *XAGE-1 – XAGE-3* genes [52]. The *GAGE-1* sequence contains an open reading frame coding for a protein of 138 amino acids. The two genes of the *GAGE* family that code for the peptide, namely *GAGE-1* and *GAGE-2*, are expressed in a significant proportion of melanomas (24%), sarcomas (25%), non-small lung cancers (19%), head and neck tumours (19%), and bladder tumours (12%). Another gene coding for the same epitope is *GAGE-8* [50]. In addition to the HLA-Cw6-restricted epitope YRPRPRRY, the HLA-A29-restricted epitope YYWPRPRRY encoded by the *GAGE-3, -4, -5, -6,* and *-7B* genes and recognised by CTL isolated from another melanoma patient has been identified [50].

During the investigation of the immunogenic properties of melanoma cells derived from the patient LB33, a variant of a melanoma cell line with a partial loss of HLA class

I expression, was found to induce the generation of a HLA-A24-restricted CTL clone recognising a new antigen called PRAME [53]. An interesting feature of this CTL clone was that it did not recognise the original melanoma cells, in spite of the fact that these cells were positive for the expression of the PRAME antigen. CTL recognition was observed only when the NK inhibitory receptor expressed by the CTL clone was blocked by antibody. In contrast to the MAGE genes, PRAME is also expressed in some normal tissues other than the testis. Except for the endometrium (which expresses up to 30% of the levels found in the LB33 melanoma cells) the levels of expression in normal tissues corresponds to less than 3%-5% of that found in melanoma cells [53]. A unique feature of the PRAME antigen among CT antigens is that, in addition to high expression in melanomas, non-small-cell lung carcinomas, sarcomas, head and neck tumours and renal carcinomas, it is also expressed in leukaemia [53,53-55], which is very rare for the other CT antigens.

Several antigens belonging to the group of testis-specific antigens expressed in tumours have been identified recently using the SEREX method (serological expression cloning of recombinant cDNA libraries of human tumours) [56]. One of them, NY-ESO-1, encoded by *CTAG* gene [57], is expressed in 23 of 67 melanoma specimens, 10 of 33 breast cancers, 4 of 16 prostate cancers, 4 of 5 bladder cancers, as well as a proportion of other tumour types, but only in 2 of 11 cultured melanoma cell lines [58]. The putative NY-ESO-1 protein consists of 180 aa and abundant in glycine residues in the N-terminal portion of the protein. In a melanoma patient, the CTL response was restricted by HLA-A2, and three peptides recognised by a melanoma-specific CTL line have been identified as SLLMWITQCFL (157-167), SLLMWITQC (157-165) and QLSLLMWIT (155-163). This antigen was also found to induce a HLA-A31-restricted CTL response in patient 586, with peptide epitopes being ASGPGGGAPR from a normal open reading frame and (L)AAQERRVPR from the alternative open reading frame [59]. In addition, MHC class II restriction recognition by CD4+ T lymphocytes has been described, with identification of three peptide epitopes [60]. The gene, homologous to *CTAG*, has recently been described using representational difference analysis [61]. This gene, called *LAGE-1*, has two alternatively spliced products of 180 and 210 amino acids. The 180 amino acid product has 84% identity with NY-ESO-1 protein and 100% identity in the region of described CTL peptide epitopes. The distribution of LAGE-1 in different tumours is similar to NY-ESO-1. Both genes are located in the q28 band of the X chromosome, close to *MAGE* genes [57,61].

Several CT antigens have been described for which T cell recognition has not yet been identified. Because of their tumour-specific expression, these antigens represent potential targets for the immunological intervention, and they will be briefly described here. They are HOM-MEL-40, SCP-1 (HOM-TES-14), TSP50, CTp11 (Table 2.1) and CT9/BRDT. HOM-MEL-40 [56] has been identified using the SEREX method. It is encoded by the *SSX-2* gene, a Krüppel-associated box-containing gene mapped to chromosome X, and is expressed in significant proportion of human melanomas (50%), colon cancers (25%), hepatocarcinomas (30%), and breast carcinoma (20%) [62]. This gene belongs to a family of 5 genes variably expressed in tumours [4]. No CTL recognition of these gene products has been described so far. The function of this antigen is not known, but the presence of a Krüppel-associated box, which probably has the function of a transcriptional repression domain [63] suggests that this factor may also be involved in the negative control of proliferation. Another antigen, HOM-TES-14, identified upon screening of a cDNA expression library enriched for testis-specific transcripts for reactivity with antibodies from the serum of a patient with renal cell carcinoma, turned out to be the synaptonemal complex protein 1 (SCP-1) [64]. SCP-1 is selectively expressed during the meiotic prophase of spermatocytes and is involved in the pairing of homologous chromosomes [65]. SCP-1 differs from other members of the class of CT antigens by its localisation on chromosome 1 and its frequent expression in malignant gliomas, breast, renal cell, and ovarian cancer. SCP-1 expression was also detected in haematological malignancies [66], which is rather rare for CT antigens. No CTL epitopes have been described so far. CTp11 [67] is a small protein of 11 kDa without homology to other CT antigens and expressed in 25-30% of melanoma and bladder carcinoma cell lines. It is encoded in the region q26.3-q27.1 of the X chromosome. TSP50 (testes-specific protease 50) is a protein with homology to protease and highly expressed in testes as well as in 28% of breast cancers [68]. The gene is localised in 3p14-p12. CT9/BRDT was identified as cancer/testis antigen in attempt to investigate, whether bromodomain testis-specific gene (BRDT), a testis-restricted member of the RING3 family of transcriptional regulators, is also expressed in cancer [69]. These authors [69] found, that by standard RT-PCR expression analysis it was possible to detect BRDT transcripts in 12 of 47 cases of non-small cell lung cancer and single cases of both squamous cell carcinoma of the head and neck (1/12) and esophagus (1/12) but not in melanoma or in cancers of the colon, breast, kidney and bladder. The authors gave a new name to this gene, CT9.

Two other antigens could be considered as CT antigens, despite the fact that they differ from classical CT antigens in that their CT-specific expression is seen only at the protein level, but not on the mRNA level. They are SART-1 and SART-3. SART-1 (squamous cell carcinoma antigen recognised by T cells) was identified as antigen expressed in squamous cell carcinomas (SCC) and recognised by HLA-A26-restricted CTLs [70]. The same gene encodes two proteins (125- and 43-kDa). The 43-kD protein was expressed in the cytosol of all the head and neck SCC tissues tested, 60% of esophageal SCCs, and half of the lung SCCs and lung adenocarcinomas, but not in leukaemia, melanomas, nor in normal tissues, normal cell lines, or normal cells except for foetal liver and testis. Four epitopes recognised by CTLs have been identified: three, restricted by HLA-A26 [70] (KGSGKMKTE (736-744), KLDEEALLK (749-757) and VLSGSGKSM (785-793)) and one, restricted by HLA-A24 [71] (EYRGFTQDF, 690-698). SART-3 was identified as a shared tumour antigen recognised by HLA-A2402-restricted and tumour-specific CTLs, using cDNA of esophageal cancer cells [72]. The protein that was expressed in the nucleus of all of the malignant tumour cell lines tested and the majority of cancer tissues with various histology, including squamous cell carcinomas, adenocarcinomas, melanomas, and leukemia cells. However, this protein was undetectable in the nucleus of any cell lines of non-malignant cells or normal tissues, except for the testis. Furthermore, this protein was expressed in the cytosol of all of the proliferating cells, including normal cells and malignant cells, but not in normal tissues, except for the testis and foetal liver. Two peptides of this protein were recognised by HLA-A2402- restricted CTLs: VYDYNCHVDL (109-118) and AYIDFEMKI (315-323). These peptides were able to induce HLA-A24-restricted and tumour-specific CTLs from peripheral blood mononuclear cells of most of HLA-A24$^+$ cancer patients tested, but not from peripheral blood mononuclear cells of any healthy donors.

DNA DEMETHYLATION AND CANCER/TESTIS ANTIGEN EXPRESSION

The mechanism of tumour-specific expression of these testis-specific genes is not known. As a possible mechanism, the role of demethylation has been investigated. It has first been demonstrated that demethylating agent 5-aza-2′-deoxycytidine can induce the expression of the *MAGE-A1* gene in MAGE-A1-negative cells [73,74]. It has therefore been proposed that *MAGE-A1* activation results from the demethylation of the promoter region, following an overall demethylation process, which occurs in many tumours. The activation effect of 5-aza-2′-deoxycytidine on gene expression has also been shown for other members of *MAGE* family [36,40] and for the gene of *GAGE* [50] and *LAGE* [61] families. The role of demethylation in the expression of *MAGE* genes in tumour cells is supported by the fact that the expression of many other testis-specific genes, whose presence was not detected in tumours, was not upregulated by 5-aza-2′-deoxycytidine treatment [75], and among *MAGE-B* genes the tumour expression have been detected only for those which are activated by 5-aza-2′-deoxycytidine treatment [36]. In addition, a good correlation between the demethylation of CpG sites in the promoter region of *MAGE-1* gene and the expression of the gene has been observed [76].

IMMUNOGENICITY OF CANCER/TESTIS ANTIGENS

From an immunological point of view, the CT antigens represent very good targets for immunotherapy. They are widely distributed in a number of tumours and present in normal tissues only in testis which is not accessible to the cells of immune system due to the lack of the direct contact of testis cells with the immune cells [77] and the lack of HLA class I expression on the surface of germ cells [78] which are the only cells in testis expressing MAGE antigens [79]. Many peptide epitopes recognised by T cells have been identified (Table 2.2). But so far, only a few patients have shown an immune response to this group of antigens (e.g. patient MZ2), suggesting an extremely low immunogenicity of the CT antigens under normal conditions.

The extremely broad specificity of the proteolytic activities in proteasomes [80] makes it rather unlikely, that it is the absence of appropriate cleavage sites in tumour-specific proteins which solely is responsible for their low immunogenicity. Another factor, which may influence presentation of antigens in amounts high enough to result in an immune response, is the structural stability of the protein. In order to be presented by the MHC class I molecules for the recognition by CTL, intracellular antigens should undergo several steps of antigen processing [81]. Important steps in this process are ubiquitination of the denatured proteins followed by the proteolytic cleavage of the polypeptide chain in proteasomes. High stability of the structures reduces the denaturation of the protein and, thus, ubiquitination as a degradation signal. Next, in order to get an access to the inner proteolytic component of the barrel-shaped proteasome, the polypeptide chain has to be unfolded [82]. The efficiency of this energy-requiring unfolding should depend on the protein structure. An α-helical conformation is known to provide the most optimal geometry for maximal amounts and strength of the hydrogen bonds formed. Therefore, highly organised proteins having a large proportion of α-helical structures are supposed to be more resistant to such unfolding. We have therefore tried to compare the predicted secondary structure of melanoma-associated antigens recognised by CTL using the computer program GOR Secondary Structure Predictions based on the predictive algorithm developed by Garnier et al. [83]. The analysis of several cancer/testis-specific and differentiation antigens is presented in Table 2.3. Obviously, the amount of α-helical structures in some cancer/testis-specific antigens (MAGE, PRAME, HOM-MEL-40, SCP-1, SART-1, SART-3, CT10, CTp11, and CT9) is significantly greater than in the group of differentiation antigens. This comparison may suggest that the proteins of the first group be supposed to have a more rigid structure, which should be more resistant to the unfolding and, subsequently, to the proteolytic cleavage in proteasomes. Therefore, we propose that these highly organised secondary structures in some CT antigens may be a possible explanation for their relatively low immunogenicity.

TABLE 2.3. Secondary structure of melanoma-associated antigens

Antigen	Number of aa	The amount (%) of a particular secondary structure			
		helical	extended	turn	coil
MAGE-A1	309	48.1	20.5	13.7	23.2
MAGE-A2	314	48.3	19.1	14.4	23.5
MAGE-A3	314	43.3	18.5	15.4	28.2
MAGE-A4	317	44.5	20.3	14.0	26.6
PRAME	509	46.0	21.5	19.5	16.2
HOM-MEL-40	188	49.4	11.6	18.0	30.2
SCP-1	976	76.6	8.2	7.7	9.2
SART-1	800	54,2	7,7	13,3	26,9
SART-3	963	58,3	15,0	14,1	14,3
CT10	373	41,5	14,6	19,3	29,1
CTp11	97	46,9	16,0	17,3	39,5
CT9	947	45,8	17,4	16,4	22,1
TSP50	385	16.5	26.6	37.1	24.1
Ny-ESO-1	180	20.7	29.3	26.2	33.5
MAGE-C1	1142	11.6	19.0	29.0	41.8
gp100	661	16.1	32.4	23.4	30.5
MART-1	118	28.4	22.5	45.1	19.6
Tyrosinase	529	27.9	17.0	33.1	25.1
TRP-1	527	20.4	25.2	34.2	23.3
TRP-2	519	13.1	27.6	50.7	15.8

For three other CT antigens – TCP50, MAGE-C1 and NY-ESO-1 - the predicted secondary structure has a low amount of α-helical structures, excluding this factor as the mechanism for their low immunogenicity. It is interesting, that these proteins contain "low-complexity" domains, existing in many proteins [84].

There is at least one example when "low-complexity" domain blocks processing and presentation of peptide epitopes present in proteins. This is the Gly-Ala repeat domain of the Epstein-Barr virus nuclear antigen 1 [85]. The mechanisms of this inhibition are not known yet (see [86]), but it may be proposed that similar mechanisms will be acting in CT proteins containing "low-complexity" domains.

This conclusion has further implications. As indicated above, initiation of a strong immune response to tumour antigens *in vivo* is an extremely rare event. Nevertheless, after being activated, CTL are capable to kill tumour cells of other patients, showing otherwise no anti-tumour response. This indicates that tumour cells express some low level of the presented antigen, probably, derived from trace amounts of not completely folded tumour-specific proteins. The limiting step may be, therefore, a priming of naive CTL which require about a 1000-fold higher concentration of antigenic peptides presented on cell surface than that required for lysis by activated CTL [87,88]. The use of dendritic cells, highly potent antigen-presenting cells [89], transfected with a construct encoding a tumour-specific protein, where its structure is modified by amino acid residue substitutions or by introducing sequences capable of disrupting long α-helical stretches in the regions outside the potential epitopes, or by removal of blocking "low-complexity" domains, may highly favour the initiation step. PEST regions that are often found in rapidly degraded proteins [90] probably serve this function and may be among good candidates for introducing into tumour proteins of interest. Nevertheless, it should be taken into consideration that some variations in amino acid sequences in the epitope flanking regions lead to generation of a cleavage position inside the epitope that may destroy the antigenic site [88]. Therefore, a proposed general approach to destabilisation of the protein structure requires the generation and testing of several artificially modified constructs as a basis for the development of tumour-specific vaccines.

CONCLUDING REMARKS

Cancer/testis antigens represent a group of antigens that are very promising for inducing immune responses for cancer-specific immunotherapy. Their appearance in tumours is a result of epigenetic changes associated with malignant transformation. Upregulation of their expression is caused by wide-range DNA demethylation, characteristic for many types of malignancies. This demethylation brings about re-expression of cancer-testis antigens in tumour cells, normally expressed only during embryogenesis and in one of immunologically privileged organs, the testis. The list of CT antigens is probably far from complete and new members are constantly appearing. Despite their apparent antigenicity, CT antigens under normal conditions are poor immunogens. The future development of immunotherapy targeted against CT antigens should be based on a) more efficient employment of dendritic cells as professional antigen-presenting cells, using different methods of their loading with tumour antigens, including transfection and fusion with tumour cells [91] and on b) modification of the primary structure of cancer/testis antigens aiming to increase their processing in proteasomes and subsequent presentation for recognition by specific T cell. In addition, targeting of as many cancer/testis antigens as possible, as well as other groups of tumour-associated antigens should be a priority in future vaccination trials in order to avoid tumour escape due to appearance of antigen-loss variants.

ACKNOWLEDGMENTS

Work in the authors' laboratory was supported by a project grant from the Danish Cancer Society and by grants from the Danish Foundation for Cancer Research.

REFERENCES

1   Boon, T. and van der Bruggen, P. Human tumor antigens recognized by T lymphocytes. J.Exp.Med., *183*: 725-729, 1996.
2.   Kirkin, A. F., Dzhandzhugazyan, K., and Zeuthen, J. Melanoma-associated antigens recognized by cytotoxic T lymphocytes. APMIS, *106*: 665-679, 1998.
3.   van der Bruggen, P., Traversari, C., Chomez, P., Lurquin, C., De Plaen, E., Van den Eynde, B. J., Knuth, A., and Boon, T. A gene encoding an antigen recognized by cytolytic T lymphocytes on a human melanoma. Science, *254*: 1643-1647, 1991.
4.   Güre, A. O., Türeci, Ö., Sahin, U., Tsang, S., Scanlan, M. J., Jäger, E., Knuth, A., Pfreundschuh, M., Old, L. J., and Chen, Y. T. *SSX*: a multigene family with several members transcribed in normal testis and human cancer. Int.J.Cancer, *72*: 965-971, 1997.
5.   Robbins, P. F., El-Gamil, M., Li, Y. F., Topalian, S. L., Rivoltini, L., Sakaguchi, K., Appella, E., Kawakami, Y., and Rosenberg, S. A. Cloning of a new gene encoding an antigen recognized by melanoma-specific HLA-A24-restricted tumor-infiltrating lymphocytes. J.Immunol., *154*: 5944-5950, 1995.
6.   De Plaen, E., Arden, K., Traversari, C., Gaforio, J. J., Szikora, J. P., De Smet, C., Brasseur, F., van der Bruggen, P., Lethé, B., and Lurquin, C. Structure, chromosomal localization, and expression of 12 genes of the *MAGE* family. Immunogenetics, *40*: 360-369, 1994.
7.   Jurk, M., Kremmer, E., Schwarz, U., Förster, R., and Winnacker, E. L. MAGE-11 protein is highly conserved in higher organisms and located predominantly in the nucleus. Int.J.Cancer, *75*: 762-766, 1998.
8.   Huang, L. Q., Brasseur, F., Serrano, A., De Plaen, E., van der Bruggen, P., Boon, T., and Van Pel, A. Cytolytic T lymphocytes recognize an antigen encoded by *MAGE-A10* on a human melanoma. J.Immunol., *162*: 6849-6854, 1999.
9.   Visseren, M. J., van der Burg, S. H., van der Voort, E. I., Brandt, R. M., Schrier, P. I., van der Bruggen, P., Boon, T., Melief, C. J. M., and Kast, W. M. Identification of HLA-A*0201-restricted CTL epitopes encoded by the tumor-specific *MAGE*-2 gene product. Int.J.Cancer, *73*: 125-130, 1997.
10.   Gaugler, B., Van den Eynde, B. J., van der Bruggen, P., Romero, P., Gaforio, J. J., De Plaen, E., Lethé, B., Brasseur, F., and Boon, T. Human gene MAGE-3 codes for an antigen recognized on a melanoma by autologous cytolytic T lymphocytes. J.Exp.Med., *179*: 921-930, 1994.
11.   Duffour, M. T., Chaux, P., Lurquin, C., Cornelis, G., Boon, T., and van der Bruggen, P. A MAGE-A4 peptide presented by HLA-A2 is recognized by cytolytic T lymphocytes. Eur.J.Immunol., *29*: 3329-3337, 1999.
12.   Tanzarella, S., Russo, V., Lionello, I., Dalerba, P., Rigatti, D., Bordignon, C., and Traversari, C. Identification of a promiscuous T-cell epitope encoded by multiple members of the *MAGE* family. Cancer Res., *59*: 2668-2674, 1999.
13.   Traversari, C., van der Bruggen, P., Luescher, I. F., Lurquin, C., Chomez, P., Van Pel, A., De Plaen, E., Amar-Costesec, A., and Boon, T. A nonapeptide encoded by human gene MAGE-1 is recognized on HLA-A1 by cytolytic T lymphocytes directed against tumor antigen MZ2-E. J.Exp.Med., *176*: 1453-1457, 1992.

14. van der Bruggen, P., Szikora, J. P., Boël, P., Wildmann, C., Somville, M., Sensi, M., and Boon, T. Autologous cytolytic T lymphocytes recognize a MAGE-1 nonapeptide on melanomas expressing HLA-Cw*1601. Eur.J.Immunol., *24*: 2134-2140, 1994.

15. Fujie, T., Tahara, K., Tanaka, F., Mori, M., Takesako, K., and Akiyoshi, T. A *MAGE-1*-encoded HLA-A24-binding synthetic peptide induces specific anti-tumor cytotoxic T lymphocytes. Int.J.Cancer, *80*: 169-172, 1999.

16. Chaux, P., Luiten, R., Demotte, N., Vantomme, V., Stroobant, V., Traversari, C., Russo, V., Schultz, E., Cornelis, G. R., Boon, T., and van der Bruggen, P. Identification of five MAGE-A1 epitopes recognized by cytolytic T lymphocytes obtained by In vitro stimulation with dendritic cells transduced with *MAGE-A1*. J.Immunol., *163*: 2928-2936, 1999.

17. Tahara, K., Takesako, K., Sette, A., Celis, E., Kitano, S., and Akiyoshi, T. Identification of a MAGE-2-encoded human leukocyte antigen-A24-binding synthetic peptide that induces specific antitumor cytotoxic T lymphocytes. Clin.Cancer Res., *5*: 2236-2241, 1999.

18. van der Bruggen, P., Bastin, J., Gajewski, T., Coulie, P. G., Boël, P., De Smet, C., Traversari, C., Townsend, A., and Boon, T. A peptide encoded by human gene MAGE-3 and presented by HLA-A2 induces cytolytic T lymphocytes that recognize tumor cells expressing MAGE-3. Eur.J.Immunol., *24*: 3038-3043, 1994.

19. Tanaka, F., Fujie, T., Tahara, K., Mori, M., Takesako, K., Sette, A., Celis, E., and Akiyoshi, T. Induction of antitumor cytotoxic T lymphocytes with a MAGE-3-encoded synthetic peptide presented by human leukocytes antigen-A24. Cancer Res., *57*: 4465-4468, 1997.

20. Herman, J., van der Bruggen, P., Luescher, I. F., Mandruzzato, S., Romero, P., Thonnard, J., Fleischhauer, K., Boon, T., and Coulie, P. G. A peptide encoded by the human *MAGE3* gene and presented by HLA-B44 induces cytolytic T lymphocytes that recognize tumor cells expressing *MAGE3*. Immunogenetics, *43*: 377-383, 1996.

21. Reynolds, S. R., Celis, E., Sette, A., Oratz, R., Shapiro, R. L., Johnston, D., Fotino, M., and Bystryn, J. C. HLA-independent heterogeneity of CD8[+] T cell responses to MAGE-3, Melan- A/MART-1, gp100, tyrosinase, MC1R, and TRP-2 in vaccine-treated melanoma patients. J.Immunol., *161*: 6970-6976, 1998.

22. Russo, V., Tanzarella, S., Dalerba, P., Rigatti, D., Rovere, P., Villa, A., Bordignon, C., and Traversari, C. Dendritic cells acquire the MAGE-3 human tumor antigen from apoptotic cells and induce a class I-restricted T cell response. Proc.Natl.Acad.Sci.U.S.A, *97*: 2185-2190, 2000.

23. Manici, S., Sturniolo, T., Imro, M. A., Hammer, J., Sinigaglia, F., Noppen, C., Spagnoli, G., Mazzi, B., Bellone, M., Dellabona, P., and Protti, M. P. Melanoma cells present a MAGE-3 epitope to CD4[+] cytotoxic T cells in association with histocompatibility leukocyte antigen DR11. J.Exp.Med., *189*: 871-876, 1999.

24. Chaux, P., Vantomme, V., Stroobant, V., Thielemans, K., Corthals, J., Luiten, R., Eggermont, A. M., Boon, T., and van der Bruggen, P. Identification of MAGE-3 epitopes presented by HLA-DR molecules to CD4[+] T lymphocytes. J.Exp.Med., *189*: 767-778, 1999.

25. Mulcahy, K. A., Rimoldi, D., Brasseur, F., Rodgers, S., Liénard, D., Marchand, M., Rennie, I. G., Murray, A. K., McIntyre, C. A., Platts, K. E., Leyvraz, S., Boon, T., and Rees, R. C. Infrequent expression of the *MAGE* gene family in uveal melanomas. Int.J.Cancer, *66*: 738-742, 1996.

26. Van Pel, A., van der Bruggen, P., Coulie, P. G., Brichard, V. G., Lethé, B., Van den Eynde, B. J., Uyttenhove, C., Renauld, J. C., and Boon, T. Genes coding for tumor antigens recognized by cytolytic T lymphocytes. Immunol.Rev., *145*: 229-250, 1995.

27. Yamashita, N., Ishibashi, H., Hayashida, K., Kudo, J., Takenaka, K., Itoh, K., and Niho, Y. High frequency of the *MAGE-1* gene expression in hepatocellular carcinoma. Hepatology, *24*: 1437-1440, 1996.

28. Chambost, H., Brasseur, F., Coulie, P., De Plaen, E., Stoppa, A. M., Baume, D., Mannoni, P., Boon, T., Maraninchi, D., and Olive, D. A tumour-associated antigen expression in human haematological malignancies. Br.J.Haematol., *84*: 524-526, 1993.

29. Shichijo, S., Tsunosue, R., Masuoka, K., Natori, H., Tamai, M., Miyajima, J., Sagawa, K., and Itoh, K. Expression of the *MAGE* gene family in human lymphocytic leukemia. Cancer Immunol.Immunother., *41*: 90-103, 1995.

30. Brasseur, F., Rimoldi, D., Liénard, D., Lethé, B., Carrel, S., Arienti, F., Suter, L., Vanwijck, R., Bourlond, A., Humblet, Y., Vacca, A., Conese, M., Lahaye, T., Degiovanni, G., Deraemaecker, R., Beauduin, M., Sastre, X., Salamon, E., Dréno, B., Jäger, E., Knuth, A., Chevreau, C., Suciu, S., Lachapelle, J. M., Pouillart, P., Parmiani, G., Lejeune, F., Cerottini, J. C., Boon, T., and Marchand, M. Expression of *MAGE* genes in primary and metastatic cutaneous melanoma. Int.J.Cancer, *63*: 375-380, 1995.

31. Eura, M., Ogi, K., Chikamatsu, K., Lee, K. D., Nakano, K., Masuyama, K., Itoh, K., and Ishikawa, T. Expression of the MAGE gene family in human head-and-neck squamous-cell carcinomas. Int.J.Cancer, *64*: 304-308, 1995.

32. Katano, M., Nakamura, M., Morisaki, T., and Fujimoto, K. Melanoma antigen-encoding gene-1 expression in invasive gastric carcinoma: correlation with stage of disease. J.Surg.Oncol., *64*: 195-201, 1997.
33. Patard, J. J., Brasseur, F., Gil-Diez, S., Radvanyi, F., Marchand, M., Francois, P., Abi-Aad, A., Van Cangh, P., Abbou, C. C., Chopin, D., and Boon, T. Expression of *MAGE* genes in transitional-cell carcinomas of the urinary bladder. Int.J.Cancer, *64* : 60-64, 1995.
34. Marchand, M., Weynants, P., Rankin, E., Arienti, F., Belli, F., Parmiani, G., Cascinelli, N., Bourlond, A., Vanwijck, R., Humblet, Y., Canon, J. L., Laurent, C., Naeyaert, J. M., Plagne, R., Deraemaecker, R., Knuth, A., Jäger, E., Brasseur, F., Herman, J., Coulie, P. G., and Boon, T. Tumor regression responses in melanoma patients treated with a peptide encoded by gene *MAGE-3*. Int.J.Cancer, *63*: 883-885, 1995.
35. Marchand, M., Van Baren, N., Weynants, P., Brichard, V., Dréno, B., Tessier, M. H., Rankin, E., Parmiani, G., Arienti, F., Humblet, Y., Bourlond, A., Vanwijck, R., Liénard, D., Beauduin, M., Dietrich, P. Y., Russo, V., Kerger, J., Masucci, G., Jäger, E., De Greve, J., Atzpodien, J., Brasseur, F., Coulie, P. G., van der Bruggen, P., and Boon, T. Tumor regressions observed in patients with metastatic melanoma treated with an antigenic peptide encoded by gene *MAGE-3* and presented by HLA- A1. Int.J.Cancer, *80*: 219-230, 1999.
36. Lurquin, C., De Smet, C., Brasseur, F., Muscatelli, F., Martelange, V., De Plaen, E., Brasseur, R., Monaco, A. P., and Boon, T. Two members of the human *MAGEB* gene family located in Xp21.3 are expressed in tumors of various histological origins. Genomics, *46*: 397-408, 1997.
37. Muscatelli, F., Walker, A. P., De Plaen, E., Stafford, A. N., and Monaco, A. P. Isolation and characterization of a *MAGE* gene family in the Xp21.3 region. Proc.Natl.Acad.Sci.U.S.A., *92*: 4987-4991, 1995.
38. Dabovic, B., Zanaria, E., Bardoni, B., Lisa, A., Bordignon, C., Russo, V., Matessi, C., Traversari, C., and Camerino, G. A family of rapidly evolving genes from the sex reversal critical region in Xp21. Mamm.Genome, *6*: 571-580, 1995.
39. Fleischhauer, K., Gattinoni, L., Dalerba, P., Lauvau, G., Zanaria, E., Dabovic, B., van Endert, P. M., Bordignon, C., and Traversari, C. The *DAM* gene family encodes a new group of tumor-specific antigens recognized by human leukocyte antigen A2-restricted cytotoxic T lymphocytes. Cancer Res., *58*: 2969-2972, 1998.
40. Lucas, S., De Smet, C., Arden, K. C., Viars, C. S., Lethé, B., Lurquin, C., and Boon, T. Identification of a new *MAGE* gene with tumor-specific expression by representational difference analysis. Cancer Res., *58*: 743-752, 1998.
41. Chen, Y. T., Güre, A. O., Tsang, S., Stockert, E., Jäger, E., Knuth, A., and Old, L. J. Identification of multiple cancer/testis antigens by allogeneic antibody screening of a melanoma cell line library. Proc.Natl.Acad.Sci.U.S.A., *95*: 6919-6923, 1998.
42. Güre, A. O., Stockert, E., Arden, K. C., Boyer, A. D., Viars, C. S., Scanlan, M. J., Old, L. J., and Chen, Y. T. CT10: A new cancer-testis (CT) antigen homologous to CT7 and the MAGE family, identified by representational-difference analysis. Int.J.Cancer, *85*: 726-732, 2000.
43. Boccaccio, I., Glatt-Deeley, H., Watrin, F., Roëckel, N., Lalande, M., and Muscatelli, F. The human *MAGEL2* gene and its mouse homologue are paternally expressed and mapped to the Prader-Willi region. Hum.Mol.Genet., *8*: 2497-2505, 1999.
44. Nakada, Y., Taniura, H., Uetsuki, T., Inazawa, J., and Yoshikawa, K. The human chromosomal gene for necdin, a neuronal growth suppressor, in the Prader-Willi syndrome deletion region. Gene, *213* : 65-72, 1998.
45. Pold, M., Zhou, J., Chen, G. L., Hall, J. M., Vescio, R. A., and Berenson, J. R. Identification of a new, unorthodox member of the MAGE gene family. Genomics, *59*: 161-167, 1999.
46. Lucas, S., Brasseur, F., and Boon, T. A new *MAGE* gene with ubiquitous expression does not code for known MAGE antigens recognized by T cells. Cancer Res., *59*: 4100-4103, 1999.
47. Boël, P., Wildmann, C., Sensi, M. L., Brasseur, R., Renauld, J. C., Coulie, P., Boon, T., and van der Bruggen, P. *BAGE*: a new gene encoding an antigen recognized on human melanomas by cytolytic T lymphocytes. Immunity, *2*: 167-175, 1995.
48. Van den Eynde, B. J., Peeters, O., De Backer, O., Gaugler, B., Lucas, S., and Boon, T. A new family of genes coding for an antigen recognized by autologous cytolytic T lymphocytes on a human melanoma. J.Exp.Med., *182*: 689-698, 1995.
49. Chen, M. E., Lin, S. H., Chung, L. W., and Sikes, R. A. Isolation and characterization of *PAGE-1* and *GAGE-7*. New genes expressed in the LNCaP prostate cancer progression model that share homology with melanoma-associated antigens. J.Biol.Chem., *273*: 17618-17625, 1998.
50. De Backer, O., Arden, K. C., Boretti, M., Vantomme, V., De Smet, C., Czekay, S., Viars, C. S., De Plaen, E., Brasseur, F., Chomez, P., Van den Eynde, B. J., Boon, T., and van der Bruggen, P. Characterization of

the *GAGE* genes that are expressed in various human cancers and in normal testis. Cancer Res., *59*: 3157-3165, 1999.

51. Brinkmann, U., Vasmatzis, G., Lee, B., Yerushalmi, N., Essand, M., and Pastan, I. *PAGE-1*, an X chromosome-linked *GAGE*-like gene that is expressed in normal and neoplastic prostate, testis, and uterus. Proc.Natl.Acad.Sci.U.S.A., *95*: 10757-10762, 1998.

52. Brinkmann, U., Vasmatzis, G., Lee, B., and Pastan, I. Novel genes in the PAGE and GAGE family of tumor antigens found by homology walking in the dbEST database. Cancer Res., *59*: 1445-1448, 1999.

53. Ikeda, H., Lethé, B., Lehmann, F., Van Baren, N., Baurain, J. F., De Smet, C., Chambost, H., Vitale, M., Moretta, A., Boon, T., and Coulie, P. G. Characterization of an antigen that is recognized on a melanoma showing partial HLA loss by CTL expressing an NK inhibitory receptor. Immunity, *6*: 199-208, 1997.

54. Van Baren, N., Chambost, H., Ferrant, A., Michaux, L., Ikeda, H., Millard, I., Olive, D., Boon, T., and Coulie, P. G. *PRAME*, a gene encoding an antigen recognized on a human melanoma by cytolytic T cells, is expressed in acute leukaemia cells. Br.J.Haematol., *102*: 1376-1379, 1998.

55. Watari, K., Tojo, A., Nagamura-Inoue, T., Nagamura, F., Takeshita, A., Fukushima, T., Motoji, T., Tani, K., and Asano, S. Identification of a melanoma antigen, PRAME, as a BCR/ABL-inducible gene. FEBS Lett., *466*: 367-371, 2000.

56. Sahin, U., Türeci, Ö., Schmitt, H., Cochlovius, B., Johannes, T., Schmits, R., Stenner, F., Luo, G., Schobert, I., and Pfreundschuh, M. Human neoplasms elicit multiple specific immune responses in the autologous host. Proc.Natl.Acad.Sci.U.S.A., *92*: 11810-11813, 1995.

57. Chen, Y. T., Boyer, A. D., Viars, C. S., Tsang, S., Old, L. J., and Arden, K. C. Genomic cloning and localization of CTAG, a gene encoding an autoimmunogenic cancer-testis antigen NY-ESO-1, to human chromosome Xq28. Cytogenet.Cell Genet., *79*: 237-240, 1997.

58. Chen, Y. T., Scanlan, M. J., Sahin, U., Türeci, Ö., Güre, A. O., Tsang, S., Williamson, B., Stockert, E., Pfreundschuh, M., and Old, L. J. A testicular antigen aberrantly expressed in human cancers detected by autologous antibody screening. Proc.Natl.Acad.Sci.U.S.A., *94*: 1914-1918, 1997.

59. Wang, R. F., Johnston, S. L., Zeng, G., Topalian, S. L., Schwartzentruber, D. J., and Rosenberg, S. A. A breast and melanoma-shared tumor antigen: T cell responses to antigenic peptides translated from different open reading frames. J.Immunol., *161*: 3598-3606, 1998.

60. Jäger, E., Jäger, D., Karbach, J., Chen, Y. T., Ritter, G., Nagata, Y., Gnjatic, S., Stockert, E., Arand, M., Old, L. J., and Knuth, A. Identification of NY-ESO-1 epitopes presented by human histocompatibility antigen (HLA)-DRB4*0101-0103 and recognized by CD4[+] T lymphocytes of patients with NY-ESO-1-expressing melanoma. J.Exp.Med., *191*: 625-630, 2000.

61. Lethé, B., Lucas, S., Michaux, L., De Smet, C., Godelaine, D., Serrano, A., De Plaen, E., and Boon, T. *LAGE*-1, a new gene with tumor specificity. Int.J.Cancer, *76*: 903-908, 1998.

62. Türeci, Ö., Sahin, U., Schobert, I., Koslowski, M., Scmitt, H., Schild, H. J., Stenner, F., Seitz, G., Rammensee, H. G., and Pfreundschuh, M. The *SSX-2* gene, which is involved in the t(X;18) translocation of synovial sarcomas, codes for the human tumor antigen HOM-MEL-40. Cancer Res., *56*: 4766-4772, 1996.

63. Margolin, J. F., Friedman, J. R., Meyer, W. K., Vissing, H., Thiesen, H. J., and Rauscher, I. I. Krüppel-associated boxes are potent transcriptional repression domains. Proc.Natl.Acad.Sci.U.S.A., *91*: 4509-4513, 1994.

64. Türeci, Ö., Sahin, U., Zwick, C., Koslowski, M., Seitz, G., and Pfreundschuh, M. Identification of a meiosis-specific protein as a member of the class of cancer/testis antigens. Proc.Natl.Acad.Sci.U.S.A., *95*: 5211-5216, 1998.

65. Meuwissen, R. L., Meerts, I., Hoovers, J. M., Leschot, N. J., and Heyting, C. Human synaptonemal complex protein 1 (SCP1): isolation and characterization of the cDNA and chromosomal localization of the gene. Genomics, *39*: 377-384, 1997.

66. Lim, S. H., Austin, S., Owen-Jones, E., and Robinson, L. Expression of testicular genes in haematological malignancies. Br.J.Cancer, *81*: 1162-1164, 1999.

67. Zendman, A. J. W., Cornelissen, I. M. A., Weidle, U. H., Ruiter, D. J., and van Muijen, G. N. P. CTp11, a novel member of the family of human cancer/testis antigens. Cancer Res., *59*: 6223-6229, 1999.

68. Yuan, L., Shan, J., De Risi, D., Broome, J., Lovecchio, J., Gal, D., Vinciguerra, V., and Xu, H. P. Isolation of a novel gene, *TSP50*, by a hypomethylated DNA fragment in human breast cancer. Cancer Res., *59*: 3215-3221, 1999.

69. Scanlan, M. J., Altorki, N. K., Gure, A. O., Williamson, B., Jungbluth, A., Chen, Y., and Old, L. J. Expression of cancer-testis antigens in lung cancer: definition of bromodomain testis-specific gene (BRDT) as a new CT gene, CT9. Cancer Lett., *150*: 155-164, 2000.

41

70. Shichijo, S., Nakao, M., Imai, Y., Takasu, H., Kawamoto, M., Niiya, F., Yang, D., Toh, Y., Yamana, H., and Itoh, K. A gene encoding antigenic peptides of human squamous cell carcinoma recognized by cytotoxic T lymphocytes. J.Exp.Med., 187: 277-288, 1998.

71. Kikuchi, M., Nakao, M., Inoue, Y., Matsunaga, K., Shichijo, S., Yamana, H., and Itoh, K. Identification of a SART-1-derived peptide capable of inducing HLA-A24-restricted and tumor-specific cytotoxic T lymphocytes. Int.J.Cancer, 81: 459-466, 1999.

72. Yang, D., Nakao, M., Shichijo, S., Sasatomi, T., Takasu, H., Matsumoto, H., Mori, K., Hayashi, A., Yamana, H., Shirouzu, K., and Itoh, K. Identification of a gene coding for a protein possessing shared tumor epitopes capable of inducing HLA-A24-restricted cytotoxic T lymphocytes in cancer patients. Cancer Res., 59: 4056-4063, 1999.

73. Weber, J., Salgaller, M., Samid, D., Johnson, B., Herlyn, M., Lassam, N., Treisman, J., and Rosenberg, S. A. Expression of the MAGE-1 tumor antigen is up-regulated by the demethylating agent 5-aza-2'-deoxycytidine. Cancer Res., 54: 1766-1771, 1994.

74. De Smet, C., De Backer, O., Faraoni, I., Lurquin, C., Brasseur, F., and Boon, T. The activation of human gene MAGE-1 in tumor cells is correlated with genome-wide demethylation. Proc.Natl.Acad.Sci.U.S.A., 93: 7149-7153, 1996.

75. De Smet, C., Martelange, V., Lucas, S., Brasseur, F., Lurquin, C., and Boon, T. Identification of human testis-specific transcripts and analysis of their expression in tumor cells. Biochem.Biophys.Res.Commun., 241: 653-657, 1997.

76. De Smet, C., Lurquin, C., Lethé, B., Martelange, V., and Boon, T. DNA methylation is the primary silencing mechanism for a set of germ line- and tumor-specific genes with a CpG-rich promoter. Mol.Cell Biol., 19: 7327-7335, 1999.

77. Barker, C. F. and Billingham, R. E. Immunologically privileged sites. Adv.Immunol., 25:1-54: 1-54, 1977.

78. Tomita, Y., Kimura, M., Tanikawa, T., Nishiyama, T., Morishita, H., Takeda, M., Fujiwara, M., and Sato, S. Immunohistochemical detection of intercellular adhesion molecule-1 (ICAM-1) and major histocompatibility complex class I antigens in seminoma. J.Urol., 149: 659-663, 1993.

79. Takahashi, K., Shichijo, S., Noguchi, M., Hirohata, M., and Itoh, K. Identification of MAGE-1 and MAGE-4 proteins in spermatogonia and primary spermatocytes of testis. Cancer Res., 55: 3478-3482, 1995.

80. Dick, L. R., Aldrich, C., Jameson, S. C., Moomaw, C. R., Pramanik, B. C., Doyle, C. K., DeMartino, G. N., Bevan, M. J., Forman, J. M., and Slaughter, C. A. Proteolytic processing of ovalbumin and beta-galactosidase by the proteasome to a yield antigenic peptides. J.Immunol., 152: 3884-3894, 1994.

81. Goldberg, A. L. and Rock, K. L. Proteolysis, proteasomes and antigen presentation. Nature, 357: 375-379, 1992.

82. Wenzel, T. and Baumeister, W. Conformational constraints in protein degradation by the 20S proteasome. Nature (Struct.Biol.), 2: 199-204, 1995.

83. Garnier, J., Gibrat, J. F., and Robson, B. GOR method for predicting protein secondary structure from amino acid sequence. Methods Enzymol., 266:540-53: 540-553, 1996.

84. Wootton, J. C. Non-globular domains in protein sequences: automated segmentation using complexity measures. Comput.Chem., 18: 269-285, 1994.

85. Levitskaya, J., Coram, M., Levitsky, V., Imreh, S., Steigerwald-Mullen, P. M., Klein, G., Kurilla, M. G., and Masucci, M. G. Inhibition of antigen processing by the internal repeat region of the Epstein-Barr virus nuclear antigen-1. Nature, 375: 685-688, 1995.

86. Levitskaya, J., Sharipo, A., Leonchiks, A., Ciechanover, A., and Masucci, M. G. Inhibition of ubiquitin/proteasome-dependent protein degradation by the Gly-Ala repeat domain of the Epstein-Barr virus nuclear antigen 1. Proc.Natl.Acad.Sci.U.S.A., 94: 12616-12621, 1997.

87. Nonacs, R., Humborg, C., Tam, J. P., and Steinman, R. M. Mechanisms of mouse spleen dendritic cell function in the generation of influenza-specific, cytolytic T lymphocytes. J.Exp.Med., 176: 519-529, 1992.

88. Niedermann, G., Butz, S., Ihlenfeldt, H. G., Grimm, R., Lucchiari, M., Hoschutzky, H., Jung, G., Maier, B., and Eichmann, K. Contribution of proteasome-mediated proteolysis to the hierarchy of epitopes presented by major histocompatibility complex class I molecules. Immunity, 2: 289-299, 1995.

89. Bell, D., Young, J. W., and Banchereau, J. Dendritic cells. Adv.Immunol., 72: 255-324, 1999.

90. Rogers, S., Wells, R., and Rechsteiner, M. Amino acid sequences common to rapidly degraded proteins: the PEST hypothesis. Science, 234: 364-368, 1986.

91. Kugler, A., Stuhler, G., Walden, P., Zöller, G., Zobywalski, A., Brossart, P., Trefzer, U., Ullrich, S., Müller, C. A., Becker, V., Gross, A. J., Hemmerlein, B., Kanz, L., Müller, G. A., and Ringert, R. H. Regression of human metastatic renal cell carcinoma after vaccination with tumor cell-dendritic cell hybrids. Nat.Med., 6: 332-336, 2000.

92. Oiso, M., Eura, M., Katsura, F., Takiguchi, M., Sobao, Y., Masuyama, K., Nakashima, M., Itoh, K., and Ishikawa, T. A newly identified *MAGE-3*-derived epitope recognized by HLA-A24-restricted cytotoxic T lymphocytes. Int.J.Cancer, *81*: 387-394, 1999.
93. Jäger, E., Chen, Y. T., Drijfhout, J. W., Karbach, J., Ringhoffer, M., Jäger, D., Arand, M., Wada, H., Noguchi, Y., Stockert, E., Old, L. J., and Knuth, A. Simultaneous humoral and cellular immune response against cancer-testis antigen NY-ESO-1: definition of human histocompatibility leukocyte antigen (HLA)-A2-binding peptide epitopes. J.Exp.Med., *187*: 265-270, 1998.
94. Aarnoudse, C. A., van den Doel, P. B., Heemskerk, B., and Schrier, P. I. Interleukin-2-induced, melanoma-specific T cells recognize CAMEL, an unexpected translation product of *LAGE-1*. Int.J.Cancer, *82*: 442-448, 1999

3
Recognition of human tumors: SEREX expression cloning to identify tumour antigens

UGUR SAHIN, GENG LI , ÖZLEM TÜRECI, and MICHAEL PFREUNDSCHUH

INTRODUCTION

The search for tumor antigens which are able to elicit specific immune responses in the tumor-bearing host is one of the cardinal quests in tumor immunology. The knowledge of their molecular nature provides us not only with potential targets for immunotherapeutic interventions against neoplastic cells, but also provides us with new disease markers and new insights into the molecular mechanisms of malignant transformation.

In the seventies and eighties of the 20th century the hybridoma technology was exploited for the identification of molecules on tumor cells which could be used as diagnostic markers or as target structures for immunotherapeutic approaches with monoclonal antibodies. While some of these efforts have yielded new therapeutic tools, such as the anti-CD20 antibody rituximab which shows considerable activity and has been licensed for the treatment of follicular lymphomas [1], forms of active immunotherapy require the identification of target structures of spontaneously occurring immune responses rather than those which elicit xenogenic immune responses and are used for the immunization of mice to generate monoclonal antibodies.

The analysis of such humoral and cellular immune responses in cancer patients had indicated for a long time that cancer specific antigens do indeed exist and are recognized by the immune system of the tumor bearing host [2]. To disclose the molecular nature of these antigens, cloning techniques were developed that used established CTL clones [3] or circulating antibodies [4] as probes for screening tumor-derived expression libraries.

R.A. Robins and R.C. Rees (eds.), Cancer Immunology, 45–57.
© 2001 Kluwer Academic Publishers. Printed in the Netherlands.

IDENTIFICATION OF HUMAN TUMOR ANTIGENS BY T-CELL CLONES

A variety of *in vitro* studies and animal tumor models demonstrated that cytotoxic T lymphocytes (CTLs) are the protagonists of an effective cytotoxic anti-tumoral immune response making them the preferred tool in the search for antigens recognized by CD8+ T-lymphocytes.

One strategy uses a biochemical approach to elute antigenic peptides bound to major histocompatibility complex class I molecules of tumor cells and fractionates them by high-pressure liquid chromatography [5]. The peptides are then tested in a target cell sensitization assay for recognition by tumor-specific cytotoxic CD8+ anti-tumor T-cell clones. After several steps of fractionation, the sequences of individual peptides recognized by the CTL are obtained by tandem mass spectrometry.

Another strategy, which was pioneered by T. Boon and colleagues [3] makes use of antigen-loss tumor cell variants or other appropriate target cells. These are transfected with recombinant DNA or cDNA libraries prepared from tumor cell lines. The transfected cells are then tested for recognition by autologous tumor-specific CTL. Once the gene is identified, the region encoding the antigenic peptide can be narrowed down by transfecting gene fragments. The amino acid sequence deduced from the nucleotide sequence of this region can be used to produce synthetic oligopeptides which are then tested in a target cell sensitization assay for recognition by the original tumor-specific CTL clone.

The latter approach has indeed endowed us with several human tumor antigens defined at the molecular level (for review see reference [6]). However, the necessity of establishing pre-characterized CTL clones with tumor-cell specific reactivity, which are difficult to obtain and to maintain, is the major limitation of CTL-based cloning approaches and was the main reason why the majority of antigens defined by these strategies were restricted to malignant melanoma.

RATIONALE FOR USING THE ANTIBODY REPERTOIRE OF CANCER PATIENTS FOR THE IDENTIFICATION OF TUMOR ANTIGENS

Even though tumor immunology has been CTL-centered in the last decade, it is now commonly accepted that immune recognition of tumors is a concerted action. A large body of evidence points to a coordinated recruitment of CD4+, CD8+ and B-cell responses against a given tumor antigen and suggests that once immune recognition of an antigen is elicited, it is not restricted to merely one effector system. Furthermore, while there are hints that the CTL repertoire of cancer patients may be deleted for many relevant CTL precursors, it is quite unlikely that a concomitant antibody response towards antigens (in particular intracellular ones) for which respective CTLs have been deleted, would also be erased [7]. Thus, circulating tumor-associated antibodies of the IgG class may be the persisting hallmark of a substantial tumor/immune system interaction and may identify such gene products to which at least cognate T-cell help, but also specific cytotoxic T-cells should exist with a high probability. Antibody responses may even help to trace back to deleted CTL specificities. Based on these rationales, we designed a novel strategy using the antibody repertoire of cancer patients for the molecular definition of antigens to be subjected subsequently to procedures of reverse T-cell immunology in order to determine epitopes which are presented by MHC class I or II molecules and are recognized by T-lymphocytes.

THE SEREX APPROACH

To identify tumor antigens recognized by the antibody repertoire of cancer patients we developed a serological cloning approach, termed SEREX (serological analysis of tumor antigens by recombinant cDNA expression cloning). It allows a systematic and unbiased search for antibody responses against proteins and the direct molecular definition of the respective tumor antigens based on their reactivity with autologous patient serum (for reviews see also references [8-10]). For SEREX, cDNA expression libraries are constructed from fresh tumor specimens, cloned into λ phage expression vectors and phages are used to transfect E. coli. Recombinant proteins expressed during the lytic infection of the bacteria are transferred onto nitrocellulose membranes, which are then incubated with diluted (1:500–1:1000) and - most importantly - extensively pre-absorbed serum from the autologous patient. Clones reactive with high-tittered antibodies are identified using an enzyme conjugated second antibody specific for human IgG. Positive clones are subcloned to monoclonality thus allowing the direct molecular characterization by DNA sequencing.

The SEREX approach is technically characterized by several features:

- There is no need for established tumor cell lines and pre-characterized CTL clones.
- The use of fresh tumor specimens restricts the analysis to genes that are expressed by the tumor cells *in vivo* and circumvents *in vitro* artifacts associated with short and long term tumor cell culture.
- The use of the polyclonal (polyspecific) patient's serum allows for the identification of multiple antigens with one screening course.
- The screening is restricted to clones against which the patient's immune system has raised high-titered IgG or/and IgA antibody responses indicating the presence of a concomitant T-helper lymphocyte response *in vivo*.
- As both the expressed antigenic protein and the coding cDNA are present in the same plaque of the phage immunoscreening assay, identified antigens can be sequenced immediately. Sequence information of excised cDNA inserts can be directly used to determine the expression spectrum of identified transcripts by Northern blot and reverse transcription polymerase chain reaction (RT-PCR).
- The release of periplasmatic proteins involved in protein folding during phage induced bacterial lysis allows at least partial folding of recombinant proteins and provides the basis for the identification of linear as well as nonlinear epitopes. This has been confirmed by the expression of transcripts which code for enzymatically active proteins (our unpublished results). In contrast, epitopes derived from

eucaryotic post-translational modification (e.g. glycosylation), are not detected by the phage immunoscreening assay.

Meanwhile a number of modifications of the original method have been implemented. Immunoglobulins which are also recombinantly expressed due to the presence of B-lymphocytes and plasma cells in the tumor specimens used for the cDNA library, may represent >90% of all "positive" clones in some libraries. They can be identified by a modified initial screening procedure whereby the nitrocellulose membrane is incubated with enzyme-conjugated anti-human IgG followed by visualization with the appropriate enzymatic color reaction prior to the incubation of the autologous patient's serum [11]. Screening of tumor cell-lines rather than fresh tumor specimen circumvents this problem and additionally provides a pure RNA-source which is not contaminated with normal stroma [12]. Subtractive approaches allow to enrich the cDNA-library for tumor specific transcripts [11]. cDNA libraries may also be prepared from sources of specific interest, such as amplified chromosomal regions obtained by microdissection [13]. Also strategies are under way, which identify first differentially expressed tumor-specific transcripts, i.e. by representational difference analysis (RDA) or differential display and subsequently subject them to "reverse SEREX" by cloning them into λ phages for the evaluation of spontaneously occurring immune responses in cancer patients (manuscript in preparation).

THE CONCEPT OF THE CANCER IMMUNOME

As stated above, the SEREX approach allows for the identification of an entire profile of antigens using the antibody repertoire of a single cancer patient. The analysis of a variety of neoplasms demonstrated that all hitherto investigated neoplasms are immunogenic in the tumor-bearing host and that immunogenicity is conferred by multiple antigens. As the anti-tumor antibody repertoires from individual cancer patients vary considerably, a large number of antigens could be identified by SEREX. The proliferation of the technology and the concerted action of the SEREX core group under the patronage of the Ludwig Institutes for Cancer Research for the coordinated analysis of different types of human cancers has allowed the systematic typing of the expressed immunogenic human cancer genome. For the systematic documentation and archivation of sequence data and immunological characteristics of identified antigens an electronical SEREX database was initiated by the Ludwig Cancer Research Institutes, which is accessible to the public (www.licr.org/SEREX.html). By December 1999, more than 1200 entries have been made into the SEREX database, the majority of them representing independent antigens. The SEREX database is not only meant as a computational interface for discovery information management but also as a tool for mapping the entire panel of gene products which elicit spontaneous immune responses in the tumor bearing autologous host, for which the name "cancer immunome" has been coined by L.J. Old (LICR, New York Branch). The cancer immunome which is defined by using spontaneously occurring immune effectors from cancer patients as probes gains increasing interest, since it has been shown that immunogenic gene products deserve particular attention. Besides their role as targets for cancer vaccination [14], identified antigens may be valuable as new molecular markers of malignant disease. The value of each of these markers or a combination of them for diagnostic or prognostic evaluation of cancer patients has to be determined by studies which correlate markers with clinical data. Furthermore, the immune system is a sensitive biodetector, which may discover structural and regulative alterations and may therefore point to gene products with significance for neoplastic transformation or tumor progression [15, 16]. The detection of common tumor associated immune responses could therefore result in the identification of common tumor-associated molecular alterations. Accordingly, to assess for each constituent of the cancer immunome whether it is relevant with regard to tumor biology, tumor immunology or tumor vaccination, a multidimensional characterization has to be pursued. Constituents of the cancer immunome picked by SEREX include known tumor antigens such as the melanoma antigens MAGE-1, MAGE-4a and tyrosinase, demonstrating that at least some of the serologically identified antigens are also targets for CTL. A second group of antigens is represented by known classical auto-antigens for which immunogenecity is associated with autoimmune diseases, such as anti-mitochondrial antibodies or antibodies to U1-snRNP. When patients without autoimmune or rheumatic disorders are selected for SEREX analysis the incidence of such antigens is 0-3%. A third group is comprised of transcripts that are either identical or highly homologous to known genes, but have not been known to elicit immune responses in humans. Kinectin, a microtubule-associated transporter of golgi vesicles or lactate dehydrogenase belong to this group. The fourth group of serologically defined antigens consists of previously unknown genes. The abundance of antigens and the fact that a large portion of them is encoded by previously unknown genes, calls for a systematic but stringent procedure to assess the association of identified transcripts and observed immune reactions with the course of the malignant disease. This evaluation of cancer-relatedness is performed by a three-step analysis which comprises a *sequence analysis* (search for tumor associated sequence alterations) with subsequent homology search, *expression studies* in neoplastic and normal tissues and the *determination of the frequency of antibodies* in sera from cancer patients and healthy controls. These preliminary data help to select those antigens to be subjected to further investigations. Based on the results of the basic analysis the SEREX antigens can be assigned to different classes (Table 3.1).

Among them is the so-called c*ancer/testis (CT) antigen class.* These proteins are selectively expressed in a variety of neoplasms (in a lineage-independent manner), but not in normal tissues except for testis. Examples are members of the MAGE gene family, which had already been defined by CTL approaches, and several new antigens such as HOM-MEL-40 and NY-ESO-1 which will be discussed in more detail below.

Differentiation antigens demonstrate a lineage-specific expression in tumors, but also in normal cells of the same origin; examples are tyrosinase and GFAP (glial fibrillary acidic protein) which are antigenic in malignant melanoma and glioma, but are also expressed in melanocytes or brain cells, respectively.

Over-expressed genes code for many tumor antigens identified by SEREX, which has an inherent methodological bias for the detection of abundant transcripts. The members of this class are expressed at low levels in normal tissues (usually detectable by RT-PCR), but are up to 100-fold overexpressed in tumors. An example is HOM-RCC-3.1.3, a new carbonic anhydrase which is overexpressed in a fraction of renal cell cancers [17]. The overexpression of a transcript may also result from gene amplification as we have demonstrated for the translation initiation factor eIF-4g in a squamous cell lung cancer [13].

Table 3.1. Categories of tumor associated antigens identified by SEREX

Class	Antigen	Homology/identity	Source
Cancer testis antigens	HOM-MEL-40	SSX-2	melanoma
Differentiation antigens	HOM-MEL-55	tyrosinase	melanoma
Overexpressed gene products	HOM-HD-21	galectin-9	Hodgkin´s
Mutated gene products	NY-COL-2	p53	colon cancer
Spice variants	HOM-HD-397	resin	Hodgkin´s
Gene amplification products	HOM-NSCLC-11	eIF-4g	lung cancer
Cancer related autoantigens	HOM-MEL-2.4	CEBPgamma	melanoma

Antigens encoded by mutated genes have been demonstrated only rarely by the serological approach, with mutated p53 being one example [18]. For SEREX detected antigens proof of an underlying mutation is technically challenging since antibody responses induced by a mutation may be directed to the wild-type backbone of the molecule and thus the wild-type allele may be picked up during the immunoscreening, so that sequencing of several independent clones from the same library as well as exclusion of polymorphisms is mandatory.

Cancer-related autoantigens are expressed ubiquitously and at a similar level in healthy as well as malignant tissues. The encoding genes are not altered in tumor samples. However, they elicit antibody responses in cancer patients, not in healthy individuals. This might result from tumor-associated post-translational modifications or changes in the antigen processing and/or presentation in tumor cells.

SEREX-IDENTIFIED ANTIGENS WITH POTENTIAL RELEVANCE FOR THE MALIGNANT PHENOTYPE

Immunogenic gene products have provided new insights into cancer associated genotypic and phenotypic alterations. The alteration of a gene product by mutation or changes in its expression pattern which evoke an immune response may also be relevant for the biology of the malignant cell. The knowledge of the functional significance of a tumor-associated antigen has also substantial importance for its evaluation as a therapeutic target. An antigen which is indispensable for a tumor cell due to its crucial role for malignant proliferation or cell survival is less prone to be lost and hence less prone to escape from a therapeutic attack.

One of the first antigens identified by SEREX was HOM-RCC-313 [17]. Our investigations established this molecule as a novel member of the carbonic anhydrase

(CA) family, so that it was designated as CA XII. We found expression of CA XII at substantial levels restricted to kidney, colon, endometrium and activated PBL. However, overexpression of this transcript was disclosed in 10% of renal cell cancers (RCC) suggesting a potential significance in this tumor type. In fact, the same transcript was cloned shortly thereafter by another group based on its downregulation by the wild-type von-Hippel-Lindau tumor suppressor gene, the loss of function of which is known to be associated with an increased incidence of RCC [19]. The observation that the invasiveness of RCC cell lines expressing CA XII may be inhibited by acetazolamid [20], establishes CA XII as a molecule worth to be further assessed for its role in kidney cancer.

The detection of HOM-Tes-14/SCP-1 [21] by SEREX revealed the aberrant expression of meiosis-specific gene products in the somatic cells of human malignancies. According to our recent studies aberrantly expressed meiosis proteins are involved in the induction of chromosomal instabilities in cancer cells.

SEREX-IDENTIFIED ANTIGENS AS DIAGNOSTIC MARKERS

Gene products with differential expression restricted to or associated with tumors are of interest for their potential value as diagnostic and prognostic markers. An interesting diagnostic aspect for which SEREX opened new avenues is the concept of serodiagnosis in cancer. The analysis of sera from patients with various malignancies and healthy controls revealed that identified antigens can be separated into different categories. Individual antigens which are only recognized by the patient's serum used for the immunoscreening as well as antigens which elicit seroresponses also in healthy controls (i. e. independent of the presence of a tumor) are of minor interest for this purpose. However, a number of identified antigens elicit strictly tumor-associated antibody responses which are detected at varying rates only in the sera of patients with tumor types selectively expressing the respective antigen. This was the case for galectin-9 [4, 11], for NY-ESO-I [22], and for several antigens cloned from colon cancer [18]. The incidence of tumor-associated antibodies in unselected tumor patients ranges between 5-50% depending on the tumor-type and the respective antigen. Our observations suggest, that to obtain an appropriate sensitivity and specificity, a set of antigens have to be assembled to a multi-antigen approach allowing for a differential serodiagnosis of cancer. Ongoing studies have to identify those gene products to be involved in such a diagnostic panel.

SEREX-IDENTIFIED ANTIGENS AS POTENTIAL CANCER VACCINES

The main idea of cancer vaccination is to induce an effective specific cytolytic and/or T-helper immune activity against tumor cells. This necessitates the availability of antigen-derived peptide epitopes capable of priming or activating specific CTL or T-helper cells. In our view serologically defined antigens are most suitable candidates for determination of such epitopes.

As stated above, anti-tumor immune responses result from a concerted immunological action which involves both cellular and humoral effector mechanisms. Since the isotype switching and the development of high-titered IgG in vivo requires cognate CD4+ T-cell help, SEREX can be instrumentalized to analyze the CD4+ T-cell repertoire against tumor antigens. With regard to CD8+ T-lymphocytes that recognize SEREX antigens, it is noteworthy that MAGE-1 and MAGE-4a which had been originally described as CTL targets have also shown up in the SEREX immunoscreening of several tumors, suggesting that at least some of the serologically identified antigens may bear epitopes that are recognized by CTL. Meanwhile, CTL responses have been determined for several SEREX-identified antigens as will be discussed later.

The search for T-lymphocyte recognized epitopes of defined molecules is an important new field of molecular tumor immunology, often referred to as "reverse T cell immunology". Because of the diversity of peptides presented by the highly polymorphic HLA alleles, this objective means an enormous challenge for each individual antigen. Our group is addressing this question in detail for members of the CT antigen class identified by SEREX. Several strategies have been pursued in the last years for this purpose.

For *the peptide approach* serologically identified antigens are scanned for peptides containing binding motifs for MHC I or MHC II alleles [23, 24] focussing on well-characterized and frequent MHC alleles. The predicted peptides are synthesized and tested for binding to the respective MHC molecules. In a next step, peptides with affinity to MHC molecules are loaded onto dendritic cells or other professional antigen-presenters and used to stimulate autologous T lymphocytes. T-cells expanded by repeated stimulation are tested for HLA restricted reactivity to antigen-positive tumor cell lines. Using this approach we have identified several HLA-A201 presented antigenic peptides for different SEREX antigens.

The whole-protein approach is based on the utilization of the full-length antigen which is either expressed in professional antigen-presenting cells by polynucleotide transfection or is fed as recombinant protein. Successful transfection of polynucleotides in dendritic cells has been described using *in vitro* translated RNA [25] or recombinant viral delivery systems [26, 27]. Dendritic cells presenting antigenic peptides after processing of endogenously expressed or exogenously loaded antigens are used for the repeated stimulation of autologous T lymphocytes. Similar to the peptide approach expanded T-lymphocytes are tested for antigen-specific reactivity and MHC-restriction. In addition, *pre-existing CTL* with tumor specific reactivity may be assessed using COS cells co-transfected with cDNA coding for serologically identified antigens together with the restriction element.

Despite the fact that reverse T cell immunology is a new terrain in tumor immunology it advances rapidly. The analysis of peptides eluted from MHC molecules by mass spectroscopy is becoming more and more sensitive and will assist in the direct identification of naturally processed peptides derived from particular antigens. Together with the typing of the immunogenic genome provided by SEREX this will shape an ever more complete picture of the repertoire of cancer-associated antigenic peptides. The knowledge derived from these studies will form the basis for rational immunotherapeutic strategies, the success and failure of which could be analyzed at the molecular level.

To avoid major side effects by destruction of non-neoplastic cells the molecular targets of the induced cytolytic activity should not be expressed or at least not recognized on tissues which are essential for the health of the vaccinated individual. With respect to specificity several classes including CT antigens, differentiation antigens, tumor-associated over expressed gene products, mutated gene products and tumor-specific splice variants may be suitable targets. Here we will focus on members of the cancer/testis antigen class.

The class of cancer/testis antigens

Analysis of tumor-specific antigens revealed a novel class of antigens with an intriguing expression pattern. A variable proportion of human tumors, ranging from 10 to 70% depending on the type of tumor express cancer/testis (CT) antigens. In normal tissues CT antigens are not expressed, except in testis. Interestingly, the prototypes of this category, MAGE [3], BAGE [28], and GAGE [29], were initially identified as targets for cytotoxic T cells. Several new members which have been added by SEREX to this category will be discussed in more detail below.

HOM-MEL-40/SSX-2

The HOM-MEL-40 antigen which was detected in a melanoma library is the first cancer/testis antigen identified by SEREX. It is encoded by the SSX-2 gene [30]. Members of the SSX gene family, SSX1 and SSX2, have been shown to be involved in the t(X;18)(p11.2; q11.2) translocation which is found in the majority of human synovial sarcomas [31] and fuses the respective SSX gene with the SYT gene from chromosome 18. We observed that the SSX genes are silenced in normal tissues except for testis but are expressed in a wide variety of human tumors. Interestingly, the transcripts expressed in neoplasms other than synovial sarcoma are all derived from non-mutated, non-translocated genes. Using homology cloning, additional members of the SSX-family were identified [32] revealing at least five genes, of which four (SSX-1, 2, 4 and 5) demonstrate a CT antigen-like expression [33]. In the meanwhile we have identified several antigenic peptides derived from SSX gene products which can sensitize specific CD8+ as well as CD4+ cells from healthy donors (unpublished results).

NY-ESO-1

By applying the SEREX methodology to esophageal squamous cell carcinoma, Chen et al. [34] identified NY-ESO-1 as a new CT antigen. NY-ESO-1 mRNA expression is detectable in a variable proportion of a wide array of human cancers, including melanomas, breast cancer, bladder cancer and prostate cancer. A homologous gene, named LAGE-1 was subsequently isolated by a subtractive cloning approach [35] demonstrating that NY-ESO-1 belongs to a gene family with at least two members.

Interestingly, after its initial cloning by SEREX, NY-ESO-1 as well as its homologue LAGE-1 were rediscovered by independent groups using tumor specific CTL or tumour-infiltrating lymphocytes (TIL) derived from melanoma patients as probes, thus disclosing several HLA-A201 and HLA-A31 restricted epitopes [36]. Notably, some of the peptide epitopes were derived from an alternative open reading frame (ORF)[37, 38]. Thus NY-ESO-1 may simultaneously be an immune target for both antibody and CTL responses in the same patient [36, 39], a posteriori confirming the notion from which our groups had started with the SEREX approach. Stockert et al. [22] observed that IgG antibody responses directed against NY-ESO-1 are present in up to 50% of antigen-expressing patients indicating that this antigen may be also an important target for CD4+ T-lymphocytes.

HOM-TES-14/SCP-1

The expression of CT antigens in tumors and testis prompted our group to modify the original SEREX technique in order to bias for the detection of members of the CT class. For this intention testis expression libraries were enriched for testis-specific transcripts by subtractive techniques and immunoscreened with allogeneic sera from cancer patients. SEREX screening using such testis-specific surrogate libraries turned out to be a successful strategy for the identification of additional CT antigens [21]. One of the identified new CT antigens was shown to be encoded by the gene coding for the synaptonemal complex protein-1 (SCP-1). SCP-1 is known to be selectively expressed during the meiotic prophase of spermatocytes and is involved in the pairing of homologous chromosomes [40], an essential step for the generation of haploid cells in meiosis I. Investigation of a broad spectrum of normal and malignant tissues revealed expression of SCP-1 transcripts and antigen selectively in a variety of neoplastic tissues and tumor cell lines. Immunofluorescence microscopy analysis with specific antiserum showed a cell cycle phase-dependent nuclear or cytoplasmic expression of SCP-1 protein in cancer cells. SCP-1 is hitherto the only CT antigen with known function.

To cope with the rapidly growing number of CT antigens, a new nomenclature has been suggested for them [41]. According to the order of their initial identification the individual genes are designated by enumeration. Since individual CT antigens are expressed only in a variable proportion of tumors, only the availability of several CTA could significantly enlarge the proportion of patients eligible for vaccination studies. In this regard it is interesting that members of a given gene family tend to be expressed in a co-regulated fashion whereas different gene families are preferentially expressed in other sets of tumors [42]. It is therefore reasonable to choose antigens from different CT families to cover as many tumors as possible. Despite the fact that SEREX enlarged the pool of available tumor antigens, the proportion of tumors for which no tumor antigen is known, is still high, particularly in frequent neoplasms such as colon and prostate cancer. Moreover, immunohistological investigations for MAGE antigens have demonstrated a heterogeneity of antigen expression even in the same tumor specimen [43]. Thus, the combined or sequential use of a whole set of several antigens in a patient would have the potential of reducing or even preventing the *in vivo* selection of antigen loss tumor cell variants and would also address the problem of a heterogeneous expression of a given antigen in an individual tumor specimen.

CONCLUSIONS AND PROSPECTS FOR THE FUTURE

The multitude of tumor-specific antigens identified by the SEREX technique has revealed that the immune recognition of human tumors by the autologous host's immune system is not impaired and opens the perspective for depicting an antigenic profile for each tumor. Together with the identification of T lymphocyte epitopes for these and other antigens a picture on the immune recognition of cancer is emerging. The knowledge of the cancer immunome provides a new basis for understanding tumor biology and for the development of new diagnostic and therapeutic strategies for cancer. The abundance of human tumor antigens will enable us to proceed with the development of polyvalent vaccines for a wide spectrum of human cancers using pure preparations of molecularly defined antigens or antigenic peptide fragments. Additionally, the study and long-term follow-up of large numbers of patients will help to determine the diagnostic and prognostic relevance of tumor-related/specific autoantibodies in patients' sera and of antigen expression in tumors, as well as the correlation with CTL responses and specific T-helpers. Finally, the knowledge of immunogenic cancer gene products will convey an improved picture of cancer associated genetic and molecular alterations.

ACKNOWLEDGEMENTS

We thank Drs. LJ.Old and Y.-T. Chen (LICR, New York) for continuing discussions.

REFERENCES

1.   Maloney DG, GrilloLopez AJ, White CA, Bodkin D, Schilder RJ, Neidhart JA, Janakiraman N, Foon KA, Liles TM, Dallaire BK, Wey K, Royston I, Davis T, and Levy R, IDEC-C2B8 (Rituximab) anti-CD20 monoclonal antibody therapy in patients with relapsed low-grade non-Hodgkin's lymphoma. Blood, 1997; 90: 2188-2195.
2.   Old LJ, Cancer Immunology - the Search for Specificity - Clowes,G.H.A. Memorial Lecture. Cancer Res, 1981; 41: 361-375.
3.   van der Bruggen P, Traversari C, Chomez P, Lurquin C, Deplaen E, van den Eynde B, Knuth A, and Boon T, A gene encoding an antigen recognized by cytolytic lymphocytes-t on a human-melanoma. Science, 1991; 254: 1643-1647.
4.   Sahin U, Tureci O, Schmitt H, Cochlovius B, Johannes T, Schmits R, Stenner F, Luo GR, Schobert I, and Pfreundschuh M, Human Neoplasms Elicit Multiple Specific Immune-Responses In the Autologous Host. Proc Natl Acad Sci U S A, 1995; 92: 11810-11813.
5.   Rotzschke O, Falk K, Deres K, Schild H, Norda M, Metzger J, Jung G, and Rammensee HG, Isolation and Analysis of Naturally Processed Viral Peptides as Recognized by Cytotoxic T-Cells. Nature, 1990; 348: 252-254.
6.   Boon T, Coulie PG, and Van den Eynde B, Tumor antigens recognized by T cells. Immunol Today, 1997; 18: 267-268.
7.   Hartley SB, Cooke MP, Fulcher DA, Harris AW, Cory S, Basten A, and Goodnow CC, Elimination of Self-Reactive Lymphocytes-B Proceeds in 2 Stages - Arrested Development and Cell-Death. Cell, 1993; 72: 325-335.
8.   Sahin U, Tureci O, and Pfreundschuh M, Serological identification of human tumor antigens. Curr Opin Immunol, 1997; 9: 709-716.
9.   Tureci O, Sahin U, and Pfreundschuh M, Serological analysis of human tumor antigens: Molecular definition and implications. Mol Med Today, 1997; 3: 342-349.

10. Tureci O, Sahin U, Zwick C, Neumann F, and Pfreundschuh M, Exploitation of the antibody repertoire of cancer patients for the identification of human tumor antigens. Hybridoma, 1999; 18: 23-28.

11. Tureci O, Schmitt H, Fadle N, Pfreundschuh M, and Sahin U, Molecular definition of a novel human galectin which is immunogenic in patients with Hodgkin's disease. J Biol Chem, 1997; 272: 6416-6422.

12. Chen YT, Gure AO, Tsang S, Stockert E, Jager E, Knuth A, and Old LJ, Identification of multiple cancer/testis antigens by allogeneic antibody screening of a melanoma cell line library. Proc Natl Acad Sci U S A, 1998; 95: 6919-6923.

13. Brass N, Heckel D, Sahin U, Pfreundschuh M, Sybrecht GW, and Meese E, Translation initiation factor eIF-4gamma is encoded by an amplified gene and induces an immune response in squamous cell lung carcinoma. Hum Mol Genet, 1997; 6: 33-39.

14. Rosenberg SA, A new era for cancer immunotherapy based on the genes that encode cancer antigens. Immunity, 1999; 10: 281-287.

15. Wolfel T, Hauer M, Schneider J, Serrano M, Wolfel C, Klehmannhieb E, Deplaen E, Hankeln T, Zumbuschenfelde KHM, and Beach D, A P16(Ink4a)-Insensitive Cdk4 Mutant Targeted by Cytolytic T- Lymphocytes in a Human-Melanoma. Science, 1995; 269: 1281-1284.

16. Wang RF, Wang X, Atwood AC, Topalian SL, and Rosenberg SA, Cloning genes encoding MHC class II-restricted antigens: Mutated CDC27 as a tumor antigen. Science, 1999; 284: 1351-1354.

17. Tureci O, Sahin U, Vollmar E, Siemer S, Gottert E, Seitz G, Parkkila AK, Shah GN, Grubb JH, Pfreundschuh M, and Sly WS, Human carbonic anhydrase XII: cDNA cloning, expression, and chromosomal localization of a carbonic anhydrase gene that is overexpressed in some renal cell cancers. Proc Natl Acad Sci U S A, 1998; 95: 7608-7613.

18. Scanlan MJ, Chen YT, Williamson B, Gure AO, Stockert E, Gordan JD, Tureci O, Sahin U, Pfreundschuh M, and Old LJ, Characterization of human colon cancer antigens recognized by autologous antibodies. Int J Cancer, 1998; 76: 652-658.

19. Ivanov SV, Kuzmin I, Wei MH, Pack S, Geil L, Johnson BE, Stanbridge EJ, and Lerman MI, Down-regulation of transmembrane carbonic anhydrases in renal cell carcinoma cell lines by wild-type von Hippel-Lindau transgenes. Proc Natl Acad Sci U S A, 1998; 95: 12596-12601.

20. Parkkila S, Rajaniemi H, Parkkila AK, Kivela J, Waheed A, Pastorekova S, Pastorek J, and Sly WS, Carbonic anhydrase inhibitor suppresses invasion of renal cancer cells in vitro. Proc Natl Acad Sci U S A, 2000; 97: 2220-2224.

21. Tureci O, Sahin U, Zwick C, Koslowski M, Seitz G, and Pfreundschuh M, Identification of a meiosis-specific protein as a member of the class of cancer/testis antigens. Proc Natl Acad Sci U S A, 1998; 95: 5211-5216.

22. Stockert E, Jager E, Chen YT, Scanlan MJ, Gout I, Karbach J, Arand M, Knuth A, and Old LJ, A survey of the humoral immune response of cancer patients to a panel of human tumor antigens. J Exp Med, 1998; 187: 1349-1354.

23. Rammensee HG, Friede T, and Stevanovic S, MHC Ligands and Peptide Motifs - First Listing. Immunogenetics, 1995; 41: 178-228.

24. Hammer J, Bono E, Gallazzi F, Belunis C, Nagy Z, and Sinigaglia F, Precise prediction of major histocompatibility complex class-ii peptide interaction based on peptide side-chain scanning. J Exp Med, 1994; 180: 2353-2358.

25. Boczkowski D, Nair SK, Snyder D, and Gilboa E, Dendritic cells pulsed with RNA are potent antigen-presenting cells in vitro and in vivo. J Exp Med, 1996; 184: 465-472.

26. Song W, Kong HL, Carpenter H, Torii H, Granstein R, Rafii S, Moore MAS, and Crystal RG, Dendritic cells genetically modified with an adenovirus vector encoding the cDNA for a model antigen induce protective and therapeutic antitumor immunity. J Exp Med, 1997; 186: 1247-1256.

27. Bronte V, Carroll MW, Goletz TJ, Wang M, Overwijk WW, Marincola F, Rosenberg SA, Moss B, and Restifo NP, Antigen expression by dendritic cells correlates with the therapeutic effectiveness of a model recombinant poxvirus tumor vaccine. Proc Natl Acad Sci U S A, 1997; 94: 3183-3188.

28. Boel P, Wildmann C, Sensi ML, Brasseur R, Renauld JC, Coulie P, Boon T, and van der Bruggen P, Bage - a New Gene Encoding an Antigen Recognized on Human Melanomas by Cytolytic T-Lymphocytes. Immunity, 1995; 2: 167-175.

29. van den Eynde B, Peeters O, Debacker O, Gaugler B, Lucas S, and Boon T, A New Family Of Genes-Coding For an Antigen Recognized By Autologous Cytolytic T-Lymphocytes On a Human-Melanoma. J Exp Med, 1995; 182: 689-698.

30. Tureci O, Sahin U, Schobert I, Koslowski M, Schmitt H, Schild HJ, Stenner F, Seitz G, Rammensee HG, and Pfreundschuh M, The SSX-2 gene, which is involved in the t(X;18) translocation of synovial sarcomas, codes for the human tumor antigen HOM-MEL-40. Cancer Res, 1996; 56: 4766-4772.

31. Clark J, Rocques PJ, Crew AJ, Gill S, Shipley J, Chan AML, Gusterson BA, and Cooper CS, Identification of Novel Genes, Syt and Ssx, Involved in the T(X18)(P11.2q11.2) Translocation Found in Human Synovial Sarcoma. Nat Genet, 1994; 7: 502-508.

32. Gure AO, Tureci O, Sahin U, Tsang S, Scanlan MJ, Jager E, Knuth A, Pfreundschuh M, Old LJ, and Chen YT, SSX: A multigene family with several members transcribed in normal testis and human cancer. Int J Cancer, 1997; 72: 965-971.

33. Tureci O, Chen YT, Sahin U, Gure AO, Zwick C, Villena C, Tsang S, Seitz G, Old LJ, and Pfreundschuh M, Expression of SSX genes in human tumors. Int J Cancer, 1998; 77: 19-23.

34. Chen YT, Scanlan MJ, Sahin U, Tureci O, Gure AO, Tsang SL, Williamson B, Stockert E, Pfreundschuh M, and Old LJ, A testicular antigen aberrantly expressed in human cancers detected by autologous antibody screening. Proc Natl Acad Sci U S A, 1997; 94: 1914-1918.

35. Lethe B, Lucas S, Michaux L, De Smet C, Godelaine D, Serrano A, De Plaen E, and Boon T, LAGE-1, a new gene with tumor specificity. Int J Cancer, 1998; 76: 903-908.

36. Jager E, Chen YT, Drijfhout JW, Karbach J, Ringhoffer M, Jager D, Arand M, Wada H, Noguchi Y, Stockert E, Old LJ, and Knuth A, Simultaneous humoral and cellular immune response against cancer-testis antigen NY-ESO-1: Definition of human histocompatibility leukocyte antigen (HLA)-A2-binding peptide epitopes. J Exp Med, 1998; 187: 265-270.

37. Aarnoudse CA, van den Doel PB, Heemskerk B, and Schrier PI, Interleukin-2-induced, melanoma-specific T cells recognize camel, an unexpected translation product of LAGE-1. Int J Cancer, 1999; 82: 442-448.

38. Wang RF, Johnston SL, Zeng G, Topalian SL, Schwartzentruber DJ, and Rosenberg SA, A breast and melanoma-shared tumor antigen: T cell responses to antigenic peptides translated from different open reading frames. J Immunol, 1998; 161: 3596-3606.

39. Jager E, Stockert E, Zidianakis Z, Chen YT, Karbach J, Jager D, Arand M, Ritter G, Old LJ, and Knuth A, Humoral immune responses of cancer patients against "Cancer- Testis" antigen NY-ESO-1: Correlation with clinical events. Int J Cancer, 1999; 84: 506-510.

40. Meuwissen RLJ, Meerts I, Hoovers JMN, Leschot NJ, and Heyting C, Human synaptonemal complex protein 1 (SCP1): Isolation and characterization of the cDNA and chromosomal localization of the gene. Genomics, 1997; 39: 377-384.

41. Old LJ and Chen YT, New paths in human cancer serology. J Exp Med, 1998; 187: 1163-1167.

42. Sahin U, Tureci O, Chen YT, Seitz G, Villena-Heinsen C, Old LJ, and Pfreundschuh M, Expression of multiple cancer/testis (CT) antigens in breast cancer and melanoma: basis for polyvalent CT vaccine strategies. Int J Cancer, 1998; 78: 387-389.

43. Hofbauer GFL, Schaefer C, Noppen C, Boni R, Kamarashev J, Nestle FO, Spagnoli GC, and Dummer R, MAGE-3 immunoreactivity in formalin-fixed, paraffin-embedded primary and metastatic melanoma - Frequency and distribution. Am J Pathol, 1997; 151: 1549-1553.

4
Recognition of human tumours: melanoma differentiation antigens

JESPER ZEUTHEN and ALEXEI F. KIRKIN

INTRODUCTION

Investigation of the immune response against human melanomas demonstrated that self-proteins belonging to lineage-specific differentiation antigens are commonly recognised by melanoma-specific cytotoxic T lymphocytes (CTL). Originally discovered for tyrosinase [1], it was later demonstrated for other melanosome proteins: gp100, Melan-A/MART-1, TRP-1 and TRP-2. A number of antigenic epitopes have been characterised in these antigens, opening up new possibilities for the immunotherapy of malignant melanomas. The first clinical trials have already been started [2-5]. In this chapter, we will concentrate on the available data concerning the characterisation of melanoma-associated differentiation antigens with focus on their immunogenic and protective properties.

CHARACTERISATION OF MELANOCYTE DIFFERENTIATION ANTIGENS

The recognition of normal melanocyte products has been demonstrated for a number of melanoma-specific CTL lines and clones and indicates the absence of strong tolerance to this group of self-proteins [6]. Several melanocyte differentiation antigens have been identified so far, representing melanosomal proteins (tyrosinase, Melan-A/MART-1, gp100, TRP-1 and TRP-2) and melanocortin 1 receptor (MC1R). Many peptide epitopes recognised by both cytotoxic T lymphocytes (CTL) and CD4$^+$ T helper cells have been identified (Table 4.1), opening new perspectives for specific immunotherapy. For identification of CTL epitopes, three main approaches has been used: a) identification of specificity of CTLs present in TIL cultures or in cultures of PBLs stimulated *in vitro* with melanoma cells; b) "reverse immunology", when predicted peptides from known antigens are used for *in vitro* immunisation and generated cultures are tested against melanoma cells;

R.A. Robins and R.C. Rees (eds.), Cancer Immunology, 59–72.

and c) identification of specificity of CTLs present in PBLs of patients immunised with protein antigens.

RECOGNITION BY CYTOTOXIC T LYMPHOCYTES

Tyrosinase

Tyrosinase is a 529-amino-acid melanosomal membrane protein previously shown to be required for the synthesis of melanin [7]. Tyrosinase was the first melanocyte differentiation antigen found to be recognised by tumour specific HLA-A2.1-restricted CTLs [1]. Two nonapeptide epitopes were later identified [8]: signal sequence 1-9 (MLLAVLYCL) and the peptide 368-376 (YMNGTMSQV). HLA-A24-restricted melanoma specific TIL 888 was also shown to recognise tyrosinase [9], but for this TIL culture the target peptide was not so far determined despite great efforts (Dr. Yutaka Kawakami, personal communication). For another HLA-A24-restricted TIL line from patient 1413, it was determined as AFLPWHRLF [10]. Several other epitopes recognised either by TIL cultures or by CTLs induced by immunisation with melanoma cells have been determined until now. They include epitope 192-200 (SEIWRDIDF) recognised by a HLA-B44-restricted CTL clone and established from the PBL of patient MZ2 [11,12], HLA-A1-restricted epitopes with core residues 243-251 (KCDICTDEY) [12], another HLA-A1-restricted epitope146-156 (SSDYVIPIGTY) [13], and HLA-B35-restricted epitope 312-320 (LPSSADVEF) [14].

The epitope 368-376, YMNGTMSQV, predicted from the amino acid sequence of the protein, was found to be slightly different from the tyrosinase epitope YMDGTMSQV identified by mass spectroscopy of peptides eluted from the HLA-A2.1 melanoma cell line [15]. This particular peptide results from posttranslational conversion of asparagine to aspartic acid. The CTL clone recognised the modified peptide much more efficiently than the unmodified peptide, indicating that the posttranslationally modified peptide in fact is the natural epitope. The possibility of a posttranslational modification of the HLA-A1-restricted peptide epitope 243-251 (KCDICTDEY) has also been suggested [12].

Screening the reactivity of CD8[+] cells, obtained after vaccination of melanoma patients with polyvalent melanoma vaccine against panel of totally 45 HLA-A2-restricted peptides from melanoma antigens, Reynolds and others [16] found response against 22 of them, including five not previously described epitopes from tyrosinase: 8-17 (CLLWSFQTSA), 214-222 (FLLRWEQEI), 482-490 (AMVGAVLTA), 487-495 (VLTALLAGL), and 490-498 (ALLAGLVSL).

In general, the generation of a tyrosinase-specific response in a melanoma patient is a relatively infrequent event and is usually seen only in patients showing a strong response against several melanoma-associated antigens (as exemplified by patients MZ2, 888 and SK29(AV)). The only data indicating its possible involvement in tumour rejection is the complete rejection of multiple melanoma metastases in patient 888 upon injection of TIL established from a resected melanoma [9] but the same TIL recognised several other antigens. Therefore other antigens than tyrosinase could constitute major rejection antigens which mediate tumour rejection caused by TIL 888.

Table 4.1. Antigenic epitopes of melanoma-associated differentiation antigens recognised by CTLs and T-helper cells

Antigen	HLA	Epitope	Sequence	References
gp100				
	A2	11-19	HLAVIGALL[a)	[16]
	A2	13-21	AVIGALLAV[a)	[16]
	A2	154-162	KTWGQYWQV	[17]
	A2	177-186	AMLGTHTMEV[b)	[18]
	A2	178-186	MLGTHTMEV[b)	[18]
	A2	209-217	ITDQVPFSV	[17]
	A2	232-241	FLRNQPLTFA[a)	[16]
	A2	280-288	YLEPGPVTA	[17]
	A2	457-466	LLDGTATLRL	[19]
	A2	476-485	VLYRYGSFSV	[17]
	A2	570-579	SLADTNSLAV[b)	[18]
	A2	585-593	IMPGQEAGL[a)	[16]
	A2	619-627	RLMKQDFSV	[13]
	A2	639-647	RLPIFCSC	[13]
	A3	17-25	ALLAVGATK	[20]
	A3	614-622	LIYRRRLMK	[13]
	A24		VYFFLPDHL[c)	[21]
	Cw8	71-78	SNDGPTLI	[22]
		70-78	ASNDGPTLI	[22]
	DR4	44-59	WNRQLYPEWTEAQRLD	[23]
Melan-A/MART-1				
	A2	27-35	AAGIGILTV	[24]
	A2	26-35	EAAGIGILTV	[25]
	A2	31-39	GILTVILGV[a)	[16]
	A2	32-40	ILTVILGVL [26]	
	A2	56-64	ALMDKSLHV[a)	[16]
	B45	24-33	AEEAAGIGIL	[27]
	B45	24-34	AEEAAGIGILT	[27]
	DR4	51-73	RNGYRALMDKSLHVGTQCALTRR	[28]
Tyrosinase				
	A1	243-251	KCDICTDEY	[12]
	A1	146-156	SSDYVIPIGTY	[13]
	A2	1-9	MLLAVLYCL	[8]
	A2	8-17	CLLWSFQTSA[a)	[16]
	A2	214-222	FLLRWEQEI[a)	[16]
	A2	369-377	YMNGTMSQV	[8]
			YMDGTMSQV[d)	[15]
	A2	482-490	AMVGAVLTA[a)	[16]
	A2	487-495	VLTALLAGL[a)	[16]
	A2	490-498	ALLAGLVSL[a)	[16]
	A24	206-214	AFLPWHRLF	[10]
	B35	312-320	LPSSADVEF	[14]
	B44	192-200	SEIWRDIDF	[11]

Table 4.1 (continued).

Antigen	HLA	Epitope	Sequence	References
Tyrosinase				
	DR4	56-70	QNILLSNAPLGPQFP	[29]
	DR4	448-462	DYSYLQDSDPDSFQD	[29]
	DR4	193-203	EIWRDIDFAHE	[30]
	DR15	386-406	FLLHHAFVDSIFEQWLQRHRP	[31]
TRP-1				
	A31	1-9[d]	MSLQRQFLR[e]	[32]
TRP-2				
	A31,A33	197-205	LLPGGRPYR	[33,34]
	A2	180-188	SVYDFFVWL	[35]
	A2	455-463	YAIDLPVSV[a]	[16]
	Cw8	387-395	ANDPIFVVL	[22]
	A*68, A*33		EVISCKLIKR[f]	[36]
MC1R				
	A2	79-87	CLALSDLLV[a]	[16]
	A2	244-253	TILLGIFFL[b] [37]	
	A2	251-259	FLCWGPFFL[a]	[16]
	A2	283-291	FLALIICNA[b]	[37]
	A2	291-299	AIIDPLIYA[b]	[37]

[a] Epitopes recognised by CTL after vaccination of patients with polyvalent melanoma vaccine.
[b] "Subdominant" epitopes – CTLs induced against peptides can kill melanoma cells expressing corresponding antigen.
[c] Antigenic peptide is coded by sequence in intron 4 of alternatively spliced *gp100* (*gp100*-in4).
[d] Natural peptide identified by elution from HLA-A2.
[e] Antigenic peptide resulted from translation of an alternative open reading frame (ORF3) of the gp75 gene.
[f] Antigenic peptide is coded by retained intron 2 of a partially spliced form of *TRP-2* (*TRP-2-INT2*).

MELAN-A/MART-1

Another melanocyte differentiation antigen, Melan-A/MART-1, was identified independently by two different groups [38,39]. This is a relatively small transmembrane protein consisting of 118 amino acid residues widely distributed in melanomas, but absent in other tumours. HLA-A2-restricted CTLs were demonstrated first and the 9-mer immunodominant peptide 27-35 with the sequence AAGIGILTV was identified and was shown to be recognised by all TIL cultures reacting against Melan-A/MART-1 [24]. Another epitope, 32-40 (ILTVILGVL) was identified by sequencing of naturally processed peptide from melanoma cells [26]. The recognition of this epitope is seen by only some Melan-A/MART-1-specific clones, which also recognise 27-35 epitope (see for example [40]). This recognition is usually less efficient, and some clones can react only by production of GM-CSF, but not by cytotoxicity or IFN-γ production [40]. The peptide 27-35 probably represents the immunodominant peptide of Melan-A/MART-1 because only this peptide was able to induce the generation of melanoma-specific CTL upon *in vitro* immunisation of PBL from melanoma patients [41]. It is interesting to note that other Melan-A/MART-1 peptides having higher affinity to the HLA-A2.1 antigen did not induce the generation of melanoma-specific CTL [42], pointing to the existence of predominantly intermediate and low affinity T cell receptors which recognise "self" antigens. In the search of the different peptides around peptide 27-35 Romero et al. have found [25] that peptide 26-35 (EAAGIGILTV) is recognised much more efficiently than the nonamer 27-35. Subsequently the same group have shown that several substitutions of amino acids in position 1 and 2 leading to the increased binding of the peptide to HLA-A2 molecule lead to further increase in their recognition by Melan-A/MART-1-specific CTL, and one of these analogues, peptide ELAGIGILTV have increased ability to induce specific CTL [43]. Two other HLA-A2-restricted epitopes (31-39, GILTVILGV, and 56-64, ALMDKSLHL) were detected after vaccination of melanoma patients with a polyvalent vaccine [16]. Two HLA-B45 epitopes, overlapping with HLA-A2-restricted epitopes, have been describes with CTLs isolated from patient SK29(AV) [27] - AEEAAGIGILT (24-34) and AEEAAGIGIL (24-33). The relative immunogenicity of Melan-A/MART-1 is thought to be the highest among the melanocyte-specific differentiation antigens, and CTL recognising this protein are easily induced after stimulation of PBLs with peptides or allogeneic melanoma cells [41,44] or expansion of TILs isolated from melanoma tumours [24,45]. On the other hand, the role of this antigen in the generation of protective immunity is probably not very significant, because the ability of different TILs to induce tumour rejection did not correlate with the recognition of Melan-A/MART-1 [17] and the immunisation of the melanoma patients with the immunodominant peptide 27-35, which increased the frequency of Melan-A/MART-1-specific CTL did not induce tumour regression [46].

GP100

The gene encoding gp100 was originally identified as a melanocyte lineage-specific antigen recognised by the antibodies NKI-beteb, HMB-50 and HMB-45, which are used as diagnostic markers for human melanoma [47]. Using TIL 1200, which induced complete regression of multiple melanoma metastases, the antigen recognised by these TILs was identified and found to be identical to the melanocyte differentiation antigen gp100 [19,48]. The 661-amino-acid gp100 glycoprotein appears to contain a signal peptide as well as a single transmembrane domain.

Five different peptide epitopes, all recognised by CTL in a HLA-A2-restricted manner, have been first identified [17,19]. The peptide epitope 280-288 (YLEPGPVTA), which was recognised by 6 of 8 different gp100-reactive TIL derived from different patients [17] was also eluted from the HLA-A2 molecule on melanoma cells and was reported to be recognised by 5/5 CTL raised from PBLs [49]. Melanoma-reactive CTL could be induced by in vitro stimulation with these gp100 peptides, but not as efficiently as with the MART-1 peptide 27-35 [50]. Subsequently additional nine epitopes of gp100 were identified. Two were recognised by HLA-A2-restricted TIL cultures (epitopes RLMKQDFSV, 619-627, and RLPIFCSC, 639-647) [13], four, also restricted by HLA-A2, were detected after vaccination with a polyvalent melanoma vaccine [16], two were recognised by HLA-A3-restricted CTL (epitopes 17-25 (ALLAVGATK) [20] and 614-622 (LIYRRRLMK) [13]) and one epitope was recognised by a HLA-Cw8-restricted TILs (nonameric form 70-78 (ASNDGPTLI) or octameric form 71-78 (SNDGPTLI)) [22]. For the epitope 639-647 (RLPIFCSC) the possibility of post-translational reduction of cysteine residues has been suggested, as a replacement of either cysteine residue with α-amino butyric acid enhanced CTL recognition [13]. Three "subdominant" HLA-A2-restricted epitopes have been detected by *in vitro* immunisation of PBLs with HLA-A2-binding peptides [18]: 178-186 (MLGTHTMEV), 177-186 (AMLGTHTMEV) and 570-579 (SLADTNSLAV). CTL generated against these peptides could induce lysis of HLA-A2-positive melanoma cells, indicating potential significance of these epitopes as immunological targets.

The HLA-A24-restricted TIL 1290 was recently found to recognise one additional antigen, a variant of the *gp100* gene that had retained the entire fourth intron of this gene, designated *gp100*-in4 [21]. The *gp100*-in4 transcript could be detected by reverse transcription-coupled PCR but could not be detected in Northern blots of melanoma RNA, indicating that it represents a relatively rare transcript. Read-through of this transcript into the region corresponding to the fourth intron gave rise to an additional 35 amino acids not found in the normal gp100 protein, and a peptide within this region (VYFFLPDHL) was shown to be recognised by a T cell subline isolated from TIL 1290. HLA-A24-matched allogeneic melanoma cell lines and melanocytes were found to be recognised by the T cell line, demonstrating that this represents a nonmutated epitope. The presence of spliced gp100 in normal melanocytes was also demonstrated by Lupetti et al. [36], stressing the classification of this antigen to the group of melanocyte differentiation antigens.

A significant correlation between T cell recognition *in vitro* and tumour regression in patients receiving TIL therapy was demonstrated for gp100 [17,51], suggesting that this protein may be a potent tumour regression antigen. However, as for tyrosinase, the same TIL cultures recognised other antigens that could induce regression, either by themselves or in combination with the CTLs recognising gp100. Nevertheless, this antigen until now probably represents the most promising HLA-A2-restricted differentiation antigen yet described for immunotherapeutic applications.

TRP-1 and TRP-2

Two other proteins involved in the biosynthesis of melanin have been shown to contain epitopes recognised by CTL. Tyrosinase-related protein-1 (TRP-1), or gp75, is responsible for the formation of a CTL epitope recognised in HLA-A31-restricted manner [52]. Attempts to identify the peptide epitope resulted in the identification of an epitope which was not in the protein sequence of TRP-1 itself but the product of an alternative reading frame (ORF3) of TRP-1 [32]. The identified peptide has the sequence MSLQRQFLR. The same HLA-A31-restricted TIL culture was used for the identification of another antigen - TRP-2 [33]. The peptide epitope of TRP-2 was identified as LLPGGRPYR (197-205). HLA-A31 belongs to the HLA-A3 supergroup [53], and it was found that both peptides are capable to bind to the members of this supergroup (HLA-A3, -A11, A31, A-33 and A68) [34]. These authors [34] have identified a TIL culture (TIL1244) from a HLA-A33-positive patient, which recognise TRP-2 peptide LLPGGRPYR presented by both HLA-A31 and –A33 molecules. These data indicate that recognition of the same epitope could be mediated in the context of several HLA class I molecules. The HLA-A2-restricted peptide 180-188 (SVYDFFVWL) from TRP-2 has been used for the induction of CTL response of PBL of HLA-A2-positive melanoma patients [35]. The generated CTLs could induce the lysis of TRP-2-positive melanomas in HLA-A2-restricted manner, indicating the possibility of the HLA-A2-restricted response against TRP-2. Another HLA-A2-restricted epitope (455-463, YAIDLPVSV) was found after vaccination of melanoma patients with a polyvalent melanoma vaccine [16]. In addition, a HLA-Cw8-restricted epitope recognised by TILs has been identified as ANDPIFVVL (residues 387-395) [22]. The interesting observation has been made with identification of another epitope of TRP-2 recognised by HLA-A*68-restricted CTL line [36]. The identified epitope, EVISCKLIKR, was found to be coded by an intronic sequence of partially spliced *TRP-2* mRNA (*TRP-2-INT2*). It is of interest, that, in contrast to the fully spliced *TRP-2* mRNA expressed in melanomas, normal skin melanocytes, and retina, the *TRP-2-INT2* mRNA could be detected at significant levels in melanomas but not in corresponding normal cells of the melanocytic lineage.

In addition to melanoma, the expression of gp75 has also been detected in a small number of renal cell carcinomas [54]. Renal cell carcinomas are also different from many other types of tumours in that they have very low levels of expression of many cancer/testis antigens with the exception of PRAME and RAGE-1 [54].

The infusion of TIL 586, recognising TRP-1 and TRP-2, plus IL-2 into the same melanoma patient from which the TIL culture was established resulted in the objective regression of tumour [55]. The question arises if these antigens have *in vivo* protective activity. TIL 586 recognises several antigens, including NY-ESO-1 [56], a recently identified cancer/testis antigen [57], therefore it is difficult to conclude, which particular antigen is most important for the tumour regression. The protective effect of TRP-2 immunisation has been recently demonstrated in experiments in mice [58]. It is interesting, that, in contrast to immunisation against TRP-1 protein [59], no development of vitiligo has been observed with immunisation against TRP-2. In addition, TRP-2 has a broader distribution in melanomas than tyrosinase or TRP-1 [60,61] and its expression correlates better with cell proliferation than with melanin content [62]. All these data may indicate that among this group of antigens, TRP-2 can have more significance for immunotherapy than tyrosinase or TRP-1.

Melanocortin 1 Receptor

Melanocortin 1 receptor (MC1R) belongs to subfamily of G-protein-coupled receptors expressed on melanomas and melanocytes. CTLs induced against three (244-253 (TILLGIFFL), 283-291 (FLALIICNA), and 291-299 (AIIDPLIYA)) out of 12 tested HLA-A2-binding peptide epitopes were able to recognise and kill HLA-A2-positive melanoma cell lines [37]. CTLs reactive with peptides of MCR1R have also been detected after immunisation of melanoma patients with a polyvalent melanoma vaccine [16]. The epitopes identified were 79-87 (CLALSDLLV), 251-259 (FLCWGPFFL) and 291-299 as above. The example of recognition of MC1R points out that several other melanocyte lineage-specific molecules could be potential targets for CTL melanoma immunotherapy.

T-HELPER EPITOPES

In general, induction of a strong CTL response requires a cooperation of CTL precursors with CD4-positive T cells. For some of melanocyte differentiation antigens epitopes inducing CD4$^+$ T cell response have recently been identified (Table 4.1). These antigens include tyrosinase [29-31], Gp100 [23,63] and MART-1 [28]. Such epitopes are probably present also in gp100, as dendritic cells loaded with recombinant gp100 can induce a strong CD4$^+$ T-helper response [64].

IMMUNOGENICITY OF MELANOCYTE DIFFERENTIATION ANTIGENS AND CONCLUDING REMARKS

Melanocyte differentiation antigens are self-proteins, and the normal mechanism of the generation of immunological tolerance should prevent the development of autoreactive T cell clones. The mechanisms of braking this tolerance for melanocyte differentiation antigens are not known. For Melan-A/MART-1 it has been suggested, that the immune response against the main peptide epitope is cross-reactive by its nature [65], [66], as many bacterial and other proteins have similar sequences. It is of interest, that peptides present in the CD2 molecule, region 214-224, have high homology with HLA-A2-binding Melan-A/MART-1 peptides:

```
Melan-A: 27 AAGIGILTVILGVL 40
            G G+L V+L   L
   CD2:   211 GAGLLLVLLVAL 222
```

The most homologous region is in the range of 32-40 epitope of Melan-A/Mart-1. According to the prediction of HLA-A2-binding peptides [67], the homologous region in CD2 molecule has at least two peptides (LLLVLLVAL and GLLLVLLVA) with a HLA-A2-binding motif. It is therefore possible that these peptides are presented on the surface of T cells. In thymus positive selection of T cells weakly recognising such peptides can take place, leading to selective proliferation of corresponding lymphocyte clones. In the periphery such clones should look like normal naïve T lymphocytes. Exactly this situation was observed during investigation of frequencies of Melan-A/MART-1-specific CTL precursors in peripheral blood employing tetramers of HLA-A2 molecules complexed with 26-35 peptides [68].

Another possible explanation is that the levels of expression of melanocyte differentiation antigens is low in normal melanocytes and is increased in tumour cells. For example it was demonstrated that at the mRNA level, gp100 expression is much higher in melanomas than in normal melanocytes [69]. In addition, normal melanocytes have a much lower reactivity with the HMB-45 monoclonal antibody detecting the gp100 protein than melanoma cells [70,71]. The mechanisms for this increase could be the same as those suggested for the expression of cancer/testis antigens in tumour cells that they are the result of wide-range DNA de-methylation [72,73]. To investigate this possibility, we have subjected the FM3.13 melanoma subline (with the loss of the expression of melanocyte differentiation antigens) to the treatment with demethylating agent 5-aza-2′-deoxycytidine (ADC), and used such melanoma cells as targets for cytotoxicicity of CTL clones directed against Melan-A/MART-1 and gp100 (clones 5/127 and 5/49 established in our lab [74]) and tyrosinase (clone IVSB, kindly provided by Dr. P. van der Bruggen, Ludwig Institute for Cancer Research, Belgium, Brussels) (Figure 4.1). Data on the reactivity of the indicated CTL clones with FM3.D subline, highly expressing differentiation antigens, are also presented. ADC treatment clearly induced the appearance of reactivity of FM3.13 melanoma subline with these CTL clones, indicating the induction of the expression of melanosomal proteins as a result of DNA demethylation. This induction has been also confirmed by the RT-PCR method (not shown). So in fact, at least some melanocyte differentiation antigens (for example gp100) behave as "neo-antigens", present in normal cells in suboptimal quantities, insufficient for the induction of immunological tolerance, but can be induced by demethylation.

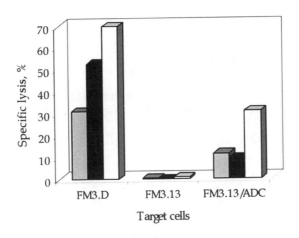

Figure 4.1. Upregulation of the lysis of FM3.13 melanoma clone after treatment with ADC by CTL clones specific against Melan-A/MART-1 (gray columns), gp100 (black columns) and tyrosinase (white columns). The CTL: target cell ration was 10.

Differentiation antigens represent an attractive target for immunotherapy, first of all because it is rather easy, compared to other tumour-associated antigens to induce immune response against them. On the other hand, only in very few cases the development of immune response against differentiation antigens has caused complete tumour rejection. One possibility for inefficiency of immune response against differentiation antigens is the low avidity of T cell recognition, and indeed the majority of peptide epitopes have low or intermediate affinity for HLA class I antigens and the corresponding peptide can activate peptide-dependent lysis of CTL clones only at relatively high concentrations [8,75]. Highly reactive T cell clones are probably inactivated due to natural mechanisms of tolerance induction. On the other hand, the presence of these low avidity T cells in large quantities may block the development of high avidity immune response against "strong" tumour-associated antigens (e.g. cancer/testis antigens), because the corresponding precursors are present at significantly lower levels. In that sense differentiation antigens behave as immunodominant. Indeed, only in the absence of differentiation antigens immune response could be induced against non-differentiation, progression-associated antigens [74]. The obvious risks for the development of autoimmunity should also be taken in consideration.

Another major obstacle for the immunotherapeutical use of the differentiation antigens is heterogeneity and instability of their expressions. This heterogeneity, best seen on the clonal level [74,76], can lead to the selection of antigen-loss variant, seen during specific immunotherapy [77,78].

The future strategies for vaccine development should probably be based on combination of differentiation antigens with other tumour-associated, e.g. cancer/testis antigens antigens (in a form which can equally induce response against different groups of antigens), in order to result in efficient induction of protective long-lasting anti-cancer immunity.

ACKNOWLEDGMENTS

Work in the authors' laboratory was supported by a project grant from the Danish Cancer Society and by grants from the Danish Foundation for Cancer Research.

REFERENCES

1. Brichard, V., Van Pel, A., Wölfel, T., Wölfel, C., De Plaen, E., Lethé, B., Coulie, P., and Boon, T. The tyrosinase gene codes for an antigen recognized by autologous cytolytic T lymphocytes on HLA-A2 melanomas. J.Exp.Med., *178*: 489-495, 1993.
2. Rosenberg, S. A., Yang, J. C., Schwartzentruber, D. J., Hwu, P., Marincola, F. M., Topalian, S. L., Restifo, N. P., Dudley, M. E., Schwarz, S. L., Spiess, P. J., Wunderlich, J. R., Parkhurst, M. R., Kawakami, Y., Seipp, C. A., Einhorn, J. H., and White, D. E. Immunologic and therapeutic evaluation of a synthetic peptide vaccine for the treatment of patients with metastatic melanoma. Nature (Med.), *4*: 321-327, 1998.
3. Clay, T. M., Custer, M. C., McKee, M. D., Parkhurst, M., Robbins, P. F., Kerstann, K., Wunderlich, J., Rosenberg, S. A., and Nishimura, M. I. Changes in the fine specificity of gp100$_{(209-217)}$-reactive T cells in patients following vaccination with a peptide modified at an HLA-A2.1 anchor residue. J.Immunol., *162*: 1749-1755, 1999.
4. Riker, A., Cormier, J., Panelli, M., Kammula, U., Wang, E., Abati, A., Fetsch, P., Lee, K. H., Steinberg, S., Rosenberg, S., and Marincola, F. Immune selection after antigen-specific immunotherapy of melanoma. Surgery, *126*: 112-120, 1999.
5. Wang, F., Bade, E., Kuniyoshi, C., Spears, L., Jeffery, G., Marty, V., Groshen, S., and Weber, J. Phase I trial of a MART-1 peptide vaccine with incomplete Freund's adjuvant for resected high-risk melanoma. Clin.Cancer Res., *5*: 2756-2765, 1999.
6. Anichini, A., Maccalli, C., Mortarini, R., Salvi, S., Mazzocchi, A., Squarcina, P., Herlyn, M., and Parmiani, G. Melanoma cells and normal melanocytes share antigens recognized by HLA-A2-restricted cytotoxic T cell clones from melanoma patients. J.Exp.Med., *177*: 989-998, 1993.
7. Bouchard, B., Fuller, B. B., Vijayasaradhi, S., and Houghton, A. N. Induction of pigmentation in mouse fibroblasts by expression of human tyrosinase cDNA. J.Exp.Med., *169*: 2029-2042, 1989.
8. Wölfel, T., Van Pel, A., Brichard, V., Schneider, J., Seliger, B., Meyer zum Büschenfelde, K.-H., and Boon, T. Two tyrosinase nonapeptides recognized on HLA-A2 melanomas by autologous cytolytic T lymphocytes. Eur.J.Immunol., *24*: 759-764, 1994.
9. Robbins, P. F., El-Gamil, M., Kawakami, Y., Stevens, E., Yannelli, J. R., and Rosenberg, S. A. Recognition of tyrosinase by tumor-infiltrating lymphocytes from a patient responding to immunotherapy [published erratum appears in Cancer Res 1994 Jul 15;54(14):3952]. Cancer Res., *54*: 3124-3126, 1994.

10. Kang, X., Kawakami, Y., El-Gamil, M., Wang, R. F., Sakaguchi, K., Yannelli, J. R., Appella, E., Rosenberg, S. A., and Robbins, P. F. Identification of a tyrosinase epitope recognized by HLA-A24-restricted, tumor-infiltrating lymphocytes. J.Immunol., *155*: 1343-1348, 1995.

11. Brichard, V. G., Herman, J., Van Pel, A., Wildmann, C., Gaugler, B., Wölfel, T., Boon, T., and Lethé, B. A tyrosinase nonapeptide presented by HLA-B44 is recognized on a human melanoma by autologous cytolytic T lymphocytes. Eur.J.Immunol., *26*: 224-230, 1996.

12. Kittlesen, D. J., Thompson, L. W., Gulden, P. H., Skipper, J. C., Colella, T. A., Shabanowitz, J. A., Hunt, D. F., Engelhard, V. H., and Slingluff, C. L. J. Human melanoma patients recognize an HLA-A1-restricted CTL epitope from tyrosinase containing two cysteine residues: implications for tumor vaccine development. J.Immunol., *160*: 2099-2106, 1998.

13. Kawakami, Y., Robbins, P. F., Wang, X., Tupesis, J. P., Parkhurst, M. R., Kang, X., Sakaguchi, K., Appella, E., and Rosenberg, S. A. Identification of new melanoma epitopes on melanosomal proteins recognized by tumor infiltrating T lymphocytes restricted by HLA-A1, - A2, and -A3 alleles. J.Immunol., *161*: 6985-6992, 1998.

14. Morel, S., Ooms, A., Pel, A. V., Wölfel, T., Brichard, V. G., van der Bruggen, P., Van den Eynde, B. J., and Degiovanni, G. A tyrosinase peptide presented by HLA-B35 is recognized on a human melanoma by autologous cytotoxic T lymphocytes. Int.J.Cancer, *83*: 755-759, 1999.

15. Skipper, J. C., Hendrickson, R. C., Gulden, P. H., Brichard, V., Van Pel, A., Chen, Y., Shabanowitz, J., Wölfel, T., Slingluff, C. L. J., Boon, T., Hunt, D. F., and Engelhard, V. H. An HLA-A2-restricted tyrosinase antigen on melanoma cells results from posttranslational modification and suggests a novel pathway for processing of membrane proteins. J.Exp.Med., *183*: 527-534, 1996.

16. Reynolds, S. R., Celis, E., Sette, A., Oratz, R., Shapiro, R. L., Johnston, D., Fotino, M., and Bystryn, J. C. HLA-independent heterogeneity of CD8[+] T cell responses to MAGE-3, Melan- A/MART-1, gp100, tyrosinase, MC1R, and TRP-2 in vaccine-treated melanoma patients. J.Immunol., *161*: 6970-6976, 1998.

17. Kawakami, Y., Eliyahu, S., Jennings, C., Sakaguchi, K., Kang, X., Southwood, S., Robbins, P. F., Sette, A., Appella, E., and Rosenberg, S. A. Recognition of multiple epitopes in the human melanoma antigen gp100 by tumor-infiltrating T lymphocytes associated with in vivo tumor regression. J.Immunol., *154*: 3961-3968, 1995.

18. Tsai, V., Southwood, S., Sidney, J., Sakaguchi, K., Kawakami, Y., Appella, E., Sette, A., and Celis, E. Identification of subdominant CTL epitopes of the GP100 melanoma-associated tumor antigen by primary in vitro immunization with peptide- pulsed dendritic cells. J.Immunol., *158*: 1796-1802, 1997.

19. Kawakami, Y., Eliyahu, S., Delgado, C. H., Robbins, P. F., Sakaguchi, K., Appella, E., Yannelli, J. R., Adema, G. J., Miki, T., and Rosenberg, S. A. Identification of a human melanoma antigen recognized by tumor-infiltrating lymphocytes associated with *in vivo* tumor rejection. Proc.Natl.Acad.Sci.U.S.A., *91*: 6458-6462, 1994.

20. Skipper, J. C., Kittlesen, D. J., Hendrickson, R. C., Deacon, D. D., Harthun, N. L., Wagner, S. N., Hunt, D. F., Engelhard, V. H., and Slingluff, C. L. J. Shared epitopes for HLA-A3-restricted melanoma-reactive human CTL include a naturally processed epitope from Pmel-17/gp100. J.Immunol., *157*: 5027-5033, 1996.

21. Robbins, P. F., El-Gamil, M., Li, Y. F., Fitzgerald, E. B., Kawakami, Y., and Rosenberg, S. A. The intronic region of an incompletely spliced *gp100* gene transcript encodes an epitope recognized by melanoma-reactive tumor-infiltrating lymphocytes. J.Immunol., *159*: 303-308, 1997.

22. Castelli, C., Tarsini, P., Mazzocchi, A., Rini, F., Rivoltini, L., Ravagnani, F., Gallino, F., Belli, F., and Parmiani, G. Novel HLA-Cw8-restricted T cell epitopes derived from tyrosinase-related protein-2 and gp100 melanoma antigens. J.Immunol., *162*: 1739-1748, 1999.

23. Li, K., Adibzadeh, M., Halder, T., Kalbacher, H., Heinzel, S., Müller, C., Zeuthen, J., and Pawelec, G. Tumour-specific MHC-class-II-restricted responses after in vitro sensitization to synthetic peptides corresponding to gp100 and Annexin II eluted from melanoma cells. Cancer Immunol.Immunother., *47*: 32-38, 1998.

24. Kawakami, Y., Eliyahu, S., Sakaguchi, K., Robbins, P. F., Rivoltini, L., Yannelli, J. R., Appella, E., and Rosenberg, S. A. Identification of the immunodominant peptides of the MART-1 human melanoma antigen recognized by the majority of HLA-A2-restricted tumor infiltrating lymphocytes. J.Exp.Med., *180*: 347-352, 1994.

25. Romero, P., Gervois, N., Schneider, J., Escobar, P., Valmori, D., Pannetier, C., Steinle, A., Wölfel, T., Liénard, D., Brichard, V., Van Pel, A., Jotereau, F., and Cerottini, J. C. Cytolytic T lymphocyte recognition of the immunodominant HLA-A*0201- restricted Melan-A/MART-1 antigenic peptide in melanoma. J.Immunol., *159*: 2366-2374, 1997.

26. Castelli, C., Storkus, W. J., Maeurer, M. J., Martin, D. M., Huang, E. C., Pramanik, B. N., Nagabhushan, T. L., Parmiani, G., and Lotze, M. T. Mass spectrometric identification of a naturally processed melanoma peptide recognized by CD8⁺ cytotoxic T lymphocytes. J.Exp.Med., *181*: 363-368, 1995.

27. Schneider, J., Brichard, V., Boon, T., Meyer zum Büschenfelde, K.-H., and Wölfel, T. Overlapping peptides of melanocyte differentiation antigen Melan-A/MART- 1 recognized by autologous cytolytic T lymphocytes in association with HLA-B45.1 and HLA-A2.1. Int.J.Cancer, *75*: 451-458, 1998.

28. Zarour, H. M., Kirkwood, J. M., Kierstead, L. S., Herr, W., Brusic, V., Slingluff, C. L., Jr., Sidney, J., Sette, A., and Storkus, W. J. Melan-A/MART-1₅₁₋₇₃ represents an immunogenic HLA-DR4-restricted epitope recognized by melanoma-reactive CD4⁺ T cells. Proc.Natl.Acad.Sci.U.S.A., *97*: 400-405, 2000.

29. Topalian, S. L., Gonzales, M. I., Parkhurst, M., Li, Y. F., Southwood, S., Sette, A., Rosenberg, S. A., and Robbins, P. F. Melanoma-specific CD4⁺ T cells recognize nonmutated HLA-DR-restricted tyrosinase epitopes. J.Exp.Med., *183*: 1965-1971, 1996.

30. Kobayashi, H., Kokubo, T., Takahashi, M., Sato, K., Miyokawa, N., Kimura, S., Kinouchi, R., and Katagiri, M. Tyrosinase epitope recognized by an HLA-DR-restricted T-cell line from a Vogt-Koyanagi-Harada disease patient. Immunogenetics, *47*: 398-403, 1998.

31. Kobayashi, H., Kokubo, T., Sato, K., Kimura, S., Asano, K., Takahashi, H., Iizuka, H., Miyokawa, N., and Katagiri, M. CD4⁺ T cells from peripheral blood of a melanoma patient recognize peptides derived from nonmutated tyrosinase. Cancer Res., *58*: 296-301, 1998.

32. Wang, R. F., Parkhurst, M. R., Kawakami, Y., Robbins, P. F., and Rosenberg, S. A. Utilization of an alternative open reading frame of a normal gene in generating a novel human cancer antigen. J.Exp.Med., *183*: 1131-1140, 1996.

33. Wang, R. F., Appella, E., Kawakami, Y., Kang, X., and Rosenberg, S. A. Identification of TRP-2 as a human tumor antigen recognized by cytotoxic T lymphocytes. J.Exp.Med., *184*: 2207-2216, 1996.

34. Wang, R. F., Johnston, S. L., Southwood, S., Sette, A., and Rosenberg, S. A. Recognition of an antigenic peptide derived from tyrosinase-related protein-2 by CTL in the context of HLA-A31 and -33. J.Immunol., *160*: 890-897, 1998.

35. Parkhurst, M. R., Fitzgerald, E. B., Southwood, S., Sette, A., Rosenberg, S. A., and Kawakami, Y. Identification of a shared *HLA-A*0201*-restricted T-cell epitope from the melanoma antigen tyrosinase-related protein 2 (TRP2). Cancer Res., *58*: 4895-4901, 1998.

36. Lupetti, R., Pisarra, P., Verrecchia, A., Farina, C., Nicolini, G., Anichini, A., Bordignon, C., Sensi, M., Parmiani, G., and Traversari, C. Translation of a retained intron in tyrosinase-related protein (TRP) 2 mRNA generates a new cytotoxic T lymphocyte (CTL)-defined and shared human melanoma antigen not expressed in normal cells of the melanocytic lineage. J.Exp.Med., *188*: 1005-1016, 1998.

37. Salazar-Onfray, F., Nakazawa, T., Chhajlani, V., Petersson, M., Kärre, K., Masucci, G., Celis, E., Sette, A., Southwood, S., Appella, E., and Kiessling, R. Synthetic peptides derived from the melanocyte-stimulating hormone receptor MC1R can stimulate HLA-A2-restricted cytotoxic T lymphocytes that recognize naturally processed peptides on human melanoma cells. Cancer Res., *57*: 4348-4355, 1997.

38. Coulie, P. G., Brichard, V., Van Pel, A., Wölfel, T., Schneider, J., Traversari, C., Mattei, S., De Plaen, E., Lurquin, C., Szikora, J. P., Renauld, J. C., and Boon, T. A new gene coding for a differentiation antigen recognized by autologous cytolytic T lymphocytes on HLA-A2 melanomas. J.Exp.Med., *180*: 35-42, 1994.

39. Kawakami, Y., Eliyahu, S., Delgado, C. H., Robbins, P. F., Rivoltini, L., Topalian, S. L., Miki, T., and Rosenberg, S. A. Cloning of the gene coding for a shared human melanoma antigen recognized by autologous T cells infiltrating into tumor. Proc.Natl.Acad.Sci.U.S.A., *91*: 3515-3519, 1994.

40. Jäger, E., Höhn, H., Karbach, J., Momburg, F., Castelli, C., Knuth, A., Seliger, B., and Maeurer, M. J. Cytotoxic T lymphocytes define multiple peptide isoforms derived from the melanoma-associated antigen MART-1/Melan-A. Int.J.Cancer, *81*: 979-984, 1999.

41. Rivoltini, L., Kawakami, Y., Sakaguchi, K., Southwood, S., Sette, A., Robbins, P. F., Marincola, F. M., Salgaller, M. L., Yannelli, J. R., and Appella, E. Induction of tumor-reactive CTL from peripheral blood and tumor-infiltrating lymphocytes of melanoma patients by in vitro stimulation with an immunodominant peptide of the human melanoma antigen MART-1. J.Immunol., *154*: 2257-2265, 1995.

42. van Elsas, A., van der Burg, S. H., van der Minne, C. E., Borghi, M., Mourer, J. S., Melief, C. J. M., and Schrier, P. I. Peptide-pulsed dendritic cells induce tumoricidal cytotoxic T lymphocytes from healthy donors against stably HLA-A*0201-binding peptides from the Melan-A/MART-1 self antigen. Eur.J.Immunol., *26*: 1683-1689, 1996.

43. Valmori, D., Fonteneau, J. F., Lizana, C. M., Gervois, N., Liénard, D., Rimoldi, D., Jongeneel, V., Jotereau, F., Cerottini, J. C., and Romero, P. Enhanced generation of specific tumor-reactive CTL in vitro by selected Melan-A/MART-1 immunodominant peptide analogues. J.Immunol., *160*: 1750-1758, 1998.

44. Stevens, E. J., Jacknin, L., Robbins, P. F., Kawakami, Y., El Gamil, M., Rosenberg, S. A., and Yannelli, J. R. Generation of tumor-specific CTLs from melanoma patients by using peripheral blood stimulated with allogeneic melanoma tumor cell lines. Fine specificity and MART-1 melanoma antigen recognition. J.Immunol., *154*: 762-771, 1995.

45. Spagnoli, G. C., Schaefer, C., Willimann, T. E., Kocher, T., Amoroso, A., Juretic, A., Zuber, M., Lüscher, U., Harder, F., and Heberer, M. Peptide-specific CTL in tumor infiltrating lymphocytes from metastatic melanomas expressing *MART-1/Melan-A, gp100* and *Tyrosinase* genes: a study in an unselected group of HLA-A2.1-positive patients. Int.J.Cancer, *64*: 309-315, 1995.

46. Cormier, J. N., Salgaller, M. L., Prevette, T., Barracchini, K. C., Rivoltini, L., Restifo, N. P., Rosenberg, S. A., and Marincola, F. M. Enhancement of cellular immunity in melanoma patients immunized with a peptide from MART-1/Melan A. Cancer J.Sci.Am., *3*: 37-44, 1997.

47. Adema, G. J., de Boer, A. J., van 't Hullenaar, R., Denijn, M., Ruiter, D. J., Vogel, A. M., and Figdor, C. G. Melanocyte lineage-specific antigens recognized by monoclonal antibodies NKI-beteb, HMB-50, and HMB-45 are encoded by a single cDNA. Am.J.Pathol., *143*: 1579-1585, 1993.

48. Bakker, A. B., Schreurs, M. W., de Boer, A. J., Kawakami, Y., Rosenberg, S. A., Adema, G. J., and Figdor, C. G. Melanocyte lineage-specific antigen gp100 is recognized by melanoma-derived tumor-infiltrating lymphocytes. J.Exp.Med., *179*: 1005-1009, 1994.

49. Cox, A. L., Skipper, J., Chen, Y., Henderson, R. A., Darrow, T. L., Shabanowitz, J., Engelhard, V. H., Hunt, D. F., and Slingluff, C. L. J. Identification of a peptide recognized by five melanoma-specific human cytotoxic T cell lines. Science, *264*: 716-719, 1994.

50. Salgaller, M. L., Afshar, A., Marincola, F. M., Rivoltini, L., Kawakami, Y., and Rosenberg, S. A. Recognition of multiple epitopes in the human melanoma antigen gp100 by peripheral blood lymphocytes stimulated *in vitro* with synthetic peptides. Cancer Res., *55*: 4972-4979, 1995.

51. Kawakami, Y., Dang, N., Wang, X., Tupesis, J., Robbins, P. F., Wang, R. F., Wunderlich, J. R., Yannelli, J. R., and Rosenberg, S. A. Recognition of shared melanoma antigens in association with major HLA-A alleles by tumor infiltrating T lymphocytes from 123 patients with melanoma. J.Immunother., *23*: 17-27, 2000.

52. Wang, R. F., Robbins, P. F., Kawakami, Y., Kang, X. Q., and Rosenberg, S. A. Identification of a gene encoding a melanoma tumor antigen recognized by HLA-A31-restricted tumor-infiltrating lymphocytes [published erratum appears in J Exp Med 1995 Mar 1;181(3):1261]. J.Exp.Med., *181*: 799-804, 1995.

53. Sidney, J., Grey, H. M., Kubo, R. T., and Sette, A. Practical, biochemical and evolutionary implications of the discovery of HLA class I supermotifs. Immunol.Today, *17*: 261-266, 1996.

54. Neumann, E., Engelsberg, A., Decker, J., Störkel, S., Jäeger, E., Huber, C., and Seliger, B. Heterogeneous expression of the tumor-associated antigens RAGE-1, PRAME, and glycoprotein 75 in human renal cell carcinoma: candidates for T-cell-based immunotherapies? Cancer Res., *58*: 4090-4095, 1998.

55. Topalian, S. L., Solomon, D., Avis, F. P., Chang, A. E., Freerksen, D. L., Linehan, W. M., Lotze, M. T., Robertson, C. N., Seipp, C. A., Simon, P., Simpson, C. G., and Rosenberg, S. A. Immunotherapy of patients with advanced cancer using tumor-infiltrating lymphocytes and recombinant interleukin-2: a pilot study. J.Clin.Oncol., *6*: 839-853, 1988.

56. Wang, R. F., Johnston, S. L., Zeng, G., Topalian, S. L., Schwartzentruber, D. J., and Rosenberg, S. A. A breast and melanoma-shared tumor antigen: T cell responses to antigenic peptides translated from different open reading frames. J.Immunol., *161*: 3598-3606, 1998.

57. Chen, Y. T., Scanlan, M. J., Sahin, U., Türeci, Ö., Güre, A. O., Tsang, S., Williamson, B., Stockert, E., Pfreundschuh, M., and Old, L. J. A testicular antigen aberrantly expressed in human cancers detected by autologous antibody screening. Proc.Natl.Acad.Sci.U.S.A., *94*: 1914-1918, 1997.

58. Bronte, V., Apolloni, E., Ronca, R., Zamboni, P., Overwijk, W. W., Surman, D. R., Restifo, N. P., and Zanovello, P. Genetic vaccination with "self" tyrosinase-related protein 2 causes melanoma eradication but not vitiligo. Cancer Res., *60*: 253-258, 2000.

59. Overwijk, W. W., Lee, D. S., Surman, D. R., Irvine, K. R., Touloukian, C. E., Chan, C. C., Carroll, M. W., Moss, B., Rosenberg, S. A., and Restifo, N. P. Vaccination with a recombinant vaccinia virus encoding a "self" antigen induces autoimmune vitiligo and tumor cell destruction in mice: requirement for CD4[+] T lymphocytes. Proc.Natl.Acad.Sci.U.S.A, *96*: 2982-2987, 1999.

60. Bouchard, B., Del, M., V, Jackson, I. J., Cherif, D., and Dubertret, L. Molecular characterization of a human tyrosinase-related-protein-2 cDNA. Patterns of expression in melanocytic cells. Eur.J.Biochem., *219*: 127-134, 1994.

61. Eberle, J., Wagner, M., and MacNeil, S. Human melanoma cell lines show little relationship between expression of pigmentation genes and pigmentary behaviour in vitro. Pigment Cell Res., *11*: 134-142, 1998.

62. Nishioka, E., Funasaka, Y., Kondoh, H., Chakraborty, A. K., Mishima, Y., and Ichihashi, M. Expression of tyrosinase, TRP-1 and TRP-2 in ultraviolet-irradiated human melanomas and melanocytes: TRP-2 protects melanoma cells from ultraviolet B induced apoptosis. Melanoma Res., *9*: 433-443, 1999.

63. Halder, T., Pawelec, G., Kirkin, A. F., Zeuthen, J., Meyer, H. E., Kun, L., and Kalbacher, H. Isolation of novel HLA-DR restricted potential tumor-associated antigens from the melanoma cell line FM3. Cancer Res., *57*: 3238-3244, 1997.

64. Cochlovius, B., Linnebacher, M., Zewe-Welschof, M., and Zöller, M. Recombinant gp100 protein presented by dendritic cells elicits a T-helper-cell response *in vitro* and *in vivo*. Int.J.Cancer, *83*: 547-554, 1999.

65. Loftus, D. J., Castelli, C., Clay, T. M., Squarcina, P., Marincola, F. M., Nishimura, M. I., Parmiani, G., Appella, E., and Rivoltini, L. Identification of epitope mimics recognized by CTL reactive to the melanoma/melanocyte-derived peptide MART-1$_{(27-35)}$. J.Exp.Med., *184*: 647-657, 1996.

66. Loftus, D. J., Squarcina, P., Nielsen, M. B., Geisler, C., Castelli, C., Odum, N., Appella, E., Parmiani, G., and Rivoltini, L. Peptides derived from self-proteins as partial agonists and antagonists of human CD8[+] T-cell clones reactive to melanoma/melanocyte epitope MART1$_{(27-35)}$. Cancer Res., *58*: 2433-2439, 1998.

67. Parker, K. C., Bednarek, M. A., and Coligan, J. E. Scheme for ranking potential HLA-A2 binding peptides based on independent binding of individual peptide side-chains. J.Immunol., *152*: 163-175, 1994.

68. Pittet, M. J., Valmori, D., Dunbar, P. R., Speiser, D. E., Liénard, D., Lejeune, F., Fleischhauer, K., Cerundolo, V., Cerottini, J. C., and Romero, P. High frequencies of naive Melan-A/MART-1-specific CD8[+] T cells in a large proportion of human histocompatibility leukocyte antigen (HLA)-A2 individuals. J.Exp.Med., *190*: 705-716, 1999.

69. Wagner, S. N., Wagner, C., Schultewolter, T., and Goos, M. Analysis of Pmel17/gp100 expression in primary human tissue specimens: implications for melanoma immuno- and gene-therapy. Cancer Immunol.Immunother., *44*: 239-247, 1997.

70. Gown, A. M., Vogel, A. M., Hoak, D., Gough, F., and McNutt, M. A. Monoclonal antibodies specific for melanocytic tumors distinguish subpopulations of melanocytes. Am.J.Pathol., *123*: 195-203, 1986.

71. Colombari, R., Bonetti, F., Zamboni, G., Scarpa, A., Marino, F., Tomezzoli, A., Capelli, P., Menestrina, F., Chilosi, M., and Fiore-Donati, L. Distribution of melanoma specific antibody (HMB-45) in benign and malignant melanocytic tumours. An immunohistochemical study on paraffin sections. Virchows Arch.A Pathol.Anat.Histopathol., *413*: 17-24, 1988.

72. Weber, J., Salgaller, M., Samid, D., Johnson, B., Herlyn, M., Lassam, N., Treisman, J., and Rosenberg, S. A. Expression of the MAGE-1 tumor antigen is up-regulated by the demethylating agent 5-aza-2'-deoxycytidine. Cancer Res., *54*: 1766-1771, 1994.

73. De Smet, C., De Backer, O., Faraoni, I., Lurquin, C., Brasseur, F., and Boon, T. The activation of human gene *MAGE-1* in tumor cells is correlated with genome-wide demethylation. Proc.Natl.Acad.Sci.U.S.A., *93*: 7149-7153, 1996.

74. Kirkin, A. F., thor Straten, P., Hansen, M. R., Barfoed, A., Dzhandzhugazyan, K. N., and Zeuthen, J. Establishment of gp100 and MART-1/Melan-A-specific cytotoxic T lymphocyte clones using in vitro immunization against preselected highly immunogenic melanoma cell clones. Cancer Immunol.Immunother., *48*: 239-246, 1999.

75. Kawakami, Y. and Rosenberg, S. A. T-cell recognition of self peptides as tumor rejection antigens. Immunol.Res., *15*: 179-190, 1996.

76. Houghton, A. N., Real, F. X., Davis, L. J., Cordon-Cardo, C., and Old, L. J. Phenotypic heterogeneity of melanoma. Relation to the differentiation program of melanoma cells. J.Exp.Med., *165*: 812-829, 1987.

77. Jäger, E., Ringhoffer, M., Karbach, J., Arand, M., Oesch, F., and Knuth, A. Inverse relationship of melanocyte differentiation antigen expression in melanoma tissues and CD8[+] cytotoxic-T-cell responses: evidence for immunoselection of antigen-loss variants in vivo. Int.J.Cancer, *66*: 470-476, 1996.

78. Jäger, E., Ringhoffer, M., Altmannsberger, M., Arand, M., Karbach, J., Jäger, D., Oesch, F., and Knuth, A. Immunoselection in vivo: independent loss of MHC class I and melanocyte differentiation antigen expression in metastatic melanoma. Int.J.Cancer, *71*: 142-147, 1997.

5
CARCINOEMBRYONIC ANTIGEN AS A VACCINE TARGET

JEFFREY SCHLOM, KWONG Y. TSANG, JAMES W. HODGE, AND JOHN W. GREINER

INTRODUCTION

The human carcinoembryonic antigen (CEA) as a target for vaccine-mediated therapy of a range of human cancers will be reviewed. The first section will provide an overview of the CEA gene family and the levels of expression of CEA in neoplastic and preneoplastic lesions, and in some normal and fetal tissues. The pros and cons of using animal models will then be discussed for (a) defining the optimal strategies for inducing an immune response and an antitumor response to a "self"-antigen such as CEA, and (b) as a prelude to clinical studies. The numerous studies that have now been carried out to define the immunogenicity of CEA in humans will then be reviewed; this will also include studies on the definition of an enhancer T-cell agonist epitope that has been shown to enhance T-cell responses to CEA. Finally, multiple strategies will be discussed that can be used to further enhance the immunogenicity of a self-antigen such as CEA, including the use of vectors containing multiple transgenes of T-cell costimulatory molecules. The potential for implementation of these strategies in vaccine clinical trials will also be discussed.

THE CEA GENE FAMILY

CEA was first described in 1965 [1,2]. The CEA gene family now consists of 29 genes that are located within the long arm of chromosome 19. The isolation of genes for the CEA family members led to their identification in 1986 as members of the immunoglobulin (Ig) supergene family [3-9 for review]. All CEA family members are glycoproteins composed of an N-terminal Ig variable region-like domain, followed by 0,2,3,4, or 6 Ig constant region-like domains of subtype A or B, and terminated by a processed hydrophobic C-terminal domain. The CEA family may be subdivided into

R.A. Robins and R.C. Rees (eds.), Cancer Immunology, 73–100.

two groups based on sequence comparisons. The first group consists of CEA and the CEA cross-reacting molecules, including nonspecific cross-reacting antigen (NCA) and biliary glycoprotein (BGP); the second group consists of the pregnancy-specific glycoproteins. The CEA subgroup is subdivided further by structural characteristics into those members attached to the outer cell membrane by glycophosphatidyl inositol (CEA, NCA, CGM-6) and those that have both transmembrane and cytoplasmic domains (BGP splice variants).

Studies have shown that CEA mediates $Ca2^+$- and temperature-independent cell aggregation [10]. Some studies have also demonstrated that CEA can function as an intercellular adhesion molecule (ICAM) [10]. However, other studies have reported that CEA may act as a signal protein that may inhibit intercellular contact in the malignant process [11].

In terms of its tissue distribution, biochemistry and molecular structure, CEA is one of the most well-characterized tumor associated antigens (TAA). At the amino acid level, CEA shares approximately 70% homology with NCA, which is found on normal granulocytes [12-14]. This immediately raises some provocative questions. Will this situation render patients tolerant to CEA and thus incapable of inducing CEA immune responses? If immune responses are generated, will this lead to autoimmune responses against normal tissues, or will the quantitative and/or qualitative differences in expression of CEA in tumor vs. normal tissues provide a therapeutic threshold for vaccine efficacy? Can immunodominant CEA peptides that share little or no homology to CEA-related molecules found on normal tissues be identified and recognized by human T cells? This review will attempt to address some of these issues.

CEA Expression

CEA is extensively expressed in the vast majority of human colorectal, gastric and pancreatic carcinomas, in approximately 50% of breast cancers and in 70% of non-small-cell lung cancers, as well as other carcinomas. To a lesser extent, CEA is also expressed on normal colon epithelium and in some fetal tissue. The relative tissue specificity of this antigen thus makes CEA an attractive target antigen for immunotherapy. In addition, since CEA has been known to function as an adhesion molecule, it might play an important role in the metastatic process by mediating the attachment of tumor cells to normal cells. Thus, immunotherapy targeted to CEA-positive tumor cells might be particularly beneficial in preventing metastasis.

The degree of CEA expression in colorectal carcinomas, adjacent "histologically normal" tissue, benign colon lesions, and colonic mucosa from healthy individuals was evaluated by quantitative radioimmunoassay (RIA) [15]. Tissues and sera from 110 patients diagnosed with primary colorectal carcinoma, 20 patients with benign colorectal disease, and 31 healthy donors were subjected to quantitative CEA analysis (Fig. 5.1). Multiple samples from tumor lesions and autologous, histologically normal mucosa (10 cm from the tumor) were obtained at the time of surgery (cancer patients) or endoscopy (patients with benign tumors and healthy volunteers). CEA content was measured in protein extracts obtained from these tissues using a quantitative RIA method. An arbitrary limit of "normality" for CEA content was established as 300 ng/mg of protein. Using this cut-off, 94.5% of carcinomas had elevated CEA levels

(Fig. 5.1). A statistically significant difference between CEA content in tumor lesions versus histologically normal mucosa from cancer patients was observed ($p= 0.001$). Moreover, CEA content was statistically higher in the normal mucosa from cancer

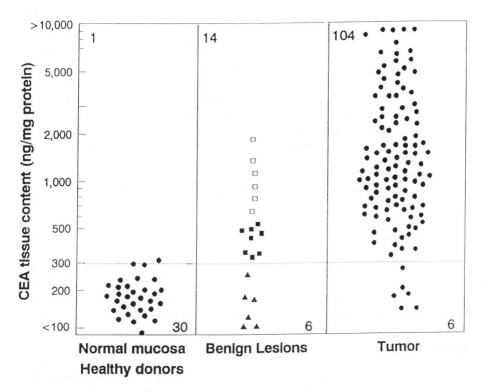

Figure 5.1. CEA content in colorectal tissues from healthy donors (n=31), in patients diagnosed with benign lesions (n=20) [i.e., hyperplastic polyps (▲); tubulovillous adenomas with low or moderate dysplasia (■); and tubulovillous adenomas with severe dysplasia (□)], and in patients diagnosed with colorectal cancer (n=110) [15].

patients versus that from healthy donors ($p= 0.005$). No statistical correlation between CEA content in carcinoma tissues and serum CEA levels (r= 0.195, $p= 0.13$) was found [15]. Therefore, in considering diagnosis or therapy with anti-CEA monoclonal antibodies (MAb) for colorectal carcinoma patients, or therapies using CEA vaccines, serum CEA levels should not be taken as the only indication of CEA expression in tumor lesions.

CEA was also evaluated in potentially premalignant colon lesions. Although fewer numbers of such lesions were available for analysis, a trend in quantitative CEA expression toward malignancy was seen [15]. All hyperplastic lesions analyzed showed CEA levels below the 300 ng/mg protein limit. However, values between 300 and 600 ng/mg protein were observed for tubulovillous adenomas with low or moderate dysplasia, and values exceeding 600 ng/mg protein were seen in tubulovillous adenomas with severe dysplasia (Fig. 5.1). The fact that CEA is overexpressed in

75

potentially premalignant lesions leaves open the potential for CEA vaccines to be administered to patients with premalignant disease to eliminate these lesions and, by extension, the risk of carcinoma development.

The quantitative differences in CEA expression in carcinoma vs. normal tissues has also been demonstrated by the clinical use of anti-CEA MAb. Numerous studies have now demonstrated the selective targeting of radiolabeled MAb to carcinoma, while little or no targeting to normal tissues was observed [16-18]. Anti-CEA MAbs have been used clinically when conjugated with the radionuclides ^{131}I, ^{90}Y and [67]Cu. Promising results have been obtained using anti-CEA MAb Fab'$_2$ fragments in colorectal cancer patients and ^{131}I-labeled MAb IgG in patients with metastatic ovarian cancer. Specifically, some disease stabilization, partial remissions and complete remissions have been observed [19-24].

Much attention has now been given to CEA as a potential target for vaccine therapy. Consequently, several animal models have been employed to determine the relative efficacies and safety of different vaccines as a prelude to clinical trials. As with the use of animal models to determine the efficacy of any type of therapy for any disease, one must consider potential advantages and pitfalls of each model.

Animal models

Much thought needs to be given to the use of appropriate model systems to determine the efficacy and safety of a given vaccine for use in humans. At first glance, animal models may appear attractive to test CEA-based vaccines. However, since human class I and class II major histocompatibility (MHC) alleles are distinct from those of any other species, it is inappropriate to try to define whether immunogenicity of a human TAA, such as CEA, in a murine model, or even a non-human primate model, will predict immunogenicity in humans. This is also true in the use of transgenic (Tg) mice containing a human tumor-antigen transgene. Such Tg mice still have murine MHC class I and II alleles as well as murine T-cell receptors (TCR) and, thus, cannot accurately predict immunogenicity in humans. Certain Tg models, however, are useful to help define the principles of the immunogenicity of a "self-antigen," such as CEA [25,26]. On the other hand, it is unclear how a specific Tg murine model reflects the human in terms of degree of expression of the gene in question during embryonic development and actual levels of expression in normal adult tissues vs. tumor tissues [27]. This is supported by recent experiments and theories further examining the concept of "tolerance" or "self" versus "non-self" [28-32].

A Tg mouse has recently been developed bearing the human MHC class I human lymphocyte antigen (HLA)-A2 transgene [33]. This has been shown to be an extremely useful and important model. However, studies have shown that a correlation does not always exist between an immune response in the HLA-A2 Tg mouse and human in vitro immune responses for some epitopes [34]. Moreover, the HLA-A2 Tg mouse still contains a murine TCR repertoire [34]. Thus, one is faced with the dilemma of finding an appropriate in vivo model to determine the immunogenicity of a given human antigen, such as CEA, and/or a specific human epitope. One point of view is that a small Phase I clinical trial to define immunogenicity of a given antigen or epitope is without equal. This, however, should absolutely not diminish the appropriate use of animal models to investigate basic concepts of vaccinology, such as advantages or disadvantages of vaccine delivery methodologies, mechanisms of T-cell costimulation, use of cytokines to enhance immune responses and the use of diversified vaccination protocols.

CEA Vaccine preclinical studies

Initial preclinical studies compared the relative degree of potency and type of immune response achieved in mice that received different types of CEA vaccines. These vaccines included native CEA protein obtained from human metastases, recombinant CEA protein expressed in baculovirus, recombinant vaccinia virus expressing the human CEA gene (rV-CEA), an anti-idiotype (Id) MAb directed against an anti-CEA MAb, a CEA polynucleotide vaccine, and a replication-defective avipox virus recombinant expressing CEA [13,35-43]. The advantage of employing cytokines such as IL-2 and granulocyte-macrophage colony-stimulating factor (GM-CSF) with anti-CEA vaccines in preclinical models has also been demonstrated [44,45]. In addition, the advantage of the use of T-cell costimulatory molecules in anti-CEA vaccines has been determined by admixing rV-CEA with recombinant competent vaccinia viruses expressing the B7-1, B7-2 or CD70 costimulatory molecule genes, or by placing both the CEA and B7-1 gene on the same vaccinia vector [46-48]. Finally, preclinical models have shown the advantage of using diversified prime and boost strategies for CEA vaccines. For example, priming with rV-CEA and boosting with either avipox-CEA or CEA protein was shown to be more efficacious than using multiple vaccinations of one of these vaccines alone [37,49].

Recently, Tg mice (designated CEA-Tg) have been developed that express CEA as a self-antigen with a tissue distribution similar to that of humans [33,50]. A recent study has compared the immune responsiveness of the CEA-Tg mice to CEA protein, administered in adjuvant, with the immune response to a recombinant vaccinia virus expressing CEA (rV-CEA) [51]. The nonvaccinated CEA-Tg mice, in contrast to conventional mice, were unresponsive to CEA, as defined by the lack of detectable CEA-specific serum antibodies and the inability to prime an *in vitro* splenic T-cell response to CEA [51]. Furthermore, vaccination with whole CEA protein in adjuvant failed to elicit either anti-CEA IgG titers or CEA-specific T-cell responses. Only weak anti-CEA IgM antibody titers were found. In contrast, CEA-Tg mice vaccinated with rV-CEA generated relatively strong anti-CEA IgG antibody titers and demonstrated evidence of Ig class switching. Those same mice also developed T_H1-type CEA-specific $CD4^+$ responses and CEA peptide-specific cytotoxic T cells. The comparison of CEA protein in adjuvant vs. rV-vector-driven CEA expression in the generation of a CEA-specific T-cell response is shown in Figure 5.2. There was a marked advantage to the use of rV-CEA. The ability to generate CEA-specific host immunity correlated with protection against challenge with CEA-expressing tumor cells. This protection against tumor growth was accomplished with no apparent immune response directed at CEA-positive normal tissues as defined by detailed histochemical and immunohistochemical analyses [51]. These results demonstrate the ability to generate an effective antitumor immune response to a self-antigen by vaccinating with a recombinant vaccinia virus

[51]. CEA-Tg mice should thus represent a suitable experimental model in which to study the effects of more aggressive vaccination strategies.

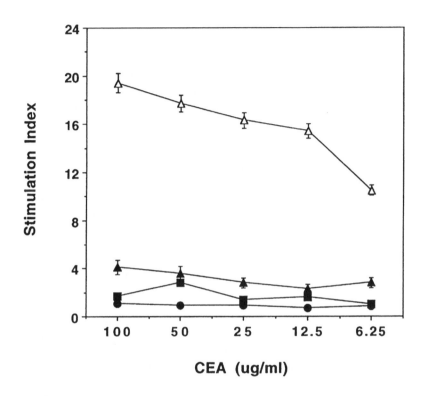

Figure 5.2. CEA-specific CD4+ proliferation responses in CEA-Tg mice. Groups of CEA-Tg mice (two to three mice/group) were vaccinated twice with 20 μg of CEA in adjuvant (▲), 10^7 pfu of V-Wyeth (wild-type) (■), or 10^7 pfu of rV-CEA (△). Control CEA-Tg mice received HBSS buffer (●). At sacrifice, spleens from each group were removed and pooled, T cells were isolated, and the lymphoproliferative assay was carried out. The stimulation index (SI) was calculated as follows: [cpm (antigen-stimulated cells)]/[cpm (unstimulated cells)]. Each data point represents the mean ± SE of triplicate determinations from a representative experiment; two to three separate experiments were carried out with similar results. Data are from reference 51.

Identification of human CEA-specific T-cell epitopes

Since the entire amino acid sequence of human CEA is known, and human HLA-A2 consensus motifs have been described, studies were undertaken to identify a series of peptides that would potentially bind human HLA-A2 molecules [52,53]. A2 was chosen since it is the most common HLA class I molecule, being represented in approximately 50% of North American Caucasians and 34% of African-Americans [54]. The peptide sequence of CEA was thus examined for matches to the consensus motifs for HLA-A2 binding peptides. Importantly, peptides were selected only if their sequence diverged sufficiently from the CEA-related NCA and BGP sequences. The amino acid sequence of human CEA (GeneBank Accession #M17303) was scanned using a predictive algorithm that combines a search for anchor residues with numerical assignments to all residues at all positions [55]. Six peptides ranging in length from 9 to 11 amino acids contained the HLA-A2 binding motif of leucine or isoleucine at position 2, and valine or leucine at the C-terminal [14]. They were given the designation carcinoembryonic antigen peptide (CAP). Another peptide, designated CAP-7, also possessed the motif for binding to HLA-A3 [56]. All peptides were selected to have minimal homology to the parallel regions of NCA and BGP after optimal alignment of the latter sequences with CEA.

The T2 cell-binding assay has been used to analyze peptides for human HLA-A2 consensus motifs [57]. In this assay, the binding of an appropriate peptide results in the upregulation of surface HLA-A2 on the T2 cells, which can be qualified via flow cytometry using an anti-HLA-A2 antibody. The CEA peptides (CAP-1 through CAP-6) scored positive for T2 binding. The order of T2 cell-peptide binding did not always correspond to the predictive algorithm [55]. Since peptide 571-579 (designated CAP-1) demonstrated the highest level of T2 binding, the peptide reflecting the NCA analog (the corresponding NCA peptide obtained after optimal alignment of NCA and CEA) was also synthesized and tested; this peptide, designated NCA-1, showed only background binding to T2 cells. The low level of binding was consistent with the fact that an amino acid substitution in NCA had abolished one of the HLA-A2 anchor residues (Arg for Leu at position 2).

Several groups have now identified CEA T-cell epitopes for a variety of human HLA alleles. One study identified a set of 34 CEA-specific peptides that fit with a specified HLA-A*0301-binding motif and a set of six peptides with high binding affinity to this allele [58]. These peptides can thus also be regarded as potential cytotoxic T lymphocyte (CTL) epitopes. In another study, some 73 CEA-derived peptides that fulfill the HLA-A*0201 motif have been described [59]. Peptides with a high binding affinity and a low peptide-MHC dissociation rate were subsequently tested for their immunogenicity in HLA-A*0201K^b Tg mice. One CEA-derived peptide was shown to induce peptide-specific CTL in these mice. In still another study, several CEA-specific CTL epitopes and CEA epitope analogs were reported [60]. Of a total of 18 motif-containing peptides (9- and 10-mer) tested for HLA-A2.1 binding, nine bound to HLA-A2.1 with an IC_{50} of 500 nM or less. Interestingly, the second highest binder peptide, reported as CEA[9_{605}] [60], actually was previously reported [14] as the CTL epitope CAP-1.

The HLA-A2.1-binding CEA peptide CAP-1 was studied for its capacity to elicit CTL using dendritic cells (DC) as antigen-presenting cells (APC). It was demonstrated that CTL could be generated *in vitro* employing the CAP-1 peptide and DC obtained from peripheral blood mononuclear cells (PBMC) of either healthy individuals or cancer patients. These CTL were capable of killing both CAP-1-pulsed targets and CEA-expressing tumor cells [61]. CTL have also been generated using CEA mRNA-transfected DC from PBMC of healthy individuals and cancer patients as APC [62]. In

CANCER IMMUNOLOGY

other studies, three of five peptides tested were found to stimulate CTL responses that recognized peptide-sensitized target cells [60]. Moreover, after restimulation with antigen and APC, killing of CEA-expressing tumor cells was demonstrated for CEA [9_{605}] (i.e., CAP-1)- and CEA[9_{691}]-specific CTL. The CTL line reactive with peptide CEA[9_{691}] was cloned and studied further in terms of specificity and recognition of various CEA-expressing tumor cells. Cloned CTL specific for CEA[9_{691}] had high, specific lytic activity toward tumor target cells (colon and gastric) that express HLA-A2 and CEA. Two analog peptides from CEA[9_{24}] were prepared and tested for binding to purified HLA-A2.1 molecules. These two analogs differed by the residue incorporated in anchor position 2. The analog peptides bound to purified HLA-A2.1 molecules with an approximately tenfold and fortyfold increased affinity as compared with the natural sequence. It was notable that although peptide CEA[9_{24}] was not capable (according to the experimental protocol) of triggering CTL responses *in vitro*, both peptide analogs were immunogenic in terms of CTL induction. CTL lines induced by both analogs specifically recognized and killed SW403 colon cancer cells expressing CEA and HLA-A2.

The HLA-A24 allele occurs in 60% of the Japanese population and frequently in the Caucasian population. CEA-encoded HLA-A24 binding peptides were tested for their capacity to elicit antitumor CTL *in vitro* [63]. CD8[+] T lymphocytes from PBMC of a healthy donor and autologous peptide-pulsed DC as APC were used. This approach resulted in the identification of two peptides, QYSWFVNGTF and TYACFVSNL, which were capable of eliciting CTL lines that lysed tumor cells expressing HLA-A24 and CEA. The cytotoxicity to tumor cells by the CTL lines was antigen-specific since it was inhibited by peptide-pulsed cold target cells as well as by anti-class I MHC and anti-CD3 MAb. Induction of CEA and HLA-A24-specific CTL has also been demonstrated by culturing human PBMC on formalin-fixed autologous adhesive PBMC loaded with CEA-bound latex beads [64]. The CTL killed CEA-producing tumor cells. Nine other A24 peptides were active to a lesser degree. The lysis observed was shown to be MHC-restricted [64]. The identification of these novel CEA epitopes for CTL also offers the opportunity to design and develop epitope-based immunotherapeutic approaches for treating both HLA-A24[+] and HLA-A2 patients who have tumors that express CEA.

CEA epitopes have also been identified employing an anti-Id MAb to a CEA MAb as immunogen [40,65]. The cDNA encoding the variable heavy and light chains of 3H1 were cloned and sequenced to study the cellular immunity invoked by the 3H1 anti-Id MAb, and the amino acid sequence of the heavy and light chains was deduced [65]. Several regions of homology in 3H1 heavy and light chain variable regions and frameworks, with the homology of CEA, were found [65]. A number of peptides were synthesized and used to stimulate PBMC from patients vaccinated with the 3H1 anti-Id MAb. Two peptides (designated LCD-2 and CEA-B) were identified by strong stimulation responses in 10 of 21 patients. No correlation with class I MHC was observed, and responding T cells were predominantly CD4[+] and of the Th$_1$-type [65].

To date, little has been reported concerning the phenotypic stability of human epitope-specific CTL to self-antigens such as CEA as a consequence of long-term *in vitro* propagation via peptide stimulation. The serial phenotypic characterization of a CTL line directed against the immunodominant CEA epitope CAP-1 has been reported

[66]. This CTL line was derived from PBMC of a patient with metastatic carcinoma who had been vaccinated with rV-CEA. The CTL line was analyzed through 20 *in vitro* cycles of stimulation with the CAP-1 peptide and IL-2 in the presence of autologous APC. The CTL line was shown to be phenotypically stable in terms of high levels of cytokine (interferon [IFN]γ, tumor necrosis factor [TNF], and GM-CSF) production, expression of homing-adhesion molecules, ability to lyse peptide-pulsed targets, and ability to lyse human carcinoma cells endogenously expressing CEA in a MHC-restricted manner. Vβ TCR gene usage was also analyzed [66]. These studies thus present a rationale for the use of long-term cultured epitope-specific human CTL that are directed against a human self-TAA for potential adoptive transfer immunotherapy protocols.

Immunogenicity of CEA in humans

The ability of a CEA vaccine to induce a CEA-specific immune response in humans is no longer in question. As seen in Table 1, a wide range of immunogens have been employed to induce CEA-specific CTL responses, T-cell lymphoproliferative responses, and antibody responses in cancer patients. The vast majority of CEA-specific CTL responses were identified employing the CAP-1 peptide to stimulate T cells and/or to pulse target cells. The following immunogens have now been shown in Phase I trials to induce CEA-specific CTL: (a) rV-CEA; (b) CAP-1-pulsed or CEA RNA-transfected DC; (c) avipox-CEA; (d) rV-CEA followed by avipox-CEA boosts and, most recently, (e) avipox-CEA-B7-1 [14,62,67-69]. The assays used to define these T-cell responses were CTL precursor frequency; ELISPOT, for IFN-γ production; and intracellular cytokine analysis. A number of groups have also shown that human CEA-specific T cells can be generated *in vitro* from PBMC of apparently healthy individuals or from cancer patients (Table 1). These studies included the use of peptide-pulsed DC [61] or RNA-transfected DC as APC [62], and the use of the CAP-1-6D enhancer agonist peptide [70,71]. It should be emphasized that in the vast majority of the studies outlined above, the CEA-specific T cells derived from either vaccinated patients or from stimulation *in vitro* were shown to be capable of lysing (a) CEA-expressing allogeneic tumors and/or autologous tumors; (b) CEA peptide-pulsed T2 cells, C1R-A2 cells, or autologous B cells; and/or (c) autologous B cells transduced with the CEA gene. All instances of lysis mentioned above were shown to be MHC-restricted. Therefore, these studies demonstrated not only the ability of CEA vaccines to induce CTL responses in patients with carcinoma, but also the ability of human carcinoma cells to process endogenous CEA, to transport CEA peptides to the cell surface in the form of MHC-peptide complexes, and to be rendered lytic by the appropriate CEA-specific CTL.

Antibody and CD4+ T-cell responses have also been demonstrated in patients that have received CEA vaccines (Table 5.1). It was demonstrated that colorectal cancer patients receiving 5FU regimens (5FU and leucovorin or levamisole) simultaneously with a CEA anti-Id vaccine in adjuvant generated high-titer polyclonal anti-CEA antibody responses that mediate antibody-dependent cell-mediated cytotoxicity [40]. Moreover, many patients generated CEA-specific CD4+ T-cell responses [40]. These studies are extremely important since they demonstrate that CEA vaccines can be administered along with at least some chemotherapeutic regimens.

Table 5.1. Immunogenicity of CEA in humans

Clinical Trials

Immunogen	Type of Immune Response	Reference
rV-CEA	CTL*	14, 66
Anti-Id	Ab, LP	40
CEA protein + GM-CSF	Ab, LP	72
CAP1-pulsed DC	CTL	62
CEA-RNA transfected DC	CTL	62
Avipox-CEA	CTL	67, 77
rV-CEA + Avipox CEA	CTL	67
Avipox CEA-B7	CTL	68, 69, 92

In vitro studies

Immunogen	Type of Immune Response	Reference
CAP1-6D agonist	CTL	70, 71
CEA peptides (A3)	CTL	58
CAP-2	CTL	73
CAP1-pulsed DC	CTL	61
CEA peptides (A2)	CTL	59, 60
CEA peptides (A24)	CTL	63

*CTL, cytotoxic T lymphocyte response; LP, lymphoproliferation (CD4+) response; antibody (Ab) response

Several studies have demonstrated the potential importance of cytokines in the clinical applications of CEA vaccines. The use of recombinant CEA protein in patients with advanced colorectal cancer, with and without the use of GM-CSF at the injection site, has been reported [72]. Rather weak responses were noted with CEA protein in adjuvant; patients receiving the vaccine in adjuvant, in the presence of GM-CSF, however, developed strong IgG anti-CEA responses and CEA-specific proliferative T-cell responses. As with all of the other CEA vaccines described above, no signs of autoimmunity were noted.

In an attempt to establish CEA-specific T-cell lines from patients who had received a CEA vaccine, PBMC were obtained from several patients with the HLA-A2 allele pre- and post-vaccination with rV-CEA. PBMC were alternately pulsed with the CAP-1 CEA peptide and interleukin (IL)-2 in the presence of autologous PMBC as APC [14]. T-cell lines could be established from five of five HLA-A2 patients from PBMC post-vaccination with rV-CEA PBMC; these T cells were cytotoxic for T2 cells when pulsed with the CAP-1 peptide and were primarily $CD8^+$ or $CD8^+/CD4^+$ double positive.

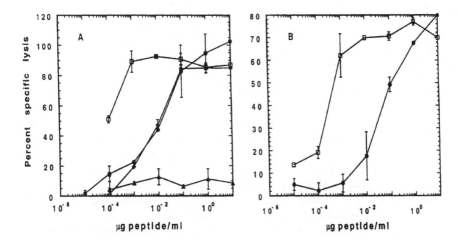

Figure 5.3. CAP-1 and analogs show different sensitivity to CEA CTL T-Vac8 cytotoxicity. T2 (A) and C1R-A2 (B) target cells were labeled with Cr_{51} and incubated in round-bottom, 96-well plates (10,000/well) with the CEA peptide CAP-1 (●) or substituted peptide CAP-1-6D (□) at the indicated concentrations. After 1 h, T-Vac8 CTL were added at E:T= 2.5, and isotope release was determined after 4 h. T-Vac8 is a CTL-derived from a patient vaccinated with rV-CEA and stimulated with CAP-1 and IL-2. All assays were done in triplicate. NCA571 (Δ) is a 9-mer peptide obtained after optimal alignment of CEA with the related gene NCA [71].

Using the same *in vitro* protocols, T-cell lines could not be established from these same patients when pre-vaccination PBMC were used. Another CEA peptide, designated CAP-2 (amino acid positions 555-563) has been employed to successfully generate CEA-specific CTL lines from a patient vaccinated with rV-CEA [73].

Phase I studies are primarily designed as toxicity studies and are traditionally conducted in patients with advanced disease. This patient population is probably the least desirable in which to examine the efficacy of a vaccine to initiate T-cell responses, since defects in TCR ζ chains and other immune defects have been reported [74-76]. Initial vaccinations with rV-CEA resulted in a clinical "take" as measured by the local erythematous reaction in 23 of 26 patients. Four of seven patients in Cohort 1 (lowest dose level) and all 19 patients in Cohorts 2 and 3 (higher vaccine dose levels) demonstrated erythema. Thus, despite the fact that all patients had previously received the smallpox vaccine, most patients displayed the classical acute manifestations of the vaccinia vaccination, confirming the capacity to be reimmunized. Lesion size correlated with the dose of rV-CEA given but was reduced with subsequent vaccinations at the same dose level. At all dose levels, no toxicity was apparent other than that normally observed with the administration of a smallpox vaccine. It thus appears that patients, even those having received a previous smallpox vaccination during childhood, can be efficiently primed to mount an immune response to CEA when administered a dose of rV-CEA of 10^7 pfu or greater.

As mentioned above, optimal preclinical results were obtained when mice first received a primary vaccination with rV-CEA and were then boosted with avipox-CEA [43]. The CEA-specific T-cell responses of patients before and after vaccination with the avipox-CEA recombinants have now been characterized [67,77]. Pre- and postvaccination PBMC of eight patients positive for the HLA-class I A2 allele, that had received avipox-CEA, were incubated with the CEA peptide CAP-1 and IL-2. Cultures could not be established, when using these methods and pre-vaccination PBMC, that had the ability to lyse C1R-A2 target cells pulsed with the CAP-1 peptide. However, T-cell cultures from seven of eight of these same patients, obtained from PBMC after avipox-CEA vaccination, were shown to lyse C1R-A2 cells only when pulsed with CAP-1. Moreover, all seven of these T-cell cultures were shown to lyse allogeneic human carcinoma cell lines (SW1463 and SW480) that were both A2$^+$ and expressed CEA (Table 5.2); an allogeneic tumor cell line (LS174T) expressing CEA that was negative for A2 expression was not lysed. HLA-A2$^+$ and CEA$^+$ autologous tumor cells were also capable of being lysed by CEA-specific T cells from one of the patients in which autologous tumor was available [77]. Analysis of this CTL line also revealed the expression of several homing and adhesion-associated molecules. Fluorescence-activated cell-sorter analysis of the T-cell lines established from patients after avipox-CEA vaccination revealed that most were CD8$^+$/CD4$^-$, but many also had a CD8$^+$/CD4$^+$ component. Analyses of T-cell receptor Vβ usage of several of the CEA-specific CTL lines showed a relatively diverse Vβ pattern.

Table 5.2. CTL activity of CEA-specific T-cell lines against human colon carcinoma cells

T-cell line[b]	%Lysis of target cell[a]		
	SW1463	SW480	LS174T
#4	19.58 (2.06)[c]	23.26 (1.79)[c]	5.55 (1.21)
#8	33.97 (5.71)[c]	51.46 (2.78)[c]	19.84 (2.26)
#11	26.96 (7.53)[c]	37.05 (4.37)[c]	7.73 (3.70)
#14	22.79 (1.62)[c]	24.63 (0.08)[c]	7.73 (3.70)
#15	11.80 (7.05)	22.51 (2.28)[c]	3.96 (0.71)
#16	27.90 (3.17)[c]	26.57 (2.49)[c]	9.34 (2.00)
#18	31.97 (7.17)[c]	27.41 (2.41)[c]	15.81 (1.23)

[a]SW1463 and SW480 are HLA-A2-positive human colon carcinoma cell lines expressing CEA. LS174T is a very low (2.1%) HLA-A2- and CEA-expressing human colon carcinoma cell. An 18-hour ^{111}In-release assay was performed. Results are expressed in percent-specific lysis at an effector:target-cell ratio of 50:1 compared with lysis obtained with LS174T cells.
[b]Each T-cell line was established from a different vaccinated patient.
[c]Statistically significant (p<0.01, two-tailed *t* test).

These studies demonstrated for the first time the ability to vaccinate cancer patients with a replication-defective avipox recombinant and derive T cells that are capable of lysing allogeneic and autologous tumor cells in a MHC-restricted manner [67,77].

Identification of a TCR enhancer agonist epitope for CEA

One strategy to enhance the immunogenicity of a self-antigen such as CEA, or indeed any antigen, would be to slightly modify a known CTL epitope such as CAP-1. The key, of course, is to ensure that the resultant CTL derived from such an analog would retain specificity for the native antigen as presented in the context of MHC on tumors. Recent studies have shown some enhanced immunogenicity *in vitro* of peptides after modification of anchor sequences to MHC [78-81]. These studies were intended to increase peptide binding to the MHC since anchor residues of those peptides were not optimal. In the case of CAP-1, however, anchor residues conformed to optimal motifs [71]; this was confirmed with binding studies. In recently described studies, a different approach has been taken to improve the immunogenicity of a CTL peptide [71]. It was proposed that by altering non-anchor amino acid residues expected to contact the TCR, one could generate a TCR agonist (i.e., an analog with substitutions at non-MHC anchor positions that stimulates CTL more efficiently than the native peptide). The rationale for this approach was derived from previous findings involving the identification of peptide antagonists [82-89]. In these studies, inhibition of the T-cell response by modified peptides was shown to be TCR-mediated and could not be explained by MHC competitive binding. By analogy, the strictest definition of a peptide TCR agonist would be an analog that increased effector function without accompanying increases in MHC binding.

Several factors were considered in deciding which positions of CAP-1 to examine for effects on TCR interactions. Sequencing and mapping experiments have defined a binding motif in which position 2 and the C-terminal (position 9 or 10) are critical for peptide presentation by HLA-A2 [90]. In addition, Tyr at position 1 has been identified as an effective secondary anchor. Therefore, CAP-1 residues at these positions were not altered. X-ray crystallographic studies of several peptides bound to soluble HLA-A2 suggest that all binding peptides assume a common conformation in the peptide binding groove [91]. When five model peptides were examined, residues 5 through 8 bulge away from the binding groove and are potentially available for binding to a TCR. Studies therefore focused on modifying these residues in an attempt to define CAP-1 analogs that would more efficiently stimulate human CEA-specific cytotoxic T cells. A panel of 80 CAP-1 analog peptides, in which the residues at positions 5 through 8 were synthesized with each of the 20 natural amino acids, were produced by PIN technology [71]. The effects of these amino acid substitutions on TCR recognition were studied using the CAP-1-specific, HLA-A2-restricted human CTL line designated V8T. V8T was generated by CAP-1 and IL-2 stimulation of PBMC from a patient vaccinated with rV-CEA [14]. For initial screening, V8T was used in a cytotoxicity assay employing C1R-A2 target cells incubated with each member of the peptide panel (at three peptide concentrations) [66]. Of the 80 single amino acid substitutions, all but six failed to activate cytotoxicity of V8T.

Subsequent studies revealed that one peptide, designated CAP-1-6D (substitution of Asn by Asp at position 6), was the best candidate agonist [71]. CAP-1-6D (YLSGADLNL) was compared to native CAP-1 in a CTL assay over a more extended range of peptide concentrations, using two different cell lines as targets. Analog CAP-1-6D was over 100 times more effective in mediating lysis by V8T than native CAP-1 (Fig. 5.3) [71]. CAP-1 and the CAP-1-6D analog were tested for binding to HLA-A2 by measuring cell surface HLA-A2 in the transport-defective human cell line T2; there were no differences in binding (Fig. 5.4) [71]. Thus, the improved effectiveness of CAP-1-6D in the CTL assays suggests a better engagement to the TCR. The CAP-1-6D

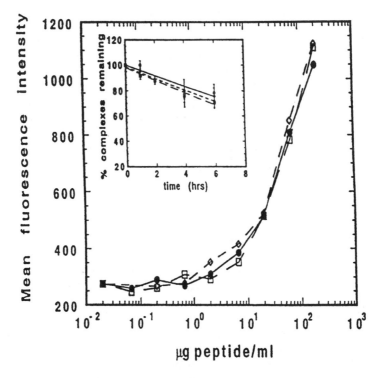

Figure 5.4. Effect of single amino acid substitutions in CAP-1 peptide on binding to and stability of HLA-A2 complexes. T2 cells were collected in serum-free medium and then incubated overnight (10^6 cells/well) with peptides CAP-1(●) or CAP-1-6D (□) at the indicated concentrations. Cells were collected and assayed for cell surface expression of functional HLA-A2 molecules by staining with conformation-sensitive MAb BB7.2. MFI was determined on a live, gated cell population. Insert: Cells were incubated with peptide at 100 μg/ml overnight, then washed free of unbound peptide and incubated at 37°C. At the indicated times, cells were stained for the presence of cell-surface peptide-HLA-A2 complexes. The error bars indicate SEM for two experiments [71].

agonist potentially could be useful in both experimental and clinical applications if it could stimulate growth of CEA-specific CTL from patients with established carcinomas more efficiently than CAP-1. Postvaccination PBMC from a cancer patient (designated Vac8) were stimulated *in vitro* with CAP-1-6D and were assayed for CTL activity against targets coated with CAP-1 or CAP-1-6D. This new line demonstrated peptide-dependent cytotoxic activity against target cells coated with either CAP-1-6D or the native CAP-1 peptide.

PBMC from patients vaccinated with rV-CEA were shown to produce CTL activity when stimulated with CAP-1, while prevaccination PBMC were negative [14,66]. New attempts to stimulate CTL activity from healthy, nonvaccinated donors using CAP-1, using this protocol, were also unsuccessful. However, CTL could be generated from healthy, nonvaccinated donors by *in vitro* stimulation with the agonist peptide CAP-1-6D [70,71]. Several peptide-specific CTL lines were obtained when generated with CAP-1-6D, but not with CAP-1. The CAP-1-6D-derived CTL were tested against a panel of human tumor cells. The CTL were shown to kill tumor targets expressing both endogenous CEA and class I HLA-A2 (Fig. 5.5) [70,71]; human tumor lines negative for either HLA-A2 or for CEA were not lysed.

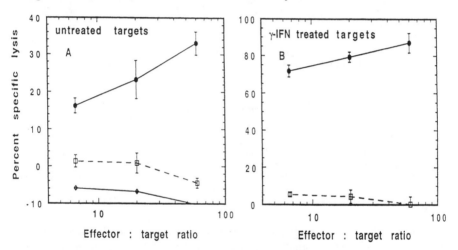

Figure 5.5. CTL generated with CAP-1-6D lyse CEA-positive, HLA-A2-positive tumors. The T-N1 CTL generated with CAP-1-6D were assayed against various tumor cell lines: SW480 (CEA+ and HLA-A2+; ●), SW1116 (CEA+ but HLA-A2-; □), and CaOV3 (CEA- but HLA-A2+; ◊). Tumor cells were cultured for 72 h in the absence (A) or presence (B) of IFN-γ, trypsinized, labeled with Cr_{51} and then incubated (5,000 cells/well) with T-N1 CTL at increasing E:T ratios. Cultures were incubated for 4 h, and the amount of isotope release was determined in a gamma counter. Values were determined from triplicate cultures [71].

The type and magnitude of cytokines produced by CAP-1-reactive CTL upon stimulation with the agonist peptide, CAP-1-6D, were compared to those obtained upon stimulation with the cognate CAP-1 peptide [70]. In addition, early events in the TCR signaling pathway were examined for differences in tyrosine phosphorylation. Upon stimulation with the agonist peptide CAP-1-6D, several different CEA-specific CTL lines exhibited a dramatic shift in the peptide dose response that resulted in as much as a 1,000-fold increase in the levels of GM-CSF (Fig. 5.6) and γ-IFN (Fig. 5.7) produced as compared with the use of CAP-1 peptide. However, levels of IL-4 and IL-10, which are associated with anti-inflammatory effects, were very low or non-existent. The cytokine profile of CAP-1- and CAP-1-6D-specific CTL is thus consistent with a Tc1-type CTL.

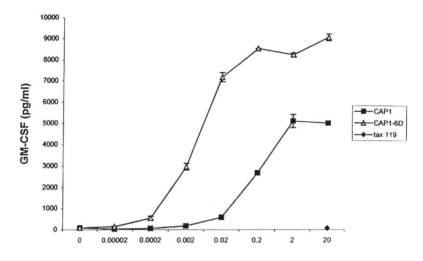

Peptide Concentration (ug/ml)

Figure 5.6. CEA-specific T-Vac8 CTL produce higher levels of GM-CSF when stimulated with CAP-1-6D agonist peptide as compared with cognate CAP-1 peptide. 1 x 10^5 T-Vac8 CTL, derived from a PBMC of a patient vaccinated with rV-CEA, were cultured with 1 x 10^5 T2 cells with either CAP-1 (■) or CAP-1-6D (Δ) at the indicated peptide concentrations in a total volume of 1 ml in each well of a 48-well plate. The Tax 119 peptide (♦) was used as a control [70].

Consistent with these findings, CEA-specific CTL showed increased tyrosine phosphorylation of TCR signaling proteins ZAP-70 and TCR ζ chains in response to both peptides. However, when CAP-1-6D was compared with the wild-type peptide, the increase in ZAP-70 phosphorylation was greater than the increase in ζ phosphorylation (Fig. 5.8). In conclusion, CTL generated with the CAP-1-6D agonist were shown capable of lysis of human carcinoma cells expressing native CEA. Thus, the ability to upregulate the production of GM-CSF, γ-IFN, TNF-α and IL-2 with the agonist peptide, as compared with CAP-1, may prove important in initiating and/or sustaining antitumor immune responses and thus potentially prove to be useful in the treatment of CEA-positive tumors.

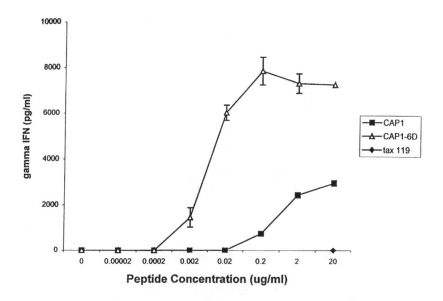

Figure 5.7. CEA-specific T-Vac8 CTL produce higher levels of γ-IFN when stimulated with CAP-1-6D (Δ) agonist as compared to native CAP-1 peptide (■). T-Vac8 CTL were cultured as described in Figure 6. Duplicate samples were assayed by specific capture ELISA (Endogen). Values are expressed as the mean +/- SEM of duplicate cultures. The Tax 119 peptide (♦) was used as a control [70].

FUTURE DIRECTIONS/T-CELL COSTIMULATION

A number of vaccines have now demonstrated the induction of CD8+ CTL, CD4+ T-cells, and antibody responses specific for CEA in humans. Several epitopes within the CEA molecule have now been identified as capable of inducing CTL responses. Moreover, the ability of human APC and human tumors to process CEA peptides, and the ability of CEA-specific CTL to lyse both allogeneic and autologous tumors in a MHC-restricted fashion, has also been established by several investigators. Thus far, these findings have been achieved principally in Phase I trials without evidence of any acute or chronic toxicity. However, the quantity (and, perhaps, quality) of T-cell responses observed in these Phase I studies is moderate at best. At this point, it is not known whether this is due to the inability of patients with advanced cancer to mount aggressive T-cell responses, to the potency of the vaccines, to dose/schedule regimens, or to a combination of these. Phase II trials in patients with less advanced disease and the use of more potent vaccines and vaccine strategies should provide answers to these questions.

One of these vaccine strategies employs the use of high intensity immune stimulation via T-cell costimulation. The activation of a T cell has been shown to require two signals via molecules present on professional APC: signal 1, via a

A

Chromium release

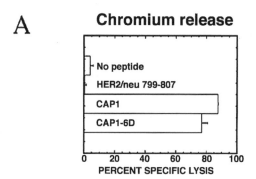

B

ZAP-70 Immunoprecipitates

C

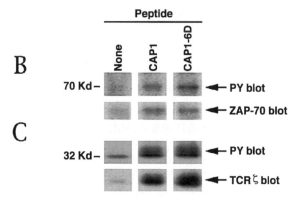

D

Phosphorylation/Unit Protein
(densitometric units)

Protein	Peptide	
	CAP1	CAP1-6D
ZAP-70	0.33	0.82
TCR-ζ	0.96	0.80

Figure 5.8. (previous page) T-Vac8 CTL generate stronger intracellular signaling with the CAP-1-6D CEA agonist peptide than with the CAP-1 native peptide. (A) Chromium-labeled T2 cells were pulsed without peptide or with 10 μg/ml peptides HER2/neu 799-807 (negative control), CAP-1 or CAP-1-6D. Rested T-Vac8 CEA-specific CTL were added at a 2.5:1 E:T ratio, and isotope release was measured after 4 hours. (B and C) Unlabeled T2 (10^6) without or with 10 μg/ml peptide were incubated for 5 min. at 37°C with rested T-Vac8 (2 x 10^6), lysed, and immunoprecipitated with anti-ZAP-70 Ab. Washed precipitates were electrophoresed, transferred to PVDF and probed with (B, top) antibody to phosphotyrosine. (B, bottom) Membrane was stripped and reprobed with anti-ZAP-70 Ab. (C, top) Brief re-exposure of (B, top) reveals phosphotyrosine state of TCR ζ chains that co-precipitated with ZAP-70. (C, bottom) Membrane was reprobed with anti-ζ Ab. (D) Densitometric analysis of panels B and C (arbitrary units) shows that when comparing CAP-1-6D to CAP-1, the increase in ZAP-70 phosphorylation exceeds the increase in ζ chain phosphorylation [70].

peptide/MHC complex, which interacts with the TCR, and signal 2, via a costimulatory molecule, which interacts with a ligand on T cells. Preclinical studies showed the advantage of employing either an admixture of rV-CEA and rV-B7-1, or rV-CEA/B7-1, in enhancing CEA-specific T-cell responses [39,40]. Moreover, Phase I clinical trials employing an avipox-CEA/B7-1 recombinant have recently been completed [68,69,92]. As with preclinical studies, the clinical studies indicated an enhancement in CEA-specific immune responses when the B7-1 costimulatory molecule gene was employed as a vaccine component.

The role of three costimulatory molecules in the activation of T cells has now been examined [93]. Poxvirus (vaccinia and avipox) vectors were employed in these studies because of their ability to efficiently express multiple transgenes. Murine cells provided with signal 1 and infected with either recombinant vaccinia or avipox vectors containing a *tri*ad of *co*stimulatory *m*olecules (B7-1/ICAM-1/leukocyte function-associated antigen [LFA]-3, designated TRICOM) induced the activation of T cells to a far greater extent than cells infected with any one or two costimulatory molecules (Fig. 5.9).

T-cells stimulated with TRICOM-vector-infected APC demonstrated enhanced cytokine levels (Fig. 5.10). Despite this T-cell "hyperstimulation" using TRICOM vectors, no evidence of apoptosis was observed in stimulated T cells (Fig. 5.11). In fact, T cells stimulated with the aid of B7.1 or TRICOM vectors actually demonstrated less apoptosis when compared with T cells stimulated by APC devoid of these vectors. Results employing the TRICOM vectors were most dramatic under conditions of either low levels of signal 1 or low stimulator cell to T-cell ratios. These studies thus demonstrate for the first time the ability of vectors to introduce three costimulatory molecules into cells, thereby activating both $CD4^+$ and $CD8^+$ T-cell populations to levels greater than those achieved with the use of only one or two costimulatory molecules [93]. This new threshold of T-cell activation has broad implications in vaccine design and development.

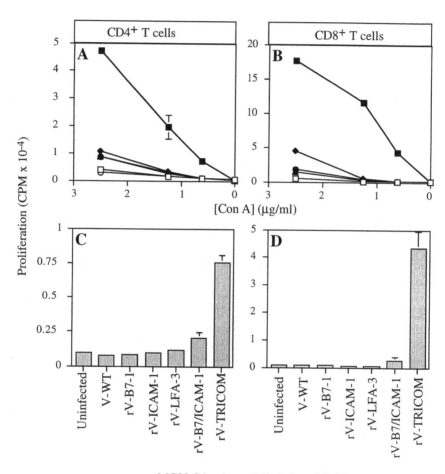

MC38 Stimulator Cells Infected With:

Figure 5.9. Effect of costimulation with TRICOM vectors on specific T-cell populations. Murine CD4+ (A) or CD8+ T cells (B) were co-cultured with uninfected MC38 colon tumor cells (○), or MC-38 cells infected with V-WT (□), rV-LFA-3 (▲), rV-ICAM-1 (●), rV-B7-1 (◆) or rV-TRICOM (■) at a 10:1 ratio for 48 hr in the presence of various concentrations of Con A as signal 1. C and D show the proliferative responses of purified CD4+ and CD8+ cells, respectively, when co-cultured in the presence of vector-infected MC38 stimulator cells at a low Con A concentration (0.625 μg/ml) as signal 1 [92].

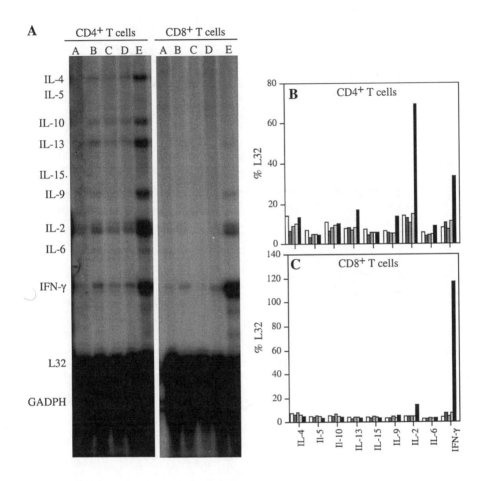

Figure 5.10. Effect of costimulation with TRICOM vector-infected APC on cytokine RNA expression. A: murine CD4+ or CD8+ T cells were co-cultured with MC38 murine colon carcinoma stimulator cells infected with V-WT (lane A), rV-B7-1(lane B), rV-ICAM-1 (lane C), rV-LFA-3 (lane D) or rV-TRICOM (lane E) at a T-cell: stimulator-cell ratio of 10:1 for 24 hr in the presence of 2.5 µg/ml Con A as signal 1. Following culture, T-cell RNA was analyzed by multiprobe RNase protection assay. The quantitative representation of results from the autoradiograph is normalized for expression of the housekeeping gene L32 in B (CD4+ cells) and C (CD8+ cells). Order of histogram bars (from left to right): MC38/V-WT, MC38/B7-1, MC38/ICAM-1, MC38/LFA-3, and MC38/TRICOM (solid histogram bar) [92].

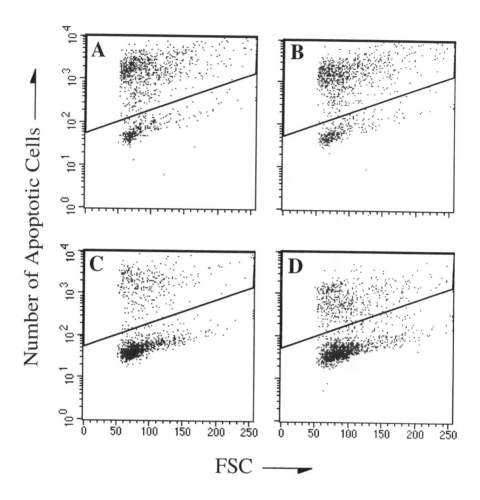

Figure 5.11. Activation of T cells with APC containing TRICOM vectors reduces T-cell apoptosis. Apoptosis of CD8+ cells activated with Con A as signal 1, and either (A) MC38, (B) MC38/V-WT, (C) MC38/B7-1, or (D) MC38/TRICOM. Each panel depicts the percentage of apoptotic cells (above line) in each group as measured by the terminal deoxynucleotidyl transferase-mediated nick-end labeling assay. FSC, forward scatter [92].

Orthopox vectors with four transgenes have now been constructed. In one such vector, the transgenes are CEA, B7-1, ICAM-1 and LFA-3, designated rV-CEA-TRICOM. CEA-Tg mice [94,95] in which the human CEA gene is expressed in normal adult gastrointestinal tissue, and whose serum is CEA-positive, were employed to determine if the rV-CEA/TRICOM vector could enhance T-cell responses to a self-antigen. T-cell responses obtained after vaccination with rV-CEA/TRICOM were substantially greater than those obtained with rV-CEA or rV-CEA/B7-1 (Table 5.3). Responses to ovalbumin and Con A were used as controls. CEA-Tg mice were also used to determine if antitumor responses to a CEA-expressing tumor could be enhanced employing a TRICOM vector. These mice were first inoculated subcutaneously with MC38 carcinoma cells expressing the CEA gene [96]. Four days later, mice were vaccinated one time at a distal site with viral recombinant or buffer. No tumors grew in mice vaccinated with rV-CEA/TRICOM, whereas tumors continued to grow in mice vaccinated with buffer, rV-CEA and rV-CEA/B7-1 (Table 5.3). Though preliminary, these results support the *in vivo* activity of TRICOM vectors.

Table 5.3. Enhanced immune response and antitumor response of rV-CEA/TRICOM in CEA transgenic (Tg) mice

	Con A	Oval	CEA	CEA	Tumor Volume	Tumor Volume
			Stimulation Index (SI)			
Immunogen	(5µg/ml)	(100 µg/ml)	(100 µg/ml)	(25 µg/ml)	Day 14	Day 35
Buffer	109	1.0	1.3	2.0	698±928	3,674±3.107
rV-CEA	123	0.9	4.9	4.0	259±0	1,112±1,685
RV-CEA/B7-1	93	1.3	7.1	4.3	150±236	2,696±1,936
RV-CEA/TRICOM	111	1.1	19.2	15.9	0±0	0±0

C57BL/6 CEA-Tg mice (5 per group) were vaccinated via skin scarification with buffer or vaccinia recombinant (10^7 pfu) one time on Day 0. On Day 30, 2 mice were killed and splenic T cells were analyzed for T-cell proliferative responses. Each value represents the SI of the mean CPM of triplicate samples versus media. Standard deviation never exceeded 10%. On Day –4, 3 mice per group were given 4×10^5 MC38 colon carcinoma cells expressing CEA. Tumor volume is given at Days 14 and 35 postvaccination.

CONCLUSION

In conclusion, numerous approaches to enhance the effectiveness of CEA vaccines are under way. The identification of agonist epitope peptides, such as CAP-1-6D, may also greatly enhance future vaccine efficacy. Since CEA is a "self" gene product, one would hypothesize the induction of only weak or moderate T-cell responses. The demonstration that an agonist epitope can enhance these responses may be crucial. Agonist epitopes can be exploited as peptide vaccines with adjuvant, with pulsed DC, or via the modification of the CEA gene to express the agonist epitope in vector-based vaccines such as vaccinia, avipox, and DNA, etc. Preclinical studies and a recent clinical trial have demonstrated that diversified vaccination protocols using two different forms of the immunogen are more potent than the repeated use of the same immunogen. The use of CEA vaccines in combination with cytokines may also be crucial. Preclinical and clinical studies have now demonstrated that the use of local GM-CSF clearly enhances CEA-specific responses. Preclinical studies also demonstrate that the use of low-dose IL-2 increases T-cell and antitumor responses. Finally, the use of T-cell costimulation may be crucial in enhancing CEA-specific T-cell responses. This can be achieved by the use of DC to present CEA or CEA peptides, or by the use of vectors engineered to express both CEA, or CEA epitopes, and one or more costimulatory molecules. A recent preclinical study employing the TRICOM vector expressing three different T-cell costimulatory molecules has shown a great enhancement of T-cell responses [93]. Thus, the use of this type of vector in concert with a self-antigen such as CEA, with or without epitope modifications, may bring host T-cell responses to a level of therapeutic efficacy. Both avipox and vaccinia vectors have now been developed containing TRICOM, along with the entire CEA gene containing the 6D modification at the CAP-1 epitope.

REFERENCES

1. Gold P and Freedman SO. Demonstration of tumor-specific antigens in human colonic carcinomata by immunological tolerance and absorption techniques. J Exp Med 1965; 121:439.
2. Gold P and Freedman SO. Specific carcinoembryonic antigens of the human digestive system. J Exp Med 1965; 122:467.
3. Gold P and Goldenberg NA. The Carcinoembryonic Antigen (CEA): Past, Present and Future. McGill J Med 1997; 3:46-66.
4. Pignatelli M, Durbin H, and Bodmer WF. Carcinoembryonic antigen functions as an accessory adhesion molecule mediating colon epithelial cell-collagen interactions. Proc Natl Acad Sci USA. 1990; 87:1541-1545.
5. Thompson JA. Molecular cloning and expression of carcinoembryonic antigen gene family members. Tumor Biol 1995; 16:10-16.
6. Schrewe H, Thompson J, Bona M, et al. Cloning of the complete gene for carcinoembryonic antigen: analysis of its promoter indicates a region conveying cell type-specific expression. Mol Cell Biol 1990; 10:2738-2748.
7. Thompson J, and Zimmerman W. The carcinoembryonic gene family: structure, expression and evolution. Tumor Biol 1988; 9:63-83.
8. Thompson JA, Pande H, Paxton RJ, et al. Molecular cloning of a gene belonging to the carcinoembryonic antigen gene family and discussion of a domain model. Proc Natl Acad Sci USA 1987; 84:2965-2969.
9. Thompson JA, Grunert F, and Zimmerman W. Carcinoembryonic antigen gene family: molecular biology and clinical perspectives. J Clin Lab Anal 1991; 5:344-366.
10. Benchimol S, Fuks A, Jothy S, et al. Carcinoembryonic antigen, a human tumor marker, functions as an intercellular adhesion molecule. Cell 1989; 57:327-334.
11. von Kleist S, Migule I, and Halla B. Possible function of CEA as cell-contact inhibitory molecule. Anticancer Res 1995; 15:1889-1894.
12. Conry RM, LoBuglio AF, Kantor J, et al. Immune response to a carcinoembryonic antigen polynucleotide vaccine. Cancer Res 1994; 54:1164-1168.

13. Kantor J, Irvine K, Abrams S, et al. Anti-tumor activity and immune responses induced by a recombinant vaccinia-carcinoembryonic antigen (CEA) vaccine. J Natl Cancer Inst 1992; 84:1084-1091.
14. Tsang KY, Zaremba S, Nieroda CA, et al. Generation of human cytotoxic T cells specific for human carcinoembryonic antigen epitopes from patients immunized with recombinant vaccinia-CEA vaccine. J Natl Cancer Inst 1995; 87:982-990.
15. Guadagni F, Roselli M, Cosimelli M, et al. Quantitative analysis of CEA expression in colorectal adenocarcinoma and serum: Lack of correlation. Int J Cancer 1997; 72:949-954.
16. Sharkey RM, Goldenberg DM, Goldenberg H, et al. Murine monoclonal antibodies against carcinoembryonic antigen: immunologica, pharmacokinetic and targeting properties in humans. Cancer Res 1990; 50:2823-2831.
17. Siccardi AG, Buraggi GL, and Callegaro L. Immunoscintigraphy of adenocarcinomas by means of radiolabeled F(ab')2 fragments of an anti-carcinoembryonic antigen monoclonal antibody: a multicenter study. Cancer Res 1989; 49:3095-3103.
18. Mach JP, Forni M, Ritschard J, et al. Use and limitations of radiolabeled anti-CEA antibodies and their fragments for photoscanning detection of human colorectal carcinomas. Oncodevelopmental Biol Med 1980; 1:49-69.
19. Juweid ME, Sharkey, RM, Behr, T, et al. Radioimmunotherapy of patients with small-volume tumors using iodine-131-labeled anti-CEA monoclonal antibody NP-4 F(ab')2. J. Nucl. Med. 1996;37(9):1504-1510.
20. Behr TM, Sharkey, RM, Juweid, ME, et al. Phase I/II clinical radioimmunotherapy with an iodine-131-labeled anti-carcinoembryonic antigen murine monoclonal antibody IgG. J. Nucl. Med. 1997;38(6):858-870.
21. Juweid ME, Hajjar, G, Swayne, LC, et al. Phase I/II trial of (131)I-MN-14F(ab)2 anti-carcinoembryonic antigen monoclonal antibody in the treatment of patients with metastatic medullary thyroid carcinoma. Cancer 1999;85(8):1828-1842.
22. Ychou M, Pelegrin, A, Faurous, P, et al. Phase-I/II radio-immunotherapy study with Iodine-131-labeled anti-CEA monoclonal antibody F6 F(ab')2 in patients with non-resectable liver metastases from colorectal cancer. Int. J. Cancer 1998;75(4):615-619.
23. Juweid M, Sharkey, RM, Alavi, A, et al. Regression of advanced refractory ovarian cancer trated with iodine-131-labeled anti-CEA monoclonal antibody. J. Nucl. Med. 1997;38(2):257-260.
24. Juweid M, Sharkey, RM, Behr, T, et al. Radioimmunotherapy of medullary thyroid cancer with iodine-131-labeled anti-CEA antibodies. J. Nucl. Med. 1996;37(6):905-911.
25. Frelinger J, Wei C, Willis R, et al. Targeted CTL-mediated immunity for prostate cancer: Development of human PSA-expressing transgenic mice. Proc Am Assoc for Cancer Res 1996; 37:3027.
26. Hasegawa T, Isobe K, Nakashima I, et al. Quantitative analysis of antigen for the induction of tolerance in carcinoembryonic antigen transgenic mice. Immunol 1992; 77: 577-581.
27. Sinclair NRS. The trouble with transgenic mice. Immunol Cell Biol 1995; 73:169-173.
28. Matzinger P. Tolerance, danger, and the extended family. Annu Rev Immunol 1994; 12:991-1045.
29. Nanda NK and Sercarz EE. Induction of anti-self-immunity to cure cancer. Cell 1995; 82:13-17.
30. Ridge JP, Fuchs EJ, and Matzinger P. Neonatal tolerance revisited: Turning on newborn T cells with dendritic cells. Science 1996; 271:1723-1726.
31. Fenton RG and Longo DL. Danger versus tolerance: Paradigms for future studies of tumor-specific cytotoxic T lymphocytes. J Natl Cancer Inst 1997; 89:272-275.
32. Tjoa BA and Kranz DM. Generation of cytotoxic T-lymphocytes to a self-peptide/class I complex: A model for peptide-mediated tumor rejection. Cancer Res 1994; 54:204-208.
33. Eades-Perner AM, van der Putten, H, Hirth A, et al. Mice transgenic for the human carcinoembryonic antigen gene maintain its spatiotemporal expression pattern. Cancer Res 1994; 54:4169-4176.
34. Theobald M, Biggs J, Dittmer D, et al.. Targeting p53 as a general tumor antigen. Proc Natl Acad Sci USA 1995; 92:11993-11997.
35. Irvine K, Kantor J, and Schlom J. Comparison of a CEA-recombinant vaccinia virus, purified CEA, and an anti-idiotypic antibody bearing the image of a CEA epitope in the treatment and prevention of CEA-expressing tumors. Vaccine Res 1993; 2:79-94.
36. Bei R, Kantor J, Kashmiri SVS, et al. Serological and biochemical characterization of recombinant baculovirus carcinoembryonic antigen. Mol Immunol 1994; 31:771-780.
37. Bei R, Kantor J, Kashmiri SVS, et al. Enhanced immune responses and anti-tumor activity by baculovirus recombinant CEA in mice primed with the recombinant vaccinia CEA. J Immunother 1994; 16:275-282.

38. Salgaller ML, Bei R, Schlom J, et al. Baculovirus recombinant expressing the human carcinoembryonic antigen gene. Cancer Res 1993; 53:2154-2161.
39. Kaufman H, Schlom J, and Kantor J. A recombinant vaccinia virus expressing human carcinoembryonic antigen (CEA). Int J Cancer 1991; 48:900-907.
40. Foon KA, John WJ, Chakraborty M, et al. Clinical and immune responses in advanced colorectal cancer patients treated with anti-idiotype monoclonal antibody vaccine that mimics the carcinoembryonic antigen. Clin Cancer Res 1997; 3:1267-1276.
41. Lou D and Kohler H. Enhanced molecular mimicry of CEA using photoaffinity crosslinked C3d peptide. Nature Biotech 1998; 16:1458-1462.
42. Conry RM, LoBuglio AF, Loechel F, et al. A carcinoembryonic antigen polynucleotide vaccine for human clinical use. Cancer Gene Ther 1995; 2:33-38.
43. Hodge JW, McLaughlin JP, Kantor JA, et al. Diversified prime and boost protocols using recombinant vaccinia virus and recombinant nonreplicating avian pox virus to enhance T-cell immunity and antitumor responses. Vaccine 1997; 16:759-768.
44. McLaughlin JP, Schlom J, Kantor JA, et al. Improved immunotherapy of a recombinant CEA vaccinia vaccine when given in combination with Interleukin-2. Cancer Res 1996; 56:2361 - 2367.
45. Kass E, Parker J, Schlom J and Greiner JW. Comparative studies of the effects of recombinant GM-CSF and GM-CSF administered via a poxvirus to enhance the concentration of antigen presenting cells in regional lymph nodes. Cytokine (In press)
46. Lorenz MGO, Kantor JA, Schlom J, et al.. Antitumor immunity elicited by a recombinant vaccinia virus expressing CD70 (CD27L). Human Gene Ther 10: 1095-1103, 1999.
47. Hodge JW, McLaughlin JP, Abrams S, et al. The admixture of a recombinant vaccinia virus containing the gene for the costimulatory molecule B7 and a recombinant vaccinia virus containing a tumor associated antigen gene results in enhanced specific T-cell responses and antitumor immunity. Cancer Res 1995; 55:3598-3603.
48. Kalus RM, Kantor JA, Gritz L, et al. The use of combination vaccinia vaccines to enhance antigen-specific T-cell immunity via T-cell costimulation. Vaccine 1999; 17:893-903.
49. Hodge JW. Carcinoembryonic antigen as target for cancer vaccines. Cancer Immunol Immunother 1996; 43:127-134.
50. Thompson JA, Eades-Perner AM, Ditter M, et al. Expression of transgenic carcinoembryonic antigen (CEA) in tumor-prone mice: an animal model for CEA-directed tumor immunotherapy. Int J Cancer 1997; 72:197-202.
51. Kass E, Schlom J, Thompson J, et al. Induction of protective host immunity to carcinoembryonic antigen (CEA), a self-antigen in CEA transgenic mice, by immunizing with a recombinant vaccinia-CEA virus. Cancer Res 1999; 59:676-683.
52. Falk K, Rotzschke O, Stevanovic S, et al. Allele-specific motifs revealed by sequencing of self-peptides eluted from MHC molecules. Nature 1991; 351:290-296.
53. Hunt DF, Henderson RA, Shabanowitz J, et al. Characterization of peptides bound to the class I MHC molecule HLA-A2.1 by mass spectometry. Science 1992; 255:1261-1263.
54. Lee J. The HLA System: A New Approach. New York: Springer-Verlag, 1990, p. 154.
55. Parker KC, Bednarek MA, and Coligan JE. Scheme for ranking potential HLA-A2 binding peptides based on independent binding of individual peptide side-chains. J Immunol 1994; 152:163-175.
56. DiBrino M, Parker KC, Shiloach J., et al. Endogenous peptides bound to HLA-A3 possess a specific combination of anchor residues that permit identification of potential antigenic peptides. Proc Natl Acad Sci USA 1993; 90:1508-1512.
57. Nijman HW, Houbiers JG, Vierboom MP, et al. Identification of peptide sequences that potentially trigger HLA-A2.1-restricted cytotoxic T lymphocytes. Eur J Immunol 1993; 23:1215-1219.
58. Bremers AJA, van der Burg SH, Kuppen PJK, et al. The use of Epstein-Barr virus-transformed B lymphocyte cell lines in a peptide-reconstitution assay: identification of CEA-related HLA-A*0301-restricted potential cytotoxic T lymphocyte epitopes. J Immunother 1995; 18:77-85.
59. Ras E, van der Burg SH, Zegveld ST, et al. Identification of potential HLA-A *0201-restricted CTL epitopes derived from the epithelial cell adhesion molecule (Ep-CAM) and the carcinoembryonic antigen (CEA). Human Immunol 1997; 53:81-89.
60. Kawashima I, Hudson SJ, Tsai V, et al. The multi-epitope approach for immunotherapy for cancer: identification of several CTL epitopes from various tumor-associated antigens expressed on solid epithelial tumors. Human Immunol 1998; 59:1-14.
61. Alters SE, Gadea JR, Sorich M, et al. Dendritic cells pulsed with CEA peptide induce CEA-specific CTL with restricted TCR repertoire. J Immunother 1998; 21:17-26.

62. Nair SK, Boczkowski D, Morse M, et al. Induction of primary carcinoembryonic antigen (CEA)-specific cytotoxic T lymphocytes in vitro using human dendritic cells transfected with RNA. Nature Biotech 1998; 16:364-369.

63. Nukaya I, Yasumoto M, Iwasaki T, et al. Identification of HLA-A24 epitope peptides of carcinoembryonic antigen which induce tumor-reactive cytotoxic T lymphocyte. Int J Cancer 1999; 80:92-97.

64. Kim C, Matsumura M, Saijo K, et al. In vitro induction of HLA-A2402-restricted and carcinoembryonic antigen-specific cytotoxic T lymphocytes on fixed autologous peripheral blood cells. Cancer Immunol Immunother 1998; 47:90-96.

65. Chatterjee SK, Tripathi PK, Chakraborty M, et al. Molecular mimicry of carcinoembryonic antigen by peptides derived from the structure of an anti-idiotype antibody. Cancer Res 1998; 58:1217-1224.

66. Tsang KY, Zhu MZ, Nieroda CA, et al. Phenotypic stability of a cytotoxic T cell line directed against an immunodominant epitope of human carcinoembryonic antigen. Clinical Cancer Res 1997; 3:2439-2449.

67. Marshall JL, Hawkins MJ, Tsang KY, et al. A phase I study in cancer patients of a replication defective avipox (ALVAC) recombinant vaccine that expresses human carcinoembryonic antigen (CEA). J Clin Oncol 1999; 17:332-337.

68. von Mehren M, Davies M, Rivera V, et al. Phase I trial with ALVAC-CEA B7-1 immunization in advanced CEA-expressing adenocarcinomas. Proc Amer Soc Clin Oncol, 1999.

69. Lee DS, Conkright W, Horig HE, et al. Preliminary results of ALVAC-CEA-B7-1 phase I vaccine trial in patients with metastatic CEA-expressing tumors. Proc Amer Soc Clin Oncol, 1999.

70. Salazar E, Zaremba S,Tsang KY, Arlen P, and Schlom J. Agonist peptide from a cytotoxic T lymphocyte epitope of human carcinoembryonic antigen stimulates production of Tc1-type cytokines and increases tyrosine phosphorylation more efficiently than cognate antigen. Int. J. Cancer 86:829-838, 2000.

71. Zaremba, S., Barzaga, E., Zhu, M.Z., Soares, N., Tsang, K.Y., and Schlom, J. Identification of an Enhancer Agonist CTL Peptide from Human Carcinoembryonic Antigen. Cancer Res. 57: 4570-4577, 1997.

72. Samanci A, Yi Q, Fagerberg J, et al. Pharmacological administration of granulocyte/macrophage-colony-stimulating factor is of significant importance for the induction of a strong humoral and cellular response in patients immunized with recombinant carcinoembryonic antigen. Cancer Immunol Immunother 1998; 47:131-142.

73. Zhu M, Zaremba S, Correale P, et al. Generation of specific anti-human carcinoembryonic antigen (CEA) cytotoxic T lymphocytes from a colon carcinoma patient immunized with recombinant vaccinia-CEA (rV-CEA) vaccine by stimulation with a CEA synthetic peptide (CAP-2) in vitro. J Immunother 1996; 19:459.

74. Mizoguchi H, O'Shea JJ, Longo DL, et al. Alterations in signal transduction molecules in T lymphocytes from tumor-bearing mice. Science 1992; 258:1795-1798.

75. Finke JH, Zea AH, Stanley J, et al. Loss of T-cell receptor z chain and p56^{lck} in T-cells infiltrating human renal cell carcinoma. Cancer Res 1993; 53:5613-5616.

76. Nakagomi H, Petersson M, Magnusson I, et al. Decreased expression of the signal-transducing z chains in tumor-infiltrating T-cells and NK cells of patients with colorectal carcinoma. Cancer Res 1993; 53:5610-5612.

77. Zhu MZ, Marshall J, Cole D, Schlom J, and Tsang KY. Specific cytolytic T-cell responses to human carcinoembryonic antigen from patients immunized with recombinant canarypox (ALVAC)-CEA vaccine. Clin. Cancer Res., 6: 24-33, 2000.

78. Parkhurst MR, Salgaller ML, Southwood S, et al. Improved induction of melanoma-reactive CTL with peptides from the melanoma antigen gp100 modified at HLA-A*0201-binding residues. J Immunol 1996; 157:2539-2548.

79. Bakker ABH, Vanderburg SH, Huubens RJF, et al. Analogs of CTL epitopes with improved MHC class-I binding capacity elicit anti-melanoma CTL recognizing the wild type epitope. Int J Cancer 1997; 70:302-309.

80. Pogue RR, Eron J, Frelinger JA, et al. Amino-terminal alteration of the HLA-A*0201-restricted human immunodeficiency virus pol peptide increases complex stability and in vitro immunogenicity. Proc Natl Acad Sci USA 1995; 92:8166-8170.

81. Lipford G, Bauer S, Wagner H, et al. Peptide engineering allows cytotoxic T cell vaccination against human papilloma virus tumor antigen E6. Immunity 1995; 84:298-303.

82. DeMagistris MT, Alexander J, Coggeshall M, et al. Antigen analog-major histocompatability complexes act as antagonists of the T cell receptor. Cell 1992; 68: 625-634.

83. Bertoletti A, Sette A, Chissari FV, et al. Natural variants of cytotoxic epitopes are T cell receptor antagonists for antiviral cytotoxic T cells. Nature 1994; 369:407-410.

84. Klenerman P, Rowland-Jones S, McAdam S, et al. Cytotoxic T cell activity antagonized by naturally occurring HIV-1 gag variants. Nature 1994; 369:403-407.

85. Kuchroo VK, Greer JM, Kaul D, et al. A single TCR antagonist peptide inhibits experimental allergic encephalomyelitis mediated by a diverse T cell repertoire. J Immunol 1994; 153:3326-3336.

86. Jameson SC and Bevan MJ. T cell receptor antagonists and partial agonists. Immunity 1995; 2:1-11.

87. Meier U-C, Kleerman P, Griffin P, et al. Cytotoxic T lymphocyte lysis inhibited by viable HIV mutants. Science 1995; 270:1360-1362.

88. Chen A, Ede NJ, Jackson DC, et al. CTL recognition of an altered peptide associated with asparagine bond rearrangement: Implications for immunity and vaccine design. J Immunol 1996; 157:1000-1005.

89. Rammensee H-G, Friede T, and Stevanovic S. MHC ligands and peptide motifs: First listing. Immunogenetics 1995; 41:178-228.

90. Madrenas J and Germain RN. Variant TCR ligands: New insights into the molecular basis of antigen-dependent signal transduction and T-cell activation. Seminars Immunol 1996; 8:83-101.

91. Madden DR, Garboczi DN, and Wiley DC. The antigenic identity of peptide-MHC complexes: A comparison of the conformations of five viral peptides presented by HLA-A2. Cell 1993; 75:693-708.

92. Von Mehren M, Arlen P, Tsang KY, et al. Pilot study of a dual gene recombinant Avipox vaccine containing both CEA and B7.1 transgenes, in patients with recurrent CEA expressing adenocarcinomas. Clin Cancer Res 2000 (In press).

93. Hodge JW, Sabzevari H, Lorenz MGO, et al. A triad of costimulatory molecules synergize to amplify T-cell activation. Cancer Res. 59:5800-5807, 1999.

94. Kass, E., Schlom, J., Thompson, J., Guadagni, F., and Greiner, J.W. Induction of protective host immunity to carcinoembryonic antigen (CEA), a self-antigen in CEA-transgenic mice, by immunizing with a recombinant vaccinia-CEA virus. Cancer Res. 59: 676-683, 1999.

95. Thomspon, J.A., Grunert, F., and Zimmerman, W. Carcinoembryonic antigen gene family: molecular biology and clinical perspectives. J. Clin. Lab. Anal. 5: 344-366, 1991.

96. Hodge, J. W., McLaughlin, J. P., Abrams, S. I., Shupert, W. L., Schlom, J. and Kantor, J. A. The admixture of a recombinant vaccinia virus containing the gene for the costimulatory molecule B7 and a recombinant vaccinia virus containing a tumor associated antigen gene results in enhanced specific T-cell responses and anti-tumor immunity. Cancer Res. 55: 3598-3603, 1995.

6
MUC1 mucin as a target for immunotherapy of cancer: Muc1 based immunotherapeutic strategies

M. SOARES AND O.J FINN

INTRODUCTION

It has been more than a 100 years since the first attempts of cancer immunotherapy were made based on the assumption that tumor cells are recognized as foreign by the immune system. Over the last decade, there has been a considerable increase in our understanding of immune responses against cancer and the antigenic structures on tumor cells that are recognized by the immune system. Tumor antigens have been classified into distinct categories: tissue-specific differentiation antigens, tumor-specific unique antigens and tumor-specific shared antigens. MUC1 belongs to both the first and the last category.. Although MUC1 is expressed on both normal tissue as well as tumors, it has been extensively studied as a tumor antigen in both basic science as well as applied research for a number of exciting reasons. Some of these include its interesting protein structure, extensive glycosylation (which is altered in tumors) increased expression on tumors and changes in cellular distribution upon malignant transformation. In addition, it is very extensively expressed on a variety of human ductal adenocarcinomas. All these facts justify its use as a candidate for tumor-specific immunotherapy. The object of this chapter is to highlight current and past data concerning experimental and clinical immunotherapy of cancer using MUC1 as the target tumor-rejection antigen.

THE MUCIN FAMILY

Mucins are typically large membrane bound or secreted glycoproteins. They are produced by epithelial cells of the gastrointestinal, respiratory and reproductive tracts. To date the mucin family includes as many as 9 different mucins [1-4] the gene for MUC1 being the first to be isolated and sequenced [2].

R.A. Robins and R.C. Rees (eds.), Cancer Immunology, 101–122.
© 2001 *Kluwer Academic Publishers. Printed in the Netherlands.*

Structurally, mucins consist of a core protein moiety (apomucin) that has numerous heavily branched oligosaccharide chains attached to serines and threonine residues via α1-3-O-glycosidic bonds. O-linked glycosylation of mucin molecules can be so extensive that the sugars could account for as much as 80% of the mass of the molecules. The protein backbones consist of numerous stretches of a tandemly repeated peptide sequence varying in length for different mucins. There is very little sequence homology in the core protein domain among the many members of the mucin family. Hence, the repeats may vary in length and sequence but they all have the serine and threonine residues necessary for O-glycosylation [5-7]. In addition, the mucin tandem repeats also have one or more proline residues that are thought to determine the specificity of the galactosamine transferase that initiates mucin oligosaccharide synthesis. The mucins do share partial homology in the N- and C-terminal domains [8, 9].

Although the mucin family is large we have focused this chapter on MUC1 for several reasons. Unlike the other mucins which have a more restricted expression primarily on normal epithelia, MUC1 has restricted expression on normal epithelia but is also overexpressed on most epithelial adenocarcinomas derived from different anatomic sites. In addition, as will be described later in the chapter, there are certain characteristics of MUC1 expression on tumors that qualify it as a tumor specific antigen. Hence, most of the immunotherapeutic approaches to date have targeted MUC1 on epithelial adenocarcinomas.

EXPRESSION AND FUNCTION OF MUC1 MUCIN

In the past, the product of the MUC1 gene has been assigned several different names including episialin, polymorphic epithelial mucin (PEM), PAS-O, human milk fat globule (HMFG) antigen, DF3 antigen. For the sake of clarity and in keeping with the Human Genome Mapping conventions, we will refer to the MUC1 gene product as MUC1.

MUC1 is expressed by epithelial cells of the breast, lung, colon, pancreas, ovary, uterus, stomach and gallbladder. It is the only member of the mucin family that is a transmembrane glycoprotein (all the others are secreted) [10, 11]. On normal ductal epithelia, MUC1 expression is polarized; i.e. it is found only on the apical surface facing into the lumen of the duct (Fig. 6.1[2]. In the adult breast, MUC1 expression increases during pregnancy and lactation and is shed into the milk [12].

MUC1 shares some basic functions with other mucin family members. These include protecting ductal epithelial cells from harsh environments caused by digestive enzymes or preventing colonization by microorganisms. In addition, MUC1 has been implicated in promoting tumor metastasis, in signal transduction and as a ligand for P- and E selectins. In mice, MUC1 expression coincides with ductal lumen formation and it is thought that MUC1 may play a role in duct formation during organogenesis in the developing embryo [12-14]. MUC1 knockout mice, however, have shown no abnormalities in duct development [15] suggesting either no role for MUC1 in this process, or considerable redundancy of molecules (perhaps other mucins) capable of this function.

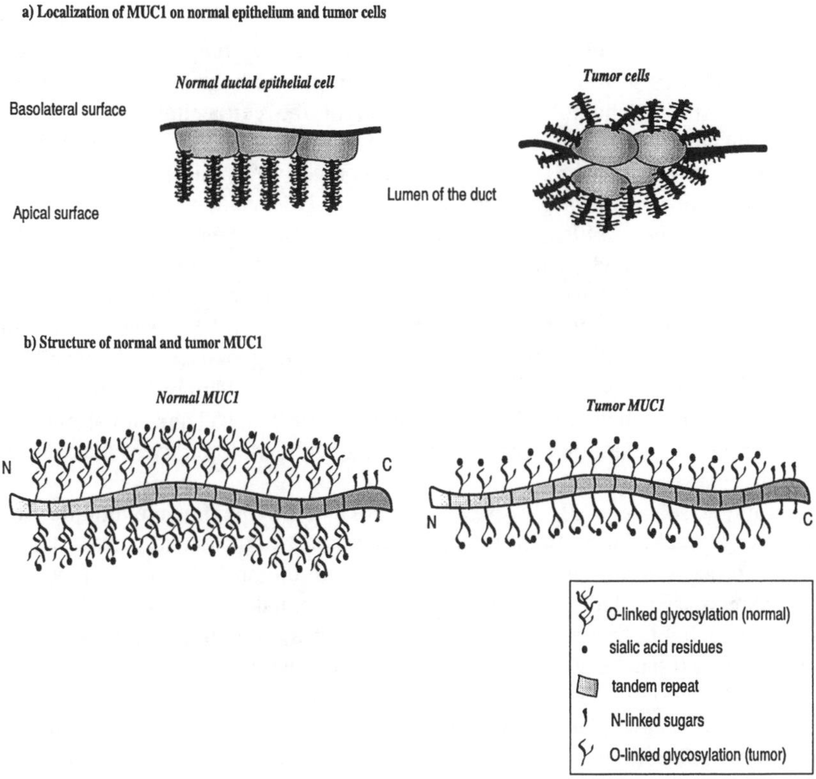

a) Localization of MUC1 on normal epithelium and tumor cells

b) Structure of normal and tumor MUC1

Figure 6.1. Schematic representation of a) Localization of MUC1 on normal epithelium and tumor cells. MUC1 on normal cells is expressed on the apical surface facing into the lumen of the duct while on tumor cells it loses its polarized expression and is expressed all over the cell. There is also an increase in the level of MUC1 expression on tumor cells. b) Structure of normal and tumor MUC1. Normal MUC1 has highly branched O-linked sugars attached to the serine and threonine residues within each tandem repeat that are terminally sialylated. On tumors, MUC1-associated O-linked sugars lack the highly branched sugar chains due to early termination of O-linked glycosylation but have terminal sialic acid residues. The figure does not show glycosylation of the five potential O-glycosylation sites within each tandem repeat region.

STRUCTURE OF MUC1 ON NORMAL AND CANCER CELLS

Domains of the MUC1 molecule

The MUC1 molecule can be divided into three regions: a large extracellular domain that makes up most of the molecule, a hydrophobic transmembrane domain and a short cytoplasmic domain. A major portion of the extracellular domain protein backbone consists of tandemly repeated sequence PDTRPAPGSTAPPAHGVTSA, 20 amino acids in length, rich in serine (10%), threonine (15%) and proline (25%). The serine and threonine residues serve as potential O-glycosylation sites [16, 17]. As a result of allelic polymorphism, the number of tandem repeats can vary anywhere between as few as 20 and as many as over 120 per allele. Thus, the length of the extracellular domain may vary greatly and in the case of the longer alleles it may extend as much as 400-500nm above the cell membrane. NMR and CD spectroscopy studies have revealed that the proline rich 20 amino acid repeated sequence forms a stable type II β-turn. At 20 amino acid intervals, there are protruding "knobs" with the PDTRP sequence on the tip of each "knob". The stability of the "knobs" and of the overall 3-D molecular structure in solution is highly influenced by the multiplicity of the repeats and degree of glycosylation [18, 19].

A unique sequence of 227 residues proximal to the transmembrane domain includes five N-glycosylation sites and a proteolytic cleavage site that is used during the intracellular processing of the molecule. Even though the protein is cut at that site, the two parts remain associated on the cell surface. C-terminal to this region is a 31 amino acid long hydrophobic transmembrane domain and a 69 amino acid long cytoplasmic domain [16, 20]. It has been shown that there are at least two discrete sequence motifs within the MUC1 molecule that specify membrane localization: one in the extracellular domain that confers apical localization and the second at the junction of the cytoplasmic and transmembrane domains that is necessary for specifying surface expression [21].

Although the major form of MUC1 is the transmembrane molecule with numerous tandem repeats, other minor forms of MUC1 do exist but their function on either normal or transformed cells remains unknown. These minor forms include secreted MUC1 and MUC1 lacking tandem repeats [22].

Glycosylation of MUC1

MUC1 expressed on normal epithelial cells is a heavily glycosylated molecule with highly branched O-linked oligosaccharide chains. Within the 20 amino acid sequence PDTRPAPGSTAPPAHGVTSA, there are five potential O-glycosylation sites, namely the three threonine and two serine residues. During O-glycosylation, N-acetylgalactosamine (Gal-Nac) is linked to serine or threonine residues, followed by the addition of galactose (Gal). The addition of Gal-Nac occurs in a sequential manner first on the two threonines and then the serine [23]. The enzyme β1-6-N-acetylglucosamine transferase then catalyzes the transfer of N-acetylglucosamine (GlcNAc) to GalNAc to form the basic core structure. In vitro glycosylation studies using MUC1 tandem repeat peptides and lysates from human breast or pancreatic tumor cell lines have shown that not all the threonine and serine residues within the tandem repeat region are glycosylated. In fact, in these studies, the threonine in the immunodominant PDTRP epitope was not glycosylated. In addition, these studies suggested that the ability of peptide residues to serve as acceptor substrates is affected by the primary amino acid sequence and by the proximity of the residue to the amino or carboxyl terminus of the peptide substrate [23-25]. In another study, Muller et al., [26] demonstrated that all five potential O-glycosylation sites within the tandem repeat region are glycosylated in purified milk MUC1. The discrepancies between these two studies might be reflective of the in vitro versus in vivo systems used to detect glycosylation patterns. The basic core structure of the MUC1 molecule is further extended to form long branched polysaccharides with relatively low concentrations of sialic acid. In addition to the O-glycosylation sites within the tandem repeat, there are five N-glycosylation sites proximal to the tandem repeat region within the extracellular domain that are all that are all glycosylated (Fig. 6.1) [20, 27].

The process of glycosylation followed by sialylation is not completed during the initial transit of newly synthesized MUC1 molecules from the ER to the plasma membrane. To generate extensively glycosylated MUC1, the molecules that reach the cell surface from the ER are repeatedly internalized and recycled through the trans-Golgi network (at least 10 times) before they are released to the outside environment as fully mature [28, 29]

Effect of malignant transformation on MUC1 expression and processing

Although the sequence of the protein backbone of MUC1 remains unchanged upon malignant transformation, there are dramatic changes that occur on the mature molecule that affect its expression pattern and glycosylation status. In adenocarcinomas, MUC1 expression on the cell surface is no longer polarized. There is also a dramatic increase in the number of MUC1 molecules produced and expressed on the surface, that can be as high as 50-fold over normal cell levels. In addition, tumor MUC1 is severely underglycosylated (Fig. 6.1). Indirect evidence to support the aberrant glycosylation of tumor MUC1 came from studies wherein the monoclonal antibody SM3 and several other MUC1-specific antibodies recognized cancer-associated MUC1 but not the normally processed glycoform secreted into the soluble fraction of milk during lactation [2]. Direct evidence was provided by studies in which Hanisch et al., [30] analyzed and compared the different MUC1 glycoforms secreted by mammary carcinoma cells (T47D) and MUC1 from a primary ductal breast carcinoma to MUC1 from human milk. Using isopycnic density gradient centrifugation they were able to demonstrate that the major glycans from tumor cell lines and from primary tumor consisted of sialylated, core type glycans that lack L-fucose, a characteristic component of peripheral oligosaccharide regions. The major glycans of tumor MUC1 ranged between trisaccharides to tetrasaccharides. Thus, there appeared to be a premature truncation of O-linked glycosylation. This aberrant glycosylation is considered to be due in part to the increased production of MUC1 requiring increased function of the glycosylation machinery, as well as to known changes in the glycosylation machinery within tumor cells. The MUC1-type O-glycan structures are greatly influenced by the expression and golgi localization of the glycosyltransferases that compete for common substrates. Thus, when the competing enzymes are located within the same golgi compartment, it is the relative activities of these enzymes that determine the glycan structure. Specifically it has been shown that there is about a 10-fold increase in the activity of α2-3-sialyl transferase and a decrease in the activity of β1-6GlcNAc- transferase in some breast cancer cell lines [31]. Changes in the activity of these enzymes lead to the premature addition of sialic acid onto the Gal residues during O-glycosylation thereby preventing further elongation of the carbohydrate side chains. The early termination of carbohydrate elongation results in the accumulation of tumor specific forms of MUC1 that bear short carbohydrates such as 3GalNAcα1-O-Ser/Thr (called Tn), Galβ1 (3GalNAcα1)-O-Ser/Thr (called T) and their sialylated forms sTn and sT [31].

IMMUNE RECOGNITION OF MUC1

For a tissue-specific or a differentiation antigen to be considered a tumor-specific antigen there must be changes in either the expression pattern or structure of the molecule on tumors that make it unique and tumor specific. Changes in the MUC1 molecule that occur upon malignant transformation of MUC1-expressing tissues are indeed noticed by the immune system. Early truncation of the oligosaccharide side chains on tumor MUC1 leads to the exposure of antigenic epitopes on the protein backbone that are recognized by B and T cells. Also, changes in the expression pattern such as its overexpression and the loss of polarization results in tumor MUC1 being abundantly expressed over the entire surface of the tumor cell. Thus the molecule is no longer sequestered within the lumen of the duct and is accessible to the effector mechanisms of the immune response. These features of tumor-associated MUC1 make it different enough from normal MUC1 such that B and T cells that recognize tumor-associated MUC1 do not recognize the fully glycosylated protein on normal ductal epithelium.

In this section of the chapter, we will describe the types of MUC1-specific immune responses that can be detected in cancer patients as well as responses that can be primed in vitro using peripheral blood lymphocytes (PBL) from cancer-free individuals.

Humoral responses to MUC1

Studies that we initially performed on sera from breast, colon and pancreatic cancer patients showed that MUC1-specific antibodies could be detected in approximately 10% of patients. We also showed that these antibodies recognized the PDTRP epitope which is at the tip of the 'immunodominant knob' present within each tandem repeat of underglycosylated tumor MUC1 molecules [32]. More sensitive ELISA assays we have developed since have detected the presence of these antibodies in most patients. Isotype analysis of the anti-MUC1 antibodies in patient serum revealed that such antibodies are primarily of the IgM isotype which is indicative of a helper T cell-independent response In fact, a majority of the antibodies to human MUC1 that have been raised in the mouse, recognize this peptide sequence confirming the immunodominance of this epitope [33].

Studies performed by others [34-36] have confirmed the presence of anti-MUC1 IgM antibodies in serum from patients with epithelial tumors such as breast, ovarian, and stomach.

The significance of an ongoing humoral response to MUC1 in cancer patients has not been fully determined. It is tempting to consider these responses potentially therapeutic in light of the expected effector functions of anti-tumor antibodies (such as direct killing of tumor cells by complement fixation, opsonization of soluble antigen and antibody-mediated cellular cytotoxicity, ADCC). In fact, circulating immune complexes of antibodies and MUC1 have been measured in sera from patients with breast cancer and have been correlated with a better clinical outcome [37, 38]. These types of observations suggest that it may be desirable to design vaccine and other immunotherapeutic approaches to elicit or amplify MUC1 specific antibodies.

Other lines of investigation that suggest potential anti-tumor effect of the humoral response are studies that have used passive antibody therapy to target tumors expressing MUC1. Radioimmunotherapy using yttrium-90 or I-131 labeled monoclonal antibodies was tested in a phase I clinical trial to treat patients with incurable metastatic breast cancer who had failed standard therapies. Therapy usually resulted in subacute or minimal acute toxicity. Approximately half the number of patients had transient clinically measurable tumor responses that lasted for upto five months post-therapy. One common problem associated with this type of therapy is that patients develop high human anti-mouse antibody titers that interfere with multicycle therapy. One way to overcome this problem is to use a "humanized" antibody [39, 40].

A radiolabelled antibody has also been tested in a phase I/II study in ovarian cancer patients following surgery and chemotherapy [41]. In this study, the monoclonal antibody HMFG-1 (which recognizes a peptide epitope within the tandem repeat region of MUC1) was radiolabelled with yttrium-90 and administered to patients intraperitoneally. No major toxicity was associated with this vaccine. On the basis of survival data from this study, it was concluded that there might be some benefit to using this type of adjuvant therapy in patients with advanced ovarian cancer. Another immunotherapeutic approach is based on bispecific antibodies (BsAbs) which redirect and trigger effector cells to kill tumors. Such antibodies have dual specificities, one for the tumor antigen and the other for the immune effector cell. Katayose et al.[42] synthesized and tested two such bispecific antibodies: MUC1xCD3 BsAb and MUC1xCD28 BsAb. In vitro experiments confirmed enhanced cytotoxicity of MUC1 expressing tumors by LAK cells. Infusion of both BsAbs followed by injection of in vitro activated LAK cells resulted in delayed tumor growth in a bile duct carcinoma (BDC)-grafted SCID mouse model.

Cytotoxic T cell responses to MUC1

In the late 1980s, it was generally accepted that T cells expressing the $\alpha\beta$-T cell receptor (TCR) recognize antigens that are processed and presented as peptide fragments in the groove of MHC molecules. Moreover, this recognition is restricted to targets that are of the same MHC haplotype as the T cell. Antigen recognition appeared to be very different in the case of cytotoxic T cells that recognized MUC1 on tumor cells. We were able to generate a cytotoxic line from the lymph node of a pancreatic cancer patient and showed that this line could recognize and kill pancreatic and breast-tumor cell lines expressing MUC1 [43]. This killing was inhibited by the MUC1-specific mAb SM-3 (that recognized the PDTRP sequence), by antibodies to the TCR-CD3 complex but not by anti-MHC class I antibodies. This suggested that the native MUC1 molecule was the antigen being recognized by the TCR in a MHC-unrestricted manner. Moreover, the epitope recognized by the CTL line was the PDTRP sequence (later shown in structural studies to be at the tip of the 'immunodominant knob'). These observations were supported by studies wherein CTL lines established using autologous or allogeneic mucin-transfected B cells killed autologous mucin-transfected B cells demonstrating that mucin, and not an alloantigen, was being recognized [44]. Moreover, in order for the MUC1-transfected B cells to be recognized, they had to be treated with a competitive inhibitor of O-linked glycosylation, phenyl-GalNAc presumably to expose the PDTRP epitope.

To explain the phenomenon of MHC-unrestricted recognition of MUC1, it was proposed that the TCRs of a single T cell could interact with multiple epitopes repeated along the extracellular domain of a single MUC1 molecule. Such high avidity interactions could potentially result in cross-linking of the TCR leading to T cell activation. Further investigation into this MHC-unrestricted recognition of MUC1 [45] revealed that MUC1 conjugated to microspheres could induce a partial T cell signal accompanied by a transient influx of Ca^{2+} but no translocation of the nuclear factor of activated T cells (NF-AT) into the nucleus or CTL proliferation. Direct recognition of MUC1 on tumor cells however, in the presence of certain accessory molecules resulted in full activation (leading to NF-AT translocation and CTL proliferation). This suggested that full T cell activation of MUC1-specific MHC unrestricted CTL requires additional intercellular interactions such as ICAM-1/LFA-1, and LFA-3/CD2

MHC-restricted responses to MUC1 have also been observed. In fact, peptide STAPPAHGV from the tandem repeat of MUC1 was shown to bind to HLA-1, -A2.1, -A3 and −A11. Secondary responses to this peptide could be detected in lymph nodes from an HLA-A11 breast cancer patient [46]. In addition, it is possible to generate CTL specific for this peptide from healthy HLA-A11 or −A1 positive donors [46, 47]. More recently, it has been shown that a peptide from the leader sequence of MUC1 can be used to prime MUC1-specific CTL from HLA-A2 positive healthy donors in vitro [48]. The MUC1 epitopes that are recognized in an MHC restricted manner are not tumor specific since they are not mutated in tumors and can potentially be presented by MHC-class I molecules on the normal epithelial in addition to tumor cells. Hence, although it is important to keep such epitopes in mind as potential targets for anti-tumor responses during immunotherapy, their utility is limited by the possibility that these responses may also target normal ductal epithelia.

Helper T cell responses to MUC1

To date, there have been no reports of MUC1-specific T helper cell responses in cancer patients. The lack of detectable T helper responses in cancer patients is surprising considering the high concentration of MUC1 that is detectable in the soluble form in sera and ascites from patients. This soluble form of MUC1 is much more glycosylated and sialilated while the underglycosylated MUC1 remains tumor associated. In our recently reported studies we have put forth a model to explain the lack of MUC1-specific T helper cell responses. We found that it was possible to prime (in vitro) class II restricted responses to MUC1 using only the unglycosylated form of MUC1 [49]. This form of MUC1 was very efficiently processed and presented by antigen presenting cells (APCs) such as dendritic cells (DC) [47]. Interestingly, using the fully glycosylated form of MUC1 (purified from patient ascites) we were unable to prime MUC1-specific MHC class II restricted responses. We found that this fully glycosylated form could be taken up by DC but remained in the early endocytic compartments and was not trafficked further into the cell to be processed and presented in the context of MHC class II molecules. Thus we believe that the lack of a detectable helper cell response in cancer patients could be explained by the inability of APCs such as DC to process the soluble form of MUC1 antigen to the immune system. This result is very significant because it also rules out potential tolerance of the helper T cell compartment to MUC1. It is obvious that supplying the underglycosylated form of the MUC1 antigen in a vaccine preparation would be expected to elicit a helper T cell response which in turn may allow expansion of both the humoral and the cytotoxic T cell response against this antigen.

TARGETING MUC1 WITH IMMUNE EFFECTOR MECHANISMS

Immune responses against MUC1 that are observed in cancer patients are a testament to the immunogenicity of this molecule. However, these existing responses are limited in their repertoire (IgM and CTL, no other IgG isotypes and no helper cells) as well as intensity (low antibody titers, low CTL frequency) and incapable of irradicating tumors in these individuals. Over the past 10 years there have been numerous attempts to enhance the existing responses or induce new immune responses against MUC1 by incorporating this antigen into various vaccine formulations. A number of studies have been carried out in animal models and in phase-I trials in humans. Although in various animals models MUC1-based vaccines have elicited a range of immune responses and in some cases protection from tumor growth, what remains a challenge is to augment MUC1-specific immune responses in cancer patients to irradicate tumors without causing massive destruction of normal tissues that express MUC1.

Animal models for testing MUC1 vaccines

Numerous studies testing vaccine formulations containing human MUC1 have been performed in conventional mice. Although this model system has been useful for determining the repertoire of MUC1-specific immune responses that could be induced, it has not been an ideal preclinical model that could predict the type of an immune response that could be expected from a cancer patient who not only might still harbor a considerable number of cancer cells, but also have MUC1 expressed on normal tissue. Human MUC1 shares very little homology to mouse MUC1 and is therefore highly immunogenic in conventional mice. How immunogenic human MUC1 can be in humans cannot be predicted from this animal model. A more relevant mouse model that has been developed is the MUC1 transgenic mouse model wherein human MUC1 is a self-antigen with an expression pattern similar to that seen in human tissues [50, 51]. In this model that is currently under study by several groups [51-55] it is possible to explore issues related to MUC1 immunogenicity, tolerance or autoimmunity, all of which could profoundly affect the choice of immunotherapy.

The chimpanzee has been a very useful animal model in which to test MUC1-based vaccines. Since chimpanzee MUC1 and human MUC1 are considered to be identical, any responses induced in this model would be expected to be induced in humans as well. Several vaccines have been tested in this model with very encouraging results. The limitations to this model however are the cost and availability of animals and the lack of transplantable tumors in the chimpanzee. Hence, while the questions of immunogenicity, tolerance and autoimmunity issues are appropriately addressed, the effect of immune responses elicited by various vaccinations on tumor rejection cannot be evaluated.

Clinical trials in cancer patients

Several phase-I clinical trials of MUC-based vaccines have been carried out over the past few years all over the world. Phase I trials are primarily carried out to test the potential toxicity of a vaccine preparation. The immune responses are evaluated only as a secondary aim. One common problem associated with phase I clinical trials is that the patients participating in these trials most often have late stage disease or have received previous therapies such as chemotherapy or radiation therapy and are often severely immunocompromised. Hence, it is very difficult to evaluate the true immunogenecity of the vaccine formulations tested. More recently, trials have been initiated in patients with early disease who are less immunocompromised. The true potential of cancer vaccines, however, including MUC1 based vaccines, will only be revealed when it becomes possible to use these in healthy young individuals at risk for development of cancer. The immune system has been harnessed through vaccinations to protect from infectious diseases, and should be able to respond the same way in cancer prevention.

MUC1 peptide-based vaccines

Use of synthetic peptides in vaccine formulations to induce either humoral or cell mediated immunity requires considerable understanding of antigenic epitopes that can be recognized by either T cells or B cells. Since B cells recognize antigen in its native form, B cell epitopes must be accessible on the soluble protein or on the surface of the tumor cell. B cell epitopes can be either a linear sequence or composed of amino acids from different parts of the molecule yielding a conformational epitope. In the case of MUC1, studies have identified the PDTRP sequence within each tandem repeat to be the immunodominant tumor-specific B cell linear epitope. However, its binding to the antibody receptors is dependent not only on the linear sequence but also on the 3D structure that this sequence assumes in the context of the longer amino acid sequence of the underglycosylated tandem repeat on tumor MUC1.

Since CTL play an important role in recognizing and killing tumor cells, it is imperative for anti-tumor peptide vaccines to include epitopes that can be recognized by CTL. These epitopes are by and large short peptides (8, 9 or 10 amino acids in length)

110

that can bind one or more human HLA Class I molecules. As mentioned before, several of such epitopes have been identified in the MUC1 sequence. In addition, and in our opinion most important, peptide vaccine must include one or more helper T-cell epitopes. These are longer peptides (12-20 amino acids in length) that bind to human HLA Class II molecules. Elicitation of a strong humoral and cell-mediated immunity requires T cell help, as does the establishment of tumor-specific memory responses. As we will discuss below, tumor-specific helper epitopes are often substituted in vaccines with heterologous proteins that can stimulate helper cells. While these may be useful in the generation of a stronger antibody or CTL response at the time of vaccination, the helper cell memory that is established is specific for the heterologous protein and will not be triggered at a later date in the case of tumor recurrence. Thus secondary anti-tumor responses will be severely compromised.

Muc1 Peptides Conjugated With Heterologous Protein Carriers

Ding et al. [56] tested a vaccine composed of MUC1 synthetic peptides containing the PDTRP epitope conjugated to a protein keyhole limpet hemocyanin (KLH) and administered to mice together with RIBI Detox adjuvant. In addition, they also tested a chimeric peptide containing two tandem repeats of a single MUC1 epitope and a tetanus toxin universal helper T cell epitope. Such immunizations were able to induce strong MUC1-specific delayed type hypersensitivity (DTH) reactions but no CTL responses. They also resulted in delayed tumor development. In a clinical trial carried out in patients with metastatic breast cancer, sixteen patients were immunization with a low dose (5µg) of a 16 amino acid MUC1 peptide conjugated to KLH and administered together with DETOX as an adjuvant. Only three patients developed weak anti-MUC1 IgG responses. In addition, seven out of eleven patients tested for MUC1 specific CTL activity showed the presence of class I restricted MUC1-specific CTL. These were shown to be restricted to HLA-A2, -A1 and A11 [57].

In other studies using peptide-carrier conjugates, immunizing mice with MUC1 peptide (containing two tandem repeats) linked with diphtheria toxoid (DT) induced a significant DTH reaction and antibody response but no CTL response. This response also resulted in delayed tumor development [58]. These mouse studies formed the basis for a phase-I clinical trial on 13 patients using MUC1 peptide-DT conjugates as the immunogen administered in increasing doses from 100µg up to 1mg of peptide. Although this trial showed that there was no significant toxicity associated with this form of immunization, the immunogenicity of the vaccine was not very impressive and was similar to what had been observed in the mouse model as far as the types of immune responses that were generated. Only weak antibody and DTH responses were detected in several patients.

In an effort to improve upon these vaccines and induce more cellular responses rather than antibody responses, efforts were made to target MUC1 to receptors on antigen presenting cells (APC) for more efficient antigen uptake and processing. For this, a MUC1 peptide sequence containing five tandem repeats was conjugated to mannan (to target the mannose receptors on APC such as macrophages and dendritic cells) and was administered to mice intraperitoneally three times at weekly intervals. It was shown that the oxidation state of the immunogen highly influenced the quality of the immune response induced. Under oxidizing conditions (which aids in the formation of Schiffs bases), immunization resulted in cellular responses characterized by high CTL precursor (CTLp) frequency, circulating CD8+ CTLs, a significant DTH response, but little antibody production. This correlated with a Th1-type response (as indicated by IFN-γ production) and significant tumor protection. In contrast, the reduced form of the immunogen induced predominantly antibody responses that had very little tumor protective effect that correlated with IL-4 production (a Th2-type response). [58, 59]). It is not clear why the oxidation status of the antigen affected the type of responses generated. A possible explanation is that processing of the immunogen is affected in some way and hence the oxidized form is targeted to the intracellular processing pathway for presentation in class I while the reduced form follows the endocytic route and is presented in class II. In addition, Apostolopoulos et al., [60] showed that coadministration of Cyclophosphamide (an immunosuppressive agent) and the oxidized form of the MUC1-mannan conjugate enhanced the CTLp frequency approximately 10-fold (from 1/84,900 without Cyclophosphamide to 1/8,100 with Cyclophosphamide). Surprisingly, in contrast to the murine studies, when cynomologus monkeys were immunized with oxidized MUC1-mannan conjugates, a predominantly humoral response was observed and no detectable CTL response [61]. Similar observations were made in a clinical trial carried out in 25 patients with metastatic breast, colon, stomach or rectal cancer. Approximately half the number of patients produced significant titers of IgG1 anti-MUC1 antibodies. T cell proliferative responses were seen in 4 out of 15 patients and CTL responses in only two out of 10 patients [62].

MUC1 peptides plus adjuvant

Another approach to enhancing the immunogenicity of MUC1 in vivo has been to coadminister MUC1 peptide with various adjuvants. These adjuvants activate APC such as macrophages and DCs which in turn enhances their APC function, resulting in increases in humoral and/or cell-mediated immunity. Taking into account the importance of cell-mediated responses in eradicating tumors, most often the adjuvants chosen are those known to skew the immune response towards a Th1 type response. In one of our studies, which was the first ever cancer peptide vaccine to be tested, a phase I clinical trial was carried out using as a 105 amino acid long synthetic MUC1 peptide (slightly longer than 5 tandem repeats) administered with BCG as the adjuvant [63]. Post immunization, the patients were monitored for enhanced MUC1-specific antibody, CTL and DTH responses. No changes in DTH and antibody responses were observed. There was an increase in the number of MUC1-specific CTL post-immunization but they were still too few to be of therapeutic value. This further emphasizes the importance of activating helper T cells in order to expand CTL and enhance CTL function

A study we carried out in the chimpanzee model was aimed at eliciting MUC1-specific cell-mediated immune responses (TH1type). Chimpanzees were immunized with the 100 amino acid synthetic MUC1 peptide admixed with recombinant LeIF (Leishmania braziliensis homologue of the eukaryotic initiation factor) as an adjuvant. As expected, such a vaccine was able to induce a CD4$^+$ response that was of the Th1 type as well as a CTL response. The animals were monitored for one year post-vaccination and there appeared to be no detectable symptoms of autoimmunity [64].

MUC1 BASED IMMUNOTHERAPEUTIC STRATEGIES

MUC1 peptides as particulate antigens

Poly (d,l-lactic-co-glycolic acid) or PLGA microspheres are made from a biodegradable biocompatible polymer and have only recently gained attention as antigen delivery systems. Their particulate nature contributes to an increased immunogenicity of antigens encapsulated in such microspheres by facilitating phagocytosis by APC. The microspheres loaded with antigen are taken up and either remain in endocytic vesicles or are released into the cytoplasm. The antigen that is released can then be processed and presented either in MHC class I or class II for presentation to both CTL and helper T cells. Newman et al. [65], used PLGA microspheres containing a 24 amino acid MUC1 peptide (from the tandem repeat region) with or without monophosphoryl lipid A(MPLA) to immunize mice. They found that immunization with MUC1 peptide loaded PLGA microspheres induced IFN-γ and no IL-4. Incorporation of MPLA into the MUC1 peptide loaded microspheres not only induced an increase in IFN-γ production but also in antibody switching to the IgG isotype. Our own experience with a 40 amino acids long MUC1 peptide (two tandem repeats) encapsulated in PLGA microspheres shows that immunization of MUC transgenic mice results in specific immunity that protects from tumor challenge (Soares et al., submitted).

Muc1 Peptides In Liposomes

Another method of enhancing antigen uptake is to use liposomes as the antigen delivery system. Liposomes containing peptide antigens are prepared by mixing the peptides with a suspension of phospholipids under conditions that form vesicles bounded by a lipid bilayer. The liposomes are thought to fuse with the cell membrane of APC thereby releasing their contents into the cytoplasm. Thus, antigens delivered by liposomes are presented primarily in the context of class I MHC. Samuel et al. [66] tested a MUC1 vaccine formulation in the mouse model for immunogenicity and anti-tumor activity. This vaccine consisted of 24 amino acid MUC1 peptide encapsulated with MPLA in multilamellar liposomes. They showed that the tumor protection mediated by the vaccine correlated with a Th1 type of response (as indicated by IFN-γ production and the production of MUC1-specific IgG2a antibodies).

MUC1 carbohydrate vaccines

As discussed previously, MUC1 on tumors is underglycosylated and new carbohydrate moieties are expressed that serve as tumor antigens. Sialyl-Tn (sTn) is one such disaccharide antigen. Initially, it was thought that carbohydrate immunogens might have certain limitations, such as inability to activate helper T cells. One way to get around the lack of helper T cell activation, has been to conjugate the carbohydrate antigen to a protein carrier. This type of vaccine would be expected to efficiently activate B cells and help them switch to various Ig isotypes and generate memory B cells. This vaccine would not be expected to induce tumor-specific memory T cells. There are recent reports in the literature that murine T cells can react specifically against carbohydrate antigens including the tumor associated Tn antigen [67, 68]. This gives carbohydrate antigens a renewed importance as tumor-specific immunogens [69, 70].

CANCER IMMUNOLOGY

A vaccine formulation consisting of the Thomsen-Friedenreich (TF) antigen conjugated to KLH administered with RIBI as an adjuvant was tested in the murine system [71]. The TF antigen is a disaccharide Gal β1-3 GalNAc carbohydrate epitope expressed on tumors. This vaccine not only induced DTH and antibody responses specific for carbohydrate determinants expressed on tumors but also appeared to confer some protection against tumors. Another carbohydrate antigen, sialyl-Tn antigen conjugated to KLH admixed with RIBI adjuvant was administered to mice and metastatic breast cancer patients. IgG responses were detected in both mice and humans, but the responses in humans were much weaker [72]. This is consistent with the notion that human MUC1 is a foreign antigen in conventional mice and would induce more potent responses than might be expected in MUC1 transgenic mice wherein human MUC1 is a self antigen. In other studies carried out in patients with breast cancer or breast, ovarian and colorectal cancer, a vaccine formulation consisting of sialyl-Tn conjugated to KLH emulsified in DETOX-B SE adjuvant, induced anti-sialyl-Tn IgG responses. There appeared to be a direct correlation between the level of the IgG antibody response and survival suggesting that such IgG antibodies have a therapeutic benefit for the patients. The exact contribution of antibody versus cellular responses towards increased patient survival is unclear since potential cellular immune responses to sTn were not analyzed in these studies [73, 74]. It has also not been convincingly shown that antibodies elicited by these vaccines crossreact with patients tumor cells, thus it is hard to postulate what effector mechanisms are at play in the tumor-specific response in these cases.

More recently, the sTn-KLH vaccine was administered multiple times to seven ovarian and 33 breast high risk stage II/III and stage IV cancer patients following high dose chemotherapy and stem cell rescue [75]. Both the cellular and humoral immune responses were studied. As seen in previous studies using this vaccine, most patients developed anti-sTn IgG responses that peaked after the fourth or fifth immunization. Seventeen patients developed proliferative responses to sTn. In addition, antigen specific IFN-γ production was detected in 11 out of 26 patients. An increase in the lytic activity against a sTn$^+$ cancer target after immunotherapy was also observed. However, the tumor specificity and MHC restriction of this response remains to be determined

MUC1 DNA vaccines

Recombinant Viral Vectors

Recombinant vaccinia virus containing MUC1 cDNA has been tested as an immunogen in both animal models as well as in humans. Use of such viral vectors to deliver antigens in vivo has certain advantages, the primary one being high levels of expression of the antigen. In addition, since the virus replicates within the infected cell, the antigen is processed and presented in MHC class I. There have been certain difficulties associated with the use of vaccinia to deliver MUC1. During viral replication, the vaccinia genome is subject to a high degree of homologous recombination that can result in the deletion of most or all MUC1 tandem repeats in which reside most important antigenic epitopes. Nevertheless, vaccinia constructs have been used to immunize mice. One such construct that maintained expression of three to four tandem

114

repeats per molecule when injected into mice induced MUC1 specific antibodies but no detectable CTL. The immunization also caused delayed tumor development [76]

In another study, Akagi et al. [77], tested in a murine model a recombinant vaccinia viral construct containing the "mini" MUC1 gene containing only ten tandem repeats in order to discourage deletions due to vaccinia recombination. In addition, they also tested an admixture of vaccinia constructs containing either the "mini" MUC1 gene (rV-MUC1) or the gene for murine costimulatory molecule B7-1 (rV-B7-1). Cytolytic responses were detected with both vaccines, however, enhanced responses were seen only with the admixture vaccine. Both vaccines conferred protection against tumor in a tumor prevention model following two administrations. Two administrations of rV-MUC1 were insufficient to confer protection against tumor in a tumor therapy model. But, when mice were primed with rV-MUC1 and rV-B7-1 followed by two administrations of rV-MUC1 there was 100% survival in the tumor therapy model. More recent efforts have been directed at enhancing the immune response to MUC1 by using vaccinia virus constructs co-expressing MUC1 and IL-2. These have been tested both in the mouse model as well as in patients with advanced breast cancer in a phase I clinical trial [78, 79].

Naked MUC1 DNA

Vaccination with naked DNA is a recently developed immunization strategy in which a plasmid coding for the antigen of interest is injected directly into the muscle. This is then taken up and expressed by muscle cells and dendritic cells. Thus, DNA vaccination offers yet another method to target the endogenous processing and presentation pathway. DNA vaccination has two major advantages: it is a method that has been shown to induce both cellular and humoral immunity and, in addition, prolonged expression of the antigen by cells that have taken up the DNA results in the generation of significant immunological memory. It is important to keep in mind that persistent expression of the antigen could also lead to a state of autoimmunity or a state of immunological unresponsiveness. Not enough has been done yet with MUC1 DNA to know the parameters of its immunogenicity.

Graham et al[80] investigated the immunostimulatory potential of naked cDNA in the mouse model. Mice were immunized intramuscularly with different doses of MUC1 cDNA and both tumor rejection and immune responses were examined. This immunization protocol resulted in tumor protection that appeared to be dose dependent (the optimal dose being 50-100 μg of DNA). Humoral responses were also seen, however, there was no correlation between tumor protection and the presence of MUC1-specific antibodies. In addition, the immunization alone was not sufficient to induce detectable MUC1-specific CTL although they were detected only in previously immunized mice post-tumor challenge.

Cellular MUC1 vaccines

Priming of an effective cellular immune response requires antigen presentation within MHC class I /II on professional APC high in co-stimulatory and adhesion molecules. Tumors are considered to be poor antigen presenting cells since they are known to express low levels of the costimulatory and adhesion molecules necessary for T cell activation [81]. Since antigen presenting cells like B cells, macrophages and dendritic cells can provide the necessary costimulatory and adhesion signals for T cell activation, they have been used as cellular vaccines designed to present MUC1 in vivo in the chimpanzee and murine model systems.

We carried out the first such study in the chimpanzee model using as a vaccine autologous EBV immortalized B cells transfected with human MUC1 cDNA [82]. The B cells were treated prior to vaccination with a potent inhibitor of O-linked glycosylation in order to expose tumor-associated epitopes on the transfected MUC1. Increases in MUC1-specific CTL precursor frequencies were observed in immunized animals. Moreover, since the response was directed at the underglycosylated form of MUC1, no toxicity associated with autoimmunity was noted presumably because normal tissue expresses the fully glycosylated form of MUC1. In addition, no MUC1-specific antibodies were detected.

In another study, we tested the efficacy of a different cellular vaccine consisting of antigen-loaded peripheral blood derived dendritic cells (generated in vitro with GM-CSF and IL-4) in the chimpanzee model [83]. In vitro-generated dendritic cells were pulsed with synthetic MUC1 peptide and then injected intravenously. Following a boost with soluble peptide plus adjuvant, the humoral and cellular responses were analyzed. Antibody responses were detected in one out of four animals but only following the boost. No MUC1-specific proliferative T cell or humoral responses were detected following the single innoculation with peptide-pulsed dendritic cells, although such responses to the other antigen (ovalbumin) used in this system were detected. The results of this study suggest that multiple boosts with peptide-pulsed DC might be necessary to induce humoral and cellular responses to the self antigen MUC1 in the chimpanzee.

A number of different cellular vaccines have been tested in the murine model as well. Initial efforts were directed at using mouse tumor cells transfected with human MUC1 cDNA to immunize mice. In one such study, immunization with MUC1-transfected mouse mammary tumor cells resulted in reduced tumor incidence when mice were challenged with the same tumor [84]. In another study, it was shown that immunization with MUC1-transfected murine 3T3-tumor cells was able to induce MUC1-specific CTL activity and confer partial protection against a subsequent challenge with the same tumor.

More recently, the choice of a cellular vaccine has been a dendritic cell modified in some way to present MUC1. We used a retroviral vector MFG-MUC1 containing MUC1 cDNA to transduce an immortalized murine dendritic cell line. This MUC1 expressing DC line was then used to immunize mice and the humoral and cell-mediated immune responses generated were analyzed. This vaccine not only induced MUC1-specific humoral responses, but also cytolytic and proliferative responses. This was the first MUC1 vaccine that was able to stimulate all three effector arms of the adaptive immune response [85]. In another approach, Gong et al. [53] tested the immunogenicity of MUC1 when presented on DC-tumor cell hybrids. This strategy is aimed at combining the potency of dendritic cells as antigen presenting cells with the multiple tumor-associated antigens on tumor cells to elicit strong tumor-specific immunity. The efficacy of this approach was measured by the strength of the anti-MUC1 response elicited. As expected, immunization led to the induction of a potent immune responses and prevention of MUC1+ tumor growth. In addition, this vaccine also caused rejection of established metastases. Both $CD4^+$ and $CD8^+$ lymphocytes appeared to be involved.

We have evaluated the potential of a cellular vaccine (DC-based) in direct comparison with previously discussed immunization approaches such as peptide plus adjuvant vaccines. MUC1 transgenic and conventional mice were immunized with 1) 140 amino acid synthetic MUC1 peptide-pulsed in vitro generated dendritic cells, 2) 140 amino acid synthetic MUC1 peptide plus adjuvant (murine GM-CSF, a cytokine previously shown to play an important role in regulating dendritic cell differentiation and function as well as increase T cell effector function), and 3) 140 amino acid synthetic MUC1 peptide coadministered with a potent adjuvant SB-AS2 that contains monophosphoryl lipid A (provided by SmithCline Beecham). As expected the three different approaches induced very different immune responses, the cellular vaccine induced primarily cell-mediated responses while the adjuvant-based vaccines induced humoral responses. In addition, it was seen that the weaker adjuvant GM-CSF induced responses only in conventional mice, while the more potent SB-AS2 induced responses in both the conventional and MUC1 transgenic mice. Tumor rejection studies using a syngeneic MUC1-expressing transplantable tumor revealed that only the peptide-pulsed DC group was capable of rejecting tumor, consistent with the induction of a TH1 type response (Soares and Finn, submitted).

CONCLUDING REMARKS

The experimental evidence presented here on MUC1-based immunotherapy illustrates some of the successes of the field of immunotherapy in animal models as well as the challenges we face in translating basic and clinical research into successful cancer therapies. The development and use of animal tumor models, such as of syngeneic tumors, spontaneously arising tumors and human tumor xenografts in immunodeficient mice, have allowed us to evaluate numerous novel anti-cancer therapies. Such studies have contributed to our understanding of the interaction between immunocompetant cells and their products on the one hand and tumor cells on the other as well as the relationship between them. MUC1 is one of the few well characterized tumor antigens. Efforts are currently being directed at discovering new ones. Most vaccination strategies to date have been based on a single tumor antigen. It is conceivable that anti-tumor vaccines consisting of more than one tumor antigen might be more effective at eliciting anti-tumor responses leading to tumor rejection. In addition, it is important to keep in mind that there are also certain host-related factors that are obstacles to the successful application of cancer vaccines, such as the immunosuppressive tumor microenvironment. Studies are being directed at overcoming such immunosuppression. It is possible that present vaccination strategies being tested will be more effective in patients with smaller tumor burdens. With the increased sensitivities of cancer screening programs, one can look toward a future wherein disease-related abnormalities are detected early in premalignant states and are treated in the clinic with preventive immunotherapeutic vaccines.

REFERENCES

1. Allen A, Physiology of the gastrointestinal tract, ed. L.R. Johnson. 1981: Raven Press. 627-629.
2. Gendler SJ, Lancaster CA, Taylorpapadimitriou J, Duhig T, Peat N, Burchell J, Pemberton L, Lalani E, and Wilson D, Molecular-Cloning and Expression of Human Tumor-Associated Polymorphic Epithelial Mucin. J Biol Chem, 1990; 265: 15286-15293.
3. Gum JR, Mucin Genes and the Proteins They Encode - Structure, Diversity, and Regulation. Am J Respir Cell Mol Biol, 1992; 7: 557-564.
4. Neutra MR and Forstner JF, *Physiology of the Gastrointestinal Tract,*, L.R. Johnson, Editor. 1987, Raven Press. p. 975-1009.
5. Griffiths B, Matthews DJ, West L, Attwood J, Povey S, Swallow DM, Gum JR, and Kim YS, Assignment of the Polymorphic Intestinal Mucin Gene (Muc2) to Chromosome-11p15. Ann Hum Genet, 1990; 54: 277-285.
6. Gum JR, Human mucin glycoproteins: Varied structures predict diverse properties and specific functions. Biochem Soc Trans, 1995; 23: 795-799.
7. Swallow DM, Gendler S, Griffiths B, Corney G, Taylorpapadimitriou J, and Bramwell ME, The Human Tumor-Associated Epithelial Mucins Are Coded by an Expressed Hypervariable Gene Locus Pum. Nature, 1987; 328: 82-84.
8. Briand JP, Andrews SP, Cahill E, Conway NA, and Young JD, Investigation of the Requirements for O-Glycosylation by Bovine Sub-Maxillary Gland Udp-N-Acetylgalactosamine - Polypeptide N-Acetylgalactosamine Transferase Using Synthetic Peptide- Substrates. J Biol Chem, 1981; 256: 2205-2207.
9. Hanover JA, Lennarz WJ, and Young JD, Synthesis of N- and O-linked glycopeptides in oviduct membrane preparations. J Biol Chem, 1980; 255: 6713-6716.
10. Seregni E, Botti C, Massaron S, Lombardo C, Capobianco A, Bogni A, and Bombardieri E, Structure, function and gene expression of epithelial mucins. Tumori, 1997; 83: 625-632.
11. Shankar V, Pichan P, Eddy RL, Tonk V, Nowak N, Sait SNJ, Shows TB, Schultz RE, Gotway G, Elkins RC, Gilmore MS, and Sachdev GP, Chromosomal localization of a human mucin gene (MUC8) and cloning of the cDNA corresponding to the carboxy terminus. Am J Respir Cell Mol Biol, 1997; 16: 232-241.
12. Braga VMM, Pemberton LF, Duhig T, and Gendler SJ, Spatial and Temporal Expression of an Epithelial Mucin, Muc-1, During Mouse Development. Development, 1992; 115: 427-437.
13. Hilkens J, Ligtenberg MJL, Vos HL, and Litvinov SV, Cell Membrane-Associated Mucins and Their Adhesion-Modulating Property. Trends Biochem Sci, 1992; 17: 359-363.
14. Lesuffleur T, Zweibaum A, and Real FX, Mucins in Normal and Neoplastic Human Gastrointestinal Tissues. Crit Rev Oncol Hematol, 1994; 17: 153-180.
15. Kardon R, Price RE, Julian J, Lagow E, Tseng SCG, Gendler SJ, and Carson DD, Bacterial conjunctivitis in Muc1 null mice. Investigative Ophthalmology & Visual Science, 1999; 40: 1328-1335.
16. Gendler SJ and Spicer AP, Epithelial Mucin Genes. Annu Rev Physiol, 1995; 57: 607-634.
17. Lancaster CA, Peat N, Duhig T, Wilson D, Taylorpapadimitriou J, and Gendler SJ, Structure and Expression of the Human Polymorphic Epithelial Mucin Gene - an Expressed Vntr Unit. Biochem Biophys Res Commun, 1990; 173: 1019-1029.
18. Fontenot JD, Mariappan SVS, Catasti P, Domenech N, Finn OJ, and Gupta G, Structure of a Tumor-Associated Antigen Containing a Tandemly Repeated Immunodominant Epitope. Journal of Biomolecular Structure & Dynamics, 1995; 13: 245-260.
19. Fontenot JD, Tjandra N, Bu D, Ho C, Montelaro RC, and Finn OJ, Biophysical Characterization of One-Tandem, 2-Tandem, and 3- Tandem Repeats of Human Mucin (Muc-1) Protein Core. Cancer Res, 1993; 53: 5386-5394.
20. Miles DW and Taylor-Papadimitriou J, Therapeutic aspects of polymorphic epithelial mucin in adenocarcinoma. Pharmacology & Therapeutics, 1999; 82: 97-106.
21. Pemberton LF, Rughetti A, TaylorPapadimitriou J, and Gendler SJ, The epithelial mucin MUC1 contains at least two discrete signals specifying membrane localization in cells. J Biol Chem, 1996; 271: 2332-2340.
22. Baruch A, Hartmann ML, ZrihanLicht S, Greenstein S, Burstein M, Keydar I, Weiss M, Smorodinsky N, and Wreschner DH, Preferential expression of novel MUC1 tumor antigen isoforms in human epithelial tumors and their tumor-potentiating function. Int J Cancer, 1997; 71: 741-749.

23. Stadie TRE, Chai WG, Lawson AM, Byfield PGH, and Hanisch FG, Studies on the Order and Site-Specificity of Galnac Transfer to Muc1 Tandem Repeats by Udp-Galnac-Polypeptide N-Acetylgalactosaminyltransferase from Milk or Mammary-Carcinoma Cells. Eur J Biochem, 1995; 229: 140-147.

24. Nishimori I, Perini F, Mountjoy KP, Sanderson SD, Johnson N, Cerny RL, Gross ML, Fontenot JD, and Hollingsworth MA, N-Acetylgalactosamine Glycosylation of Muc1 Tandem Repeat Peptides by Pancreatic Tumor-Cell Extracts. Cancer Res, 1994; 54: 3738-3744.

25. Nishimori I, Johnson NR, Sanderson SD, Perini F, Mountjoy K, Cerny RL, Gross ML, and Hollingsworth MA, Influence of Acceptor Substrate Primary Amino-Acid-Sequence on the Activity of Human Udp-N-Acetylgalactosamine-Polypeptide N- Acetylgalactosaminyltransferase - Studies with the Muc1 Tandem Repeat. J Biol Chem, 1994; 269: 16123-16130.

26. Muller S, Goletz S, Packer N, Gooley A, Lawson AM, and Hanisch FG, Localization of O-glycosylation sites on glycopeptide fragments from lactation-associated MUC1 - All putative sites within the tandem repeat are glycosylation targets in vivo. J Biol Chem, 1997; 272: 24780-24793.

27. Xing PX, Prenzoska J, and McKenzie IFC, Epitope Mapping of Anti-Breast and Antiovarian Mucin Monoclonal-Antibodies. Mol Immunol, 1992; 29: 641-650.

28. Litvinov SV and Hilkens J, The Epithelial Sialomucin, Episialin, Is Sialylated During Recycling. J Biol Chem, 1993; 268: 21364-21371.

29. Pimental RA, Julian J, Gendler SJ, and Carson DD, Synthesis and intracellular trafficking of Muc-1 and mucins by polarized mouse uterine epithelial cells. J Biol Chem, 1996; 271: 28128-28137.

30. Hanisch FG, Stadie TRE, Deutzmann F, and PeterKatalinic J, MUC1 glycoforms in breast cancer - Cell line T47D as a model for carcinoma-associated alterations of O-glycosylation. Eur J Biochem, 1996; 236: 318-327.

31. Brockhausen I, Yang JM, Burchell J, Whitehouse C, and Taylorpapadimitriou J, Mechanisms Underlying Aberrant Glycosylation of Muc1 Mucin in Breast-Cancer Cells. Eur J Biochem, 1995; 233: 607-617.

32. Kotera Y, Fontenot JD, Pecher G, Metzgar RS, and Finn OJ, Humoral Immunity against a Tandem Repeat Epitope of Human Mucin Muc-1 in Sera from Breast, Pancreatic, and Colon-Cancer Patients. Cancer Res, 1994; 54: 2856-2860.

33. Xing PX, Tjandra JJ, Stacker SA, Teh JG, Thompson CH, McLaughlin PJ, and McKenzie IFC, Monoclonal-Antibodies Reactive with Mucin Expressed in Breast- Cancer. Immunol Cell Biol, 1989; 67: 183-195.

34. Petrarca C, Casalino B, von Mensdorff-Pouilly S, Rughetti A, Rahimi H, Scambia G, Hilgers J, Frati L, and Nuti M, Isolation of MUC1-primed B lymphocytes from tumour-draining lymph nodes by immunomagnetic beads. Cancer Immunology Immunotherapy, 1999; 47: 272-277.

35. Richards ER, Devine PL, Quin RJ, Fontenot JD, Ward BG, and McGuckin MA, Antibodies reactive with the protein core of MUC1 mucin are present in ovarian cancer patients and healthy women. Cancer Immunology Immunotherapy, 1998; 46: 245-252.

36. Rughetti A, Turchi V, Ghetti CA, Scambia G, Panici PB, Roncucci G, Mancuso S, Frati L, and Nuti M, Human B-Cell Immune-Response to the Polymorphic Epithelial Mucin. Cancer Res, 1993; 53: 2457-2459.

37. Gourevitch MM, von Mensdorff-Pouilly S, Litvinov SV, Kenemans P, Vankamp GJ, Verstraeten AA, and Hilgers J, Polymorphic Epithelial Mucin (Muc-1)-Containing Circulating Immune-Complexes in Carcinoma Patients. Br J Cancer, 1995; 72: 934-938.

38. von Mensdorff-Pouilly S, Gourevitch MM, Kenemans P, Verstraeten AA, Litvinov SV, vanKamp GJ, Meijer S, Vermorken J, and Hilgers J, Humoral immune response to polymorphic epithelial mucin (MUC-1) in patients with benign and malignant breast tumours. Eur J Cancer, 1996; 32A: 1325-1331.

39. DeNardo SJ, Richman CM, Goldstein DS, Shen S, Salako Q, Kukis DL, Meares CF, Yuan A, Welborn JL, and DeNardo GL, Yttrium-90/indium-111-DOTA-peptide-chimeric L6: Pharmacokinetics, dosimetry and initial results in patients with incurable breast cancer. Anticancer Res, 1997; 17: 1735-1744.

40. DeNardo SJ, Ogrady LF, Richman CM, Goldstein DS, Odonnell RT, DeNardo DA, Kroger LA, Lamborn KR, Hellstrom KE, Hellstrom I, and DeNardo GL, Radioimmunotherapy for advanced breast cancer using I-131-ChL6 antibody. Anticancer Res, 1997; 17: 1745-1751.

41. Hird V, Maraveyas A, Snook D, Dhokia B, Soutter WP, Meares C, Stewart JSW, Mason P, Lambert HE, and Epenetos AA, Adjuvant Therapy of Ovarian-Cancer with Radioactive Monoclonal- Antibody. Br J Cancer, 1993; 68: 403-406.

42. Katayose Y, Kudo T, Suzuki M, Shinoda M, Saijyo S, Sakurai N, Saeki H, Fukuhara K, Imai K, and Matsuno S, MUC1-specific targeting immunotherapy with bispecific antibodies: Inhibition of xenografted human bile duct carcinoma growth. Cancer Res, 1996; 56: 4205-4212.

43. Jerome KR, Barnd DL, Bendt KM, Boyer CM, Taylorpapadimitriou J, McKenzie IFC, Bast RC, and Finn OJ, Cytotoxic Lymphocytes-T Derived from Patients with Breast Adenocarcinoma Recognize an Epitope Present on the Protein Core of a Mucin Molecule Preferentially Expressed by Malignant-Cells. Cancer Res, 1991; 51: 2908-2916.

44. Jerome KR, Domenech N, and Finn OJ, Tumor-Specific Cytotoxic T-Cell Clones from Patients with Breast and Pancreatic Adenocarcinoma Recognize Ebv-Immortalized B-Cells Transfected with Polymorphic Epithelial Mucin Complementary-DNA. J Immunol, 1993; 151: 1654-1662.

45. Magarian-Blander J, Ciborowski P, Hsia S, Watkins SC, and Finn OJ, Intercellular and intracellular events following the MHC- unrestricted TCR recognition of a tumor-specific peptide epitope on the epithelial antigen MUC1. J Immunol, 1998; 160: 3111-3120.

46. Domenech N, Henderson RA, and Finn OJ, Identification of an Hla-A11-Restricted Epitope from the Tandem Repeat Domain of the Epithelial Tumor-Antigen Mucin. J Immunol, 1995; 155: 4766-4774.

47. Hiltbold EM, Alter MD, Ciborowski P, and Finn OJ, Presentation of MUC1 tumor antigen by class I MHC and CTL function correlate with the glycosylation state of the protein taken up by dendritic cells. Cell Immunol, 1999; 194: 143-149.

48. Brossart P, Heinrich KS, Stuhler G, Behnke L, Reichardt VL, Stevanovic S, Muhm A, Rammensee HG, Kanz L, and Brugger W, Identification of HLA-A2-restricted T-cell epitopes derived from the MUC1 tumor antigen for broadly applicable vaccine therapies. Blood, 1999; 93: 4309-4317.

49. Hiltbold EM, Ciborowski P, and Finn OJ, Naturally processed class II epitope from the tumor antigen MUC1 primes human CD4(+) T cells. Cancer Res, 1998; 58: 5066-5070.

50. Peat N, Gendler SJ, Lalani EN, Duhig T, and Taylorpapadimitriou J, Tissue-Specific Expression of a Human Polymorphic Epithelial Mucin (Muc1) in Transgenic Mice. Cancer Res, 1992; 52: 1954-1960.

51. Rowse GJ, Tempero RM, VanLith ML, Hollingsworth MA, and Gendler SJ, Tolerance and immunity to MUC1 in a human MUC1 transgenic murine model. Cancer Res, 1998; 58: 315-321.

52. Gong JL, Chen DS, Kashiwaba M, Li YQ, Chen L, Takeuchi H, Qu H, Rowse GJ, Gendler SJ, and Kufe D, Reversal of tolerance to human MUC1 antigen in MUC1 transgenic mice immunized with fusions of dendritic and carcinoma cells. Proc Natl Acad Sci U S A, 1998; 95: 6279-6283.

53. Gong JL, Chen DS, Kashiwaba M, and Kufe D, Induction of antitumor activity by immunization with fusions of dendritic and carcinoma cells. Nat Med, 1997; 3: 558-561.

54. Tempero RM, Rowse GJ, Gendler SJ, and Hollingsworth MA, Passively transferred anti-MUC1 antibodies cause neither autoimmune disorders nor immunity against transplanted tumors in MUC1 transgenic mice. Int J Cancer, 1999; 80: 595-599.

55. Tempero RM, VanLith ML, Morikane K, Rowse GJ, Gendler SJ, and Hollingsworth MA, CD4(+) lymphocytes provide MUC1-specific tumor immunity in vivo that is undetectable in vitro and is absent in MUC1 transgenic mice. J Immunol, 1998; 161: 5500-5506.

56. Ding L, Lalani E, Reddish M, Koganty R, Wong T, Samuel J, Yacyshyn MB, Meikle A, Fung PYS, Taylorpapadimitriou J, and Longenecker BM, Immunogenicity of Synthetic Peptides Related to the Core Peptide Sequence Encoded by the Human Muc1 Mucin Gene - Effect of Immunization on the Growth of Murine Mammary Adenocarcinoma Cells Transfected with the Human Muc1 Gene. Cancer Immunology Immunotherapy, 1993; 36: 9-17.

57. Reddish MA, MacLean GD, Koganty RR, Kan-Mitchell J, Jones V, Mitchell MS, and Longenecker BM, Anti-MUC1 class I restricted CTLs in metastatic breast cancer patients immunized with a synthetic MUC1 peptide. Int J Cancer, 1998; 76: 817-823.

58. Apostolopoulos V, Pietersz GA, Xing PX, Lees CJ, Michael M, Bishop J, and McKenzie IFC, The Immunogenicity of Muc1 Peptides and Fusion Protein. Cancer Lett, 1995; 90: 21-26.

59. Apostolopoulos V, Pietersz GA, and McKenzie IFC, Cell-mediated immune responses to MUC1 fusion protein coupled to mannan. Vaccine, 1996; 14: 930-938.

60. Apostolopoulos V, Popovski V, and McKenzie IFC, Cyclophosphamide enhances the CTL precursor frequency in mice immunized with MUC1-Mannan fusion protein (M-FP). J Immunother, 1998; 21: 109-113.

61. Vaughan HA, Ho DWM, Karanikas VA, Ong CS, Hwang LA, Pearson JM, McKenzie IFC, and Pietersz GA, Induction of humoral and cellular responses in cynomolgus monkeys immunised with mannan-human MUC1 conjugates. Vaccine, 1999; 17: 2740-2752.

62. Karanikas V, Hwang LA, Pearson J, Ong CS, Apostolopoulos V, Vaughan H, Xing PX, Jamieson G, Pietersz G, Tait B, Broadbent R, Thynne G, and McKenzie IFC, Antibody and T cell responses of

patients with adenocarcinoma immunized with mannan-MUC1 fusion protein. J Clin Invest, 1997; 100: 2783-2792.

63.   Goydos JS, Elder E, Whiteside TL, Finn OJ, and Lotze MT, A phase I trial of a synthetic mucin peptide vaccine induction of specific immune reactivity in patients with adenocarcinoma. J Surg Res, 1996; 63: 298-304.

64.   Barratt-Boyes SM, Vlad A, and Finn OJ, Immunization of chimpanzees with tumor antigen MUC1 mucin tandem repeat peptide elicits both helper and cytotoxic T-cell responses. Clin Cancer Res, 1999; 5: 1918-1924.

65.   Newman KD, Sosnowski DL, Kwon GS, and Samuel J, Delivery of MUC1 mucin peptide by poly(d,l-lactic-co-glycolic acid) microspheres induces type 1 T helper immune responses. J Pharm Sci, 1998; 87: 1421-1427.

66.   Samuel J, Budzynski WA, Reddish MA, Ding L, Zimmermann GL, Krantz MJ, Koganty RR, and Longenecker BM, Immunogenicity and antitumor activity of a liposomal MUC1 peptide-based vaccine. Int J Cancer, 1998; 75: 295-302.

67.   GalliStampino L, Meinjohanns E, Frische K, Meldal M, Jensen T, Werdelin O, and Mouritsen S, T-cell recognition of tumor-associated carbohydrates: The nature of the glycan moiety plays a decisive role in determining glycopeptide immunogenicity. Cancer Res, 1997; 57: 3214-3222.

68.   Springer GF, T and Tn, general carcinoma autoantigens. Science, 1984; 224: 1198-1206.

69.   Kieber-Emmons T, Luo P, Qiu JP, Chang TY, O IS, Blaszczyk-Thurin M, and Steplewski Z, Vaccination with carbohydrate peptide mimotopes promotes anti-tumor responses. Nat Biotechnol, 1999; 17: 660-665.

70.   Lo-Man R, Bay S, Vichier-Guerre S, Deriaud E, Cantacuzene D, and Leclerc C, A fully synthetic immunogen carrying a carcinoma-associated carbohydrate for active specific immunotherapy. Cancer Res, 1999; 59: 1520-1524.

71.   Henningsson CM, Selvaraj S, Maclean GD, Suresh MR, Noujaim AA, and Longenecker BM, T-Cell Recognition of a Tumor-Associated Glycoprotein and Its Synthetic Carbohydrate Epitopes - Stimulation of Anticancer T- Cell Immunity Invivo. Cancer Immunology Immunotherapy, 1987; 25: 231-241.

72.   Longenecker BM, Reddish M, Koganty R, and Maclean GD, Immune-Responses of Mice and Human Breast-Cancer Patients Following Immunization with Synthetic Sialyl-Tn Conjugated to Klh Plus Detox Adjuvant. Ann N Y Acad Sci, 1993; 690: 276-291.

73.   MacLean GD, Miles DW, Rubens RD, Reddish MA, and Longenecker BM, Enhancing the effect of THERATOPE STn-KLH cancer vaccine in patients with metastatic breast cancer by pretreatment with low-dose intravenous cyclophosphamide. J Immunother, 1996; 19: 309-316.

74.   MacLean GD, Reddish MA, Koganty RR, and Longenecker BM, Antibodies against mucin-associated sialyl-Tn epitopes correlate with survival of metastatic adenocarcinoma patients undergoing active specific immunotherapy with synthetic STn vaccine. J Immunother, 1996; 19: 59-68.

75.   Sandmaier BM, Oparin DV, Holmberg LA, Reddish MA, MacLean GD, and Longenecker BM, Evidence of a cellular immune response against sialyl-Tn in breast and ovarian cancer patients after high-dose chemotherapy, stem cell rescue, and immunization with theratope STn-KLH cancer vaccine. J Immunother, 1999; 22: 54-66.

76.   Acres RB, Hareuveni M, Balloul JM, and Kieny MP, Vaccinia Virus Muc1 Immunization of Mice - Immune-Response and Protection against the Growth of Murine Tumors Bearing the Muc1 Antigen. J Immunother, 1993; 14: 136-143.

77.   Akagi J, Hodge JW, McLaughlin JP, Gritz L, Mazzara G, Kufe D, Schlom J, and Kantor JA, Therapeutic antitumor response after immunization with an admixture of recombinant vaccinia viruses expressing a modified MUC1 gene and the murine T-cell costimulatory molecule B7. J Immunother, 1997; 20: 38-47.

78.   Balloul JM, Acres RB, Geist M, Dott K, Stefani L, Schmitt D, Drillien R, Spehner D, McKenzie I, Xing PX, and Kieny MP, Recombinant Muc-1 Vaccinia Virus - a Potential Vector for Immunotherapy of Breast-Cancer. Cell Mol Biol, 1994; 40: 49-59.

79.   Scholl S, Acres RB, Schatz C, Kieny MP, Balloul JM, Vincent-Salomon A, Deneux L, Tartour E, Fridman H, and Pouillart P, The polymorphic epithelial mucin (MUC1): a phase I clinical trial testing the tolerance and immunogenicity of a vaccina virus-MUC1-IL2 construct in breast cancer. Breast Cancer Res Treat, 1997; 46: 67.

80.   Graham RA, Burchell JM, Beverley P, and TaylorPapadimitriou J, Intramuscular immunisation with MUC1 cDNA can protect C57 mice challenged with MUC1-expressing syngeneic mouse tumour cells. Int J Cancer, 1996; 65: 664-670.

81. Chen LP, Linsley PS, and Hellstrom KE, Costimulation of T-Cells for Tumor-Immunity. Immunol Today, 1993; 14: 483-486.
82. Pecher G and Finn OJ, Induction of cellular immunity in chimpanzees to human tumor- associated antigen mucin by vaccination with MUC-1 cDNA- transfected Epstein-Barr virus immortalized autologous B cells. Proc Natl Acad Sci U S A, 1996; 93: 1699-1704.
83. Barratt-Boyes SM, Kao H, and Finn OJ, Chimpanzee dendritic cells derived in vitro from blood monocytes and pulsed with antigen elicit specific immune responses in vivo. J Immunother, 1998; 21: 142-148.
84. Graham R, Stewart L, Peat N, Beverley P, and Taylor-Papadimitriou J, MUC1-based immunogens for tumour therapy:development of murine model systems. Tumor Target, 1995; 1: 211-221.
85. Henderson RA, Konitsky WM, Barratt-Boyes SM, Soares M, Robbins PD, and Finn OJ, Retroviral expression of MUC-1 human tumor antigen with intact repeat structure and capacity to elicit immunity in vivo. J Immunother, 1998; 21: 247-256.

7
Recognition of human tumours: viral antigens as immunological targets for cytotoxic T cells

STEPHEN MAN

ABSTRACT

It has been estimated that some 15% of human cancers are associated with viral infection and the use of more sensitive molecular techniques may well reveal more. Preventing viral infection using prophylactic vaccines would dramatically decrease cancer incidence, particularly in developing countries. However viral infection *per se* is not sufficient in itself to cause cancer and other host cell related events are required for cell transformation. Thus cancers may take decades to become manifest. This time delay means that the true efficacy of prophylactic vaccines will not be established for at least a decade. In the meantime, the global burden of virally associated cancers increases annually and alternative therapies are required. The enormous progress in immunology and recombinant DNA technology now allows the design of biological therapies based on the use of T lymphocytes. In this chapter recent research on cytotoxic T lymphocyte recognition of viruses associated with human cancer will be reviewed. This will be placed in the context of human clinical trials.

INTRODUCTION

The destructive power of host cell-mediated immunity (CMI) is illustrated by the rapid rejection of organ grafts transplanted from an unrelated donor, however tumours growing within the host are largely ignored by the immune system. Research in the last several years has been focussed on inducing an anti-tumour response analogous to the allograft response. The use of immunotherapy or therapy based on manipulation of host immunity has the theoretical advantage that the specificity of the immune system can be used to destroy tumour cells while leaving healthy cells unharmed. In this respect it should produce fewer side effects than conventional radiotherapy and chemotherapy treatments. However immunological approaches to the treatment of cancer have been

123

R.A. Robins and R.C. Rees (eds.), Cancer Immunology, 123–145.
© 2001 *Kluwer Academic Publishers. Printed in the Netherlands.*

largely unsuccessful (reviewed in [1]). Many of the early attempts were very crude in nature, as there was little knowledge of tumour antigens or of the types of immune response required. In the last decade there has been enormous progress in the knowledge of how immune effector cells recognise foreign antigens, how they become activated and how they function *in vivo*. This knowledge now allows the prospect of rationally designed therapies based on immune responses against human tumours. Certain virally associated cancers provide particularly attractive models in this regard as tumour cells will express viral antigens which are tumour specific yet foreign to the host. These antigens are largely expressed intracellularly so CD8$^+$ cytotoxic T lymphocytes (CTL) have been the effector cell of most interest. Research has focussed on methods to boost the numbers of tumour specific CTL in cancer patients either by vaccination or adoptive therapy. This chapter will focus on recent research on CTL recognition of virally encoded tumour antigens with the emphasis on human studies.

CYTOTOXIC T LYMPHOCYTES-INDUCTION AND ACTIVATION

Cytotoxic T lymphocytes (CTL) usually (although not exclusively) express the cell-surface marker CD8, and play a vital role in the clearance of virally infected cells. The major effector function of CD8$^+$ T lymphocytes is thought to be direct killing of virally infected cells however non-cytolytic mechanisms can also operate [2]. Regardless of the mechanisms used by CD8$^+$ T cells (which are often generically referred to as CTL), the host benefits from decreased viral spread and morbidity. CTL recognise foreign viral antigens on the surface of virally infected cells in the form of short peptides bound to major histocompatibility complex (MHC) class I molecules (or human leucocyte antigens (HLAs) in man) [3, 4]. These foreign peptides are 8–10 amino acids long and are generated by the proteolysis of viral proteins in the cytoplasm of a virus-infected cell. These peptides are then transported from the cytosol into the endoplasmic reticulum where they bind to newly synthesised MHC class I molecules. A complex of MHC class I and antigenic peptide plus β_2 microglobulin (β_2m) then migrates to the cell surface where recognition by a CTL bearing a T-cell receptor (TCR) of the appropriate specificity can take place (reviewed in [5]). MHC class I molecules are expressed on the surface of all nucleated cells, therefore anti-viral CTLs are a powerful effector mechanism for the clearance of virally infected cells.

Activation of CTLs from naïve precursors requires recognition of foreign antigens on so-called 'professional' antigen-presenting cells (APCs), such as macrophages, activated B lymphocytes (B cells) and dendritic cells. All of these cells express; high levels of both MHC class I and MHC class II molecules, are able to process exogenous antigens, and are rich in the co-stimulation molecules (such as B7-1) that are important for T-cell activation. Defining tumour antigens recognised by CTL and optimising CTL activation are key considerations for design of vaccines or adoptive transfer protocols.

CTL have been shown in many animal models to protect against tumour challenge. This has been accomplished either by; inducing protective CTL responses in animals using a variety of vaccine formulations (reviewed in [6]), or by adaptively transferring CTL grown *in vitro* (reviewed in [7]). There have been fewer reports however, of the efficacy of CTL in animals with established tumours [8, 9]. The latter situation is one most relevant to the human clinical situation, and as few animal models mimic human disease exactly, there is a need for more well designed clinical trials.

A large variety of prototypic cancer vaccines have been developed in an attempt to induce or boost anti-tumour CTL activity *in vivo*. The presence of clearly identified viral gene products which are tumour specific allows the use of a variety of recombinant vaccine delivery systems including; vaccinia virus [10] (or related/modified poxviruses [10]), adenovirus [11], and DNA plasmids [12]. Alternatively the vaccines could comprise soluble proteins or peptides either injected directly or pulsed onto host dendritic cells prior to injection [13].

An alternative approach is isolate tumour specific CTL from the host, preferably at an early stage of disease, for expansion *in vitro* and subsequent re-infusion. The identification of virally associated tumour antigens allows rapid selection of specific (and therapeutic) CTL *in vitro*. The best example of this approach has been the treatment of Epstein Barr virus induced tumours in bone marrow transplant patients (see below). However the growth of large numbers of lymphocytes is technically demanding and requires a hospital setting to be useful.

EPSTEIN BARR VIRUS ASSOCIATED TUMOURS

Epstein Barr Virus (EBV) is a human gamma herpesvirus with a marked tropism for B-lymphocytes, and persists as a life-long asymptomatic infection in most individuals. Paradoxically it is also one of the most efficient growth transforming viruses known and is associated with development of several human cancers. EBV is highly immunogenic and both humoral and cell mediated responses are important in controlling the virus in healthy virus carriers. How the virus persists in the face of such strong host immune responses continues to be extensively studied.

Study of the CTL response against EBV has made major contributions to understanding how CTL recognise foreign antigens in general [14]. This is largely because EBV immunologists are blessed with a system in which 90% of the general population are infected, providing a large pool of donors. Importantly EBV readily transforms B-lymphocytes *in vitro*. These B-lymphoblastoid cell lines (B-LCL) express eight latent proteins that are highly immunogenic, thus providing a renewable source of autologous antigen presenting cells (APCs) to restimulate CTL. As will be seen later, this is in direct contrast to the majority of other tumour systems in which supply of patient material is limited and tumour cells are difficult to grow and poorly immunogenic.

The EBV proteins expressed in B-LCL can be divided into those that are expressed in the nucleus (EBNAs 1, 2, 3a, 3b, 3c) and those expressed in the membrane (LMP1 and LMP2). Apart from the special case of EBNA1, CTL responses against all proteins have been described, although it appears that the EBNA 3 proteins are immunodominant [14]. A large number of CTL peptide epitopes restricted by multiple HLA alleles have been defined [14] including those which appear to have mutated as mechanism of viral escape [15].

CANCER IMMUNOLOGY

Immunoblastic lymphomas

Immunoblastic lymphomas (IL) or lymphoproliferative diseases are a significant problem for immunosuppressed patients such as those who are HIV-infected or recipients of allogeneic organ transplants. Fatal EBV-associated IL can occur in up to 25% of children receiving bone marrow transplants (BMT) from HLA mismatched or unrelated donors [16]. Since the onset of IL appears to reflect the loss of EBV specific T cells in those patients, reconstitution of these responses using adoptive immunotherapy has the potential to control disease. This strategy has been employed with encouraging results in two studies. In the first, five patients who developed EBV lymphoproliferative disease (after receiving T cell depleted allogeneic BMT) [17] were treated with infusions of peripheral blood mononuclear cells (PBMC) from BM donors. It was assumed that since the donors were EBV seropositive that the blood contained populations of EBV specific CD4$^+$ and CD8$^+$ T cells. In this study adoptive therapy was associated with a complete clinical and pathological regression of the EBV IL in all 5 patients within 30 days, and 3 of patients became long-term survivors. However acute and chronic graft versus host disease (GVHD) was observed in the patients perhaps as a result of transferring relatively impure cell populations (monocytes and NK cells were also present in the PBMC). In concurrent studies [16, 18] polyclonal EBV specific CTL reactivated *in vitro*, were used for adoptive transfer. These EBV specific CTL were tagged by retrovirally infecting cells with a neomycin marker that could be detected by PCR. To date a total of 39 BMT recipients have been tested with 4 doses of cells of 10^7 –5x10^7 cells/m^2 [16]. In 12 of patients, EBV specific CTL numbers increased up to 32-fold after infusion and CTL were detected in blood for up to 18 weeks. In 6 patients high EBV DNA levels in PBL fell by 3 to 5 log$_{10}$ within 3 weeks of CTL infusion. Although in the majority of cases CTL were used to prevent EBV lymphomas, in two patients who did not receive prophylaxis, adoptive transfer of stored donor CTL were used to successful treat established lymphomas. In one patient there were complications of local inflammation at site of CTL infusion, requiring mechanical ventilation. However this patient remains well at 24 months [16].

The studies described above have illustrated the capacity of adoptively transferred T lymphocytes to treat a virus-associated malignancy, with complete tumour regression being observed in some patients. They were remarkable in that the epitope specificities of the transferred T cells were not known. These studies in BMT patients are being extended to patients with IL who have received solid organ grafts [19, 20]. It is now possible to use cloned CD8$^+$ CTL with precisely defined epitope specificity and known T cell receptor usage. Indeed, the use of purified CTL clones might abrogate the GVHD observed or prevent local inflammation. However it is equally possible that synergy between CD4$^+$ and CD8$^+$ T cells, or multiple CTL specificities are required for maximum efficacy. EBV specific CTL could be generated from 98% of BMT donors tested [16], but is unlikely to be the case for other viruses associated with cancer. Even so the immunodominant CTL specificities that occur naturally and are easily reactivated *in vitro* may not be the ones most clinically effective.

126

Burkitt's lymphoma

Burkitt's lymphoma (BL) is a childhood tumour which is rare in the developed world but occurs at high incidence in the malarial belts of Africa and New Guinea, where it affects about 10 in every 100,000 children per year. The tumour is one of the fast growing tumours in man, with a cell doubling time of around 24 hours. This property may explain the successful use of chemotherapy in the treatment of this tumour, although access to this treatment may be limited in developing countries. The fast growing nature and geographical incidence of BL would suggest that it is unsuitable for a CTL immunotherapy approach. However a vaccine designed to induce strong CTL responses against BL cells, and delivered to children before or immediately after EBV infection could abrogate the development of BL tumours. The main problem with this scenario is that it is extremely difficult to get CTL responses against BL cells as by contrast to B-LCL, BL cell lines are non-immunogenic *in vitro*. EBV specific CTL are unable to recognise and kill BL cell lines [21], unless the cells are loaded with the appropriate EBV peptide epitope. This evasion of CTL surveillance is due to several features of BL cells. Firstly BL cells are poor APC in that they express low levels of "accessory" molecules such as ICAM-1 and LFA-3 [22] which function in cell:cell adhesion and T cell co-stimulation. Furthermore by contrast to B-LCL, BL cells only express 1 EBV latent gene product, EBNA1. Until recently it was impossible to detect any EBNA1 specific CTL responses. This is largely because EBNA1 is not processed endogenously like the other latent proteins, due to intrinsic properties of its structure. EBNA1 contains internal glycine alanine repeat domains which prevent endogenous antigen processing [23]. These domains have a generic effect in that known CTL epitopes engineered into recombinant EBNA1 constructs also fail to be processed and recognised by CTL [23]. Antigen processing is further hampered in BL cells by the low levels of TAP/TAP2 genes compared to B-LCL [24], together with co-ordinate low level expression of HLA class I genes. Interestingly in spite of these obstacles, EBNA1 specific CTL can be detected at low frequency in the PBMC of seropositive donors [25]. Priming of these CTL is likely to occur through exogenous presentation of EBNA1 proteins however these same peptide epitopes are unlikely to be displayed by BL cells in vivo, precluding the use of these CTL for immunotherapy [25].

NPC and Hodgkin's lymphoma

Nasopharyngeal carcinoma (NPC) is a malignant epithelial tumour of the post-nasal space and is strongly associated with EBV infection, both in high incidence (SouthEast Asia) and low incidence areas. In contrast to BL, NPC is a disease of older age groups suggesting a slow development and opportunity for immune intervention. CTL recognising EBV proteins on B-LCL can be readily derived from NPC patients [26] suggesting that NPC despite CTL surveillance. NPC cells have a similar phenotype to BL cells, with EBNA1 being constitutively expressed. Unlike BL, however, there is also expression in NPCs of other latent proteins such as LMP2, EBNA3a, 3b and 3c. The expression of LMP1 is only seen in a proportion of NPCs, and it should be noted that the EBNA 3 proteins are downregulated. Another cancer associated with EBV, albeit to a weaker extent, is Hodgkin's lymphoma (HL) [27]. This incidence of this disease is widespread and unlike BL and NPC the incidence is not restricted to certain geographical region. HL tumours are unusual in that the malignant cells of the tumour, the Reed-Sternberg (RS) lymphoid cells only form part of the total mass. The HL cells have a restricted pattern of EBV gene expression similar to that of NPC, with EBNA1, LMP1, LMP2 expressed at reasonable levels and EBNA3 proteins downregulated. Clearly LMP1 and LMP2 would be good targets for potentially immunotherapeutic CTL in NPC and HL. However LMP1 and LMP2 are only weakly immunogenic, and CTL responses against these proteins are sub-dominant to those against the EBNA3 proteins [28]. Thus the expression of LMP1 and LMP2 is not necessarily detrimental to the tumour cells. Additionally the tumour cells may also produce cytokines such as IL10 [29] which could suppress local CTL responses [30]. However a recent study has demonstrated that IL10 does not suppress EBV specific CTL responses against HL cells *in vitro*, supporting the possibility of CTL based immunotherapy against HL. Despite the weak immunogenicity of LMP1 and LMP2, CTL responses against these proteins could be selected and boosted by selective restimulation in vitro either with the whole proteins [31] or with synthetic peptides [32]. Recently a pilot study of adoptive therapy with HL has been completed with EBV specific CTL (including some with LMP2a) derived from the PBMC of HL patients [33]. This was not a study for clinical efficacy but did illustrate the feasibility of the approach.

Vaccines for EBV associated malignancies

Besides the cancers described above, there are a large number of diseases associated with EBV, so prevention of EBV infection would have a significant impact on human health world-wide. The EBV glycoprotein gp340 is an attractive vaccine candidate, as it is known to be the target of neutralising antibody responses in man. Many different types of vaccine formulation based on Gp340 have been developed and small scale trials in tamarins [34] and human subjects [35] have been completed. The encouraging results warrant the support of large scale trials however the true efficacy of these vaccines may take decades to realise.

For reasons discussed later in this chapter the adoptive immunotherapy approach used for IL may not be applicable to other EBV-related malignancies. For these, efforts have largely concentrated on research into vaccines designed to elicit CTL *in vivo*. Clinical trials based on delivery of synthetic peptides with either oil based (Montanide ISA 720) or cell based (dendritic cells) adjutants are underway (A. Rickinson personal communication). A more recent approach is to combine the epitope specific approach with a virus delivery system forming so called "poly-epitope" vaccines. These constructs have been shown to present the appropriate CTL epitopes to human CTL *in vitro* [36] and to induce HLA restricted CTL in HLA-A2 transgenic mice *in vivo* [37]. It is likely that this approach will soon enter clinical trials. Meanwhile the bottleneck on translating CTL research into clinical trials has allowed researchers to switch their attention to other aspects of EBV immunology such as the role of CD4$^+$ T cells.

HUMAN PAPILLOMAVIRUS (HPV) ASSOCIATED TUMOURS

Papillomaviruses are small DNA viruses that infect cutaneous or mucosal epithelial tissue and cause a variety of proliferative lesions. This lesion may progress to malignancy, and human papillomaviruses have been isolated from a variety of human cancers. However the most significant and best-studied association is that between HPV and carcinoma of the cervix (CaCx), with HPV being found in >99.4% of CaCx cases studied [38].

At least 75 distinct HPV types have been isolated from various human tissue biopsies with a subset (~25) which are sexually transmitted and cause disease in the male and female genital tract [39]. These HPVs can be categorised according to their potential to cause malignancy as low risk, intermediate risk or high risk. HPV types 6 (HPV-6) and 11 (HPV-11), for example, are associated with low-risk disease, such as genital warts. By contrast, high-risk HPVs, such as HPV-16, HPV-18, HPV-31, HPV-33 and HPV-45, are associated with high-grade cervical intraepithelial lesions (CIN3) and invasive cancer. HPV-16 and HPV-18 are the types most commonly detected [38]. Papillomaviruses are strictly epitheliotropic viruses, and the target cell of infection is the keratinocyte [40]. Only keratinocytes (or cells with the potential for keratinocyte maturation) are infected, and synthesis of viral capsid proteins and viral particle assembly occurs only in the terminally differentiating keratinocyte [41]. HPVs can induce immortalization in primary cultures of human and rodent cells. The principal transforming genes of the high-risk viruses are E6 and E7. They have both been shown to have immortalizing properties in human foreskin keratinocytes [42]. The detection of integrated viral DNA sequences in cervical neoplasia is frequently associated with malignant progression, integration being more common in carcinomas than in the preinvasive state, cervical intraepithelial neoplasia (CIN) [43, 44]. Continued expression of E6 and E7 is mandatory for the maintenance of the malignant phenotype of cell lines from cervical cancer [45].

CaCx is a major disease worldwide with nearly 500,000 new cases diagnosed each year. There is overwhelming epidemiological evidence that HPV infection is the major but not exclusive risk factor for development of cervical cancer [38]. HPV infection is common among young sexually active women, but only a minority have evidence of viral persistence or develop CIN [46]. This suggests that, as for other virus-associated cancers, additional environmental, genetic or immunological factors influence the progression of disease. Cervical smear testing and treatment for pre-invasive cervical intraepithelial neoplasia (CIN3) have reduced the overall incidence of cervical cancer in the UK and other developed countries [47]. Nevertheless women treated for CIN3 still have a 20-fold higher risk of developing cervical cancer than the general population [48, 49]. Therefore current therapies are limited, both by economic constraints in developing countries and their ineffectiveness in recurrent diseases, requiring development of novel approaches to the disease. Two immunological approaches have been taken. The first has been the development of prophylactic vaccines aimed at inducing neutralising antibodies against viral capsid proteins (L1 and L2) to prevent infection [50]. Such vaccines would have great impact in developing countries where 80% of cervical cancers arise. These vaccines are in the first stages of clinical testing, however treatments are still needed for those women who have already have CaCx. The persistent and obligate expression of HPV E6 and E7 genes in tumour cells offers the prospect of targeted immunotherapies for CaCx.

T cell responses against HPV

Our knowledge of the immune response to HPV has been limited because the virus cannot easily be grown *in vivo* or *in vitro*, and few virions are isolated from genital lesions [41]. Studies of the immune response have relied on the development of recombinant viral proteins or synthetic viral peptides. Even so it has been difficult to establish reliable serological assays to monitor infection and diagnosis is often based on overt disease symptoms or use of molecular techniques. As a noncytopathic virus, HPV may manage to evade the immune system by remaining within keratinocytes in the epithelium, which are poor antigen presenting cells [51]. No inflammation accompanies infection and replication, which may prevent an effective immune response [52]. If antigens are not presented by migrating professional APCs or within lymphoid organs, they are ignored by T cells, and tolerance may be induced instead [53]. None of these reasons would obviate the use of CTL in immunotherapy they would argue against the presence of naturally occurring immune responses [54]. There is evidence however that natural cell-mediated immunity can control this persistent virus infection: HPV associated cervical lesions are more prevalent in immunosuppressed individuals [55-58]; regression of papillomavirus induced warts is associated with lymphocytic infiltration in man [59] and animal models [60-62]; peritumoural lymphocytic infiltration correlates with improved prognosis in squamous cervical cancer [63].

Cytotoxic T cell responses in HPV infection

HPV-specific CTLs can be readily induced in rodent models after injection of the animals with recombinant viruses containing HPV genes [64] or rodent cells transfected with HPV genes [65]. Furthermore, such HPV-specific CTLs can protect against subsequent challenge with tumour cells transfected with HPV genes [65, 66]. Until recently it has been difficult to detect HPV specific T cell responses in man, with a consensus that HPVs are able to evade the human immune system and establish a state of immune tolerance [54, 67]. This view did not, however, hinder the development of vaccines designed to elicit HPV-specific immunity (see below). Early clinical trials of such vaccines were set up in the absence of any data that CMI responses occurred naturally in human HPV infection or, indeed, were relevant to human cervical disease.

One of the first demonstrations that HPV antigens could be recognised by human CTL used HLA*0201 binding peptides to induce peptide-specific CTLs *in vitro* from healthy donors [68]. Some of these CTLs were able to recognise a human HLA*0201$^+$ CaCx cell line (CaSki) that had been transformed by HPV-16, suggesting that at least some of the peptide specific CTLs also recognised endogenously processed HPV epitopes. This approach was extended to the study of patients with CIN3 and CaCx; CTL responses against the same peptides could be shown using PBMC [69, 70] and also T cells isolated from cervical biopsy specimens [71]. No CTL responses were seen in healthy volunteers, suggesting the responses were disease related. By contrast, another study using the same peptides was unable to detect CTLs using similar restimulation protocols [72]. The variation in detection rates between studies may reflect differences in protocols, patient groups or both. Recently, fluorescent tetrameric complexes (tetramers) comprising HLA-A*0201 and the HPV16 E7$_{11-20}$ peptide epitope have been used to address these issue. It was found that the HPV tetramer$^+$ CD8$^+$ T cells could be detected in the PBMC of both patients and healthy volunteers [73]. But these frequencies were very low (1/1260-42004) when compared to the frequencies of CTL recognising immunodominant epitopes of EBV (up to 1/25, [74]) or influenza A (up to 1/500, [75]). The frequencies of HPV tetramer$^+$ cells in patient PBMC but not healthy volunteers could be boosted by subsequent *in vitro* restimulation, confirming previous reports that CTL against this epitope could only be generated from patients [69, 70]. HPV tetramer$^+$ CD8$^+$ were virtually undetectable in some patients suggesting that for these patients it would be very difficult to generate CTL against this epitope *in vitro*. This HPV tetramer proved to be an efficient means of isolating monospecific populations of CD8$^+$ CTL to derive lines and clones. These CTL were able to recognise endogenous HPV antigens presented by the CaCx cell line CaSki. Others have used CaSki as an APC to generate CTL from patients PBMC that recognise HPV E6 and E7 antigens in the context of HLA-A*0201 [70]. Interestingly these CTL did not recognise the peptides that had previously been shown to be immunogenic to patients [69, 70].

More recently full-length HPV E6/E7 proteins have been used to detect HPV specific CTL responses in PBMC from patients with cervical neoplasia. APC infected with recombinant adenoviruses encoding HPV 16 E6 and E7, and HPV-18 E6 and E7 were used to demonstrate HPV specific CTL responses in patients with premalignant CIN3 [76] but not in healthy volunteers. This suggested that these CTL responses were disease related so the same protocols were used on a cohort of 38 Dutch patients with varying stages of CIN. This cohort was carefully monitored for the presence of HPV-16 and regularly screened for the status of their CIN. It was found that HPV specific CTL responses could be most readily detected in those patients with high grade lesions or CaCx but not in patients who had cleared HPV-16 (H.Bontkes, submitted for publication). Soluble HPV-16 E6 and E7 proteins have also been used to detect HPV specific CTL among CIN patients [77, 78] but healthy controls were not tested so it was difficult to assess whether these T cell responses were disease specific [77]. More efficient HPV specific CTL generation can be achieved by allowing dendritic cells to present the soluble proteins [78, 79]. Such approaches might be suitable for generating primary HPV specific CTL suitable for adoptive immunotherapy.

The low frequency of HPV specific CTL in blood might reflect a localisation of CTL to the cervix. Both CD4$^+$ and CD8$^+$ T cells can be readily derived from cervical biopsy material [71, 80]. HPV specific CTL were found to be present at higher frequencies in tumour compared to blood [71], and activated CD8$^+$ T cells expressing perforin can be detected immunohistochemically in cervical tumours [81]. This is not unique to CaCx, as melanoma specific CTL are considerably enriched in tumours or tumour infiltrated lymph nodes [82]. Whether the CD8$^+$ T cells that have infiltrated tumour are functionally active is not known. In this regard, detailed analyses of the function and specificity of CTL in both tumour and blood will be crucial.

Overall, the studies of CTL function in humans with HPV-associated cervical disease suggest that naturally occurring HPV-specific CTLs do occur, although their role in disease is unknown. For immunotherapeutic purposes, dendritic cells expressing

HPV antigens might be the most efficient means to restimulate low frequency CTL responses or generate primary CTL responses. By contrast to EBV, very few peptide epitopes have been defined for HPV. This necessitates the use of full-length genes for restimulation of CTL and has the incorporation of full-length, potential oncogenes into vaccines has safety implications. The dearth of peptide epitopes also limits the use of recently developed techniques such as tetramers, intracellular cytokine (ICC) staining and ELISPOT assays to increase the sensitivity of HPV CTL detection [83]. Detection of HPV specific CTL responses has been on an operational basis, as these have mostly relied on the use of recombinant viral gene products and APC. However the HPV epitopes processed and presented by tumour cells may be different. For successful immunotherapy of CaCx, future studies of HPV specific CTL must be based on strategies that target specifically those epitopes that are expressed on CaCx cells.

Vaccines and clinical trials

The laboratory studies reviewed above show that the HPV proteins are immunogenic to human T cells. This provides the basis for clinical investigations to establish whether HPV specific T cells will be therapeutic in cancer patients. Two approaches can be considered. First, vaccines could be developed to boost or induce HPV specific CTL responses *in vivo*. The efficacy of such vaccines would be limited in patients with advanced disease due to immunosuppression [84] however it might be of benefit in patients with early stage or premalignant disease. Vaccines could also be used as an adjunct to conventional treatment. e.g. in patients with minimum residual disease after surgery. Second, adoptive T cell therapy could be attempted in-patients with advanced cancer. This is the most direct way of addressing the likely effectiveness of HPV specific CTL. However it has been difficult to detect, generate and propagate these CTL, so no trials with adoptive T cell therapy have been reported to date. By contrast there have been several prototypic therapeutic vaccines that have been tested in clinical trials.

Recombinant viral vaccines

The most extensively tested vaccine designed to elicit therapeutic T cell responses in vivo, has been one based on a recombinant vaccinia virus construct (TA-HPV). This live vaccine consists of the E6 and E7 proteins of the two HPV types (HPV-16 and HPV-18) most commonly associated with cervical cancer [85]. The pros and cons of using vaccinia virus as an immunotherapeutic agent have been discussed in detail elsewhere [86, 87], but the rationale behind its design was as follows:

- Vaccinia virus has been used extensively in humans as the vaccine that eradicated smallpox.
- Vaccinia virus elicits strong humoral and T cell responses in animal models.
- Vaccinia virus is a lytic virus preventing the persistent expression of potential oncogenes in human cells.
- The E7 gene products have been mutated to reduce Rb binding and abolish co-transformation activity in rat fibroblast assays [85].

- The E6 and E7 gene products were orientated and fused to to minimise the likelihood of recombination with any natural HPV strain present within the patient.

The safety, and immunogenicity of TA-HPV was investigated in a phase I/II trial of 8 patients with advanced or recurrent cervical cancer   [88]. All patients produced detectable anti-vaccinia IgG antibodies after vaccination confirming successful "take" of the vaccine. HPV-specific CTL responses were measured in 6 patients by stimulation of patient PBMC *in vitro* using replication deficient recombinant adenoviruses encoding HPV16 E6/E7 and HPV18 E6/E7. PBMC from only 3/6 of the patients tested for HPV specific CTL, responded to control stimuli such as mitogens, mixed lymphocyte culture and recall antigens. Only these 3 patient samples were deemed evaluable and from these, HPV specific CTL could only be detected from the PBMC of 1 patient. These CTL were detected 9 weeks after vaccination, after restimulation with HPV18 E/E7 adenoviruses *in vitro*. Interestingly the operationally defined HPV18 specific CTL response was a transient one, as no CTL responses could be detected at 14 or 20 weeks post-vaccination. The HPV-18 specific CTL detected at week 9 were not present before vaccination, and the tumour biopsy from this patient was HPV-16 positive and HPV-18 negative, suggesting that the CTL response was a result of immunisation with TA-HPV. While no therapeutic effect can be ascribed to vaccination on the basis of this study (7 patients died from disease), anecdotally patient 6 has remained well and tumour free, some 5 years after the study (vaccinated July 1994).

To circumvent possible immunosuppression in CaCx patients [84, 89], a further trial using TA-HPV was performed on 12 patients with premalignant CIN3. Pre-existing HPV18 specific CTL responses could be detected in 2 patients, and vaccination induced HPV-18 specific CTL responses in a further 3 patients [90]. A large-scale trial of TA-HPV involving 29 early stage cervical cancer patients from around Europe is in progress. To date HPV specific CTL responses resulting from vaccination have been shown for 4 patients, confirming the results previously seen in the UK (J.Hickling personal communication). All together 49 patients have been immunised with TA-HPV, with HPV specific CTL responses detected in 8 patients following vaccination. The direct clinical effect of this vaccine remains to be evaluated, however the trials described above demonstrate that HPV-specific CTL responses can be readily induced by vaccination.

The HPV specific CTL responses induced by vaccination were found to be of low magnitude and transient, when compared to strong memory CTL responses against common viruses such as influenza A or EBV. However the CTL response was only measured in blood and it is possible that this response does not mirror the responses at sites of disease where HPV transformed tissue is present . At the time of writing, approval has been granted for a new clinical trial to systematically investigate HPV specific T cell responses in the cervix and the blood after TA-HPV immunisation.

Peptide vaccines

The identification of the molecular nature of antigens recognized by CTL on both virally induced and other cancers allows the development of vaccines containing the minimal essential components that may elicit T cell responses [91]. For HPV this has the major advantage that expression of these peptides would not have the same oncogenic potential as full-length HPV E6, E7 proteins. Furthermore peptide vaccines would be simpler to manufacture and transport than those based on recombinant viral vectors. Based on impressive results with eliciting protective CTL using synthetic peptides in a murine model [92], a clinical trial was initiated using a vaccine consisting of two HLA-A*0201 binding peptides from HPV-16 E7, together with a "helper" peptide designed to stimulate CD4$^+$ T cell responses [93]. To date no HPV peptide specific CTL have been detected after vaccination, although clear responses against the helper peptide were shown (Offringa, personal communication 1999).

One of the problems faced when using peptide vaccines is the HLA polymorphism exhibited by the outbred human population. For instance in the clinical trial described above, recruitment was limited to patients who were HPV-16$^+$ and HLA-A*0201$^+$. In practical terms this means defining multiple peptides for each HLA allele [94]. Sequence variation within HPV types may also influence the selection of peptide epitopes used in vaccines [95]. A more fundamental problem is the possibility of inducing tolerance rather than immunity as a result of peptide immunisation. This has been shown in murine models with tumour growth being promoted rather than inhibited as a result of peptide immunisation [96, 97]. This effect could be abrogated if the peptide was delivered on the surface of dendritic cells [98] or if the peptide was expressed as a minigene in a recombinant virus [99]. These two strategies are likely to be the next tested in clinical trials.

Bacterial fusion protein vaccines

Theoretically, these would overcome some of the problems described with peptide vaccines, but have the disadvantage of being more difficult to purify. The advantages are these vaccines would be suitable for all HLA types and might encompass both CD8 and CD4 epitopes. In Australia,, five patients with late stage disease were immmunized three times with escalating doses of HPV 16 E7 as a glutathione-S-transferase (GST) bacterial fusion protein in Algammulin adjuvant. All patients demonstrated antibody to E7, and 2 out of 3 evaluable patients had proliferative T cell responses to GST-E7 and E7 peptides [100]. Recently a prototype vaccine consisting of a fusion of hsp70 protein and HPV-16 E7 has been reported showing responses in animal models [101]. It is likely this vaccine will soon enter clinical trials.

Potential Pitfalls for CTL based immunotherapy of CaCX

It is clear that from the number of laboratories now working on T cell mediated responses against HPV that an increasing number of clinical trials will be initiated. While no clinical effect can so far be attributed to the presence of HPV specific CTL, the trials have provided much useful information with regard to design of assays, vaccine formulations and dosage. The lack of an appropriate animal model for HPV associated genital cancer means that clinical trials (for all their flaws) will be the way forward. Nevertheless certain theoretical concerns have been raised about the likely effectiveness of T cell mediated therapy specifically with relationship to the properties of the HPV transformed cell (reviewed in [67]). Such properties include HLA class I downregulation [102], lack of co-stimulatory molecules [103], low levels of HPV antigen expression [104] and production of immunosuppressive cytokines [105]. The

134

expression of HPV antigens in epithelial cells could lead to systemic tolerance as has been demonstrated in animal models [106]. However these are not insurmountable obstacles and could be addressed by laboratory studies. For instance it could be argued that previous studies demonstrate that if at least one HLA allele is expressed by 80% of tumours [102] this should be sufficient for CTL recognition in the majority of cases. HPV specific CTL generated after restimulation with full-length HPV16 E6/E7 proteins recognize a multitude of MHC class I/HPV peptide combinations [76]. Judicious vaccination and/or selective expansion of CTL *in vitro* will allow CTL of the correct specificity to be selected. There is also the possibility that down-regulation of HLA molecules on tumour cells may result in generation of novel immune responses against the tumour [107]. Low levels of HPV antigens in conjunction with the low levels of co-stimulatory molecules might prevent CTL priming, however activated CTL need considerably lower levels of antigen to realise their effector function [108]. Again *in vitro* methods of generating high-affinity CTL able to lyse HPV tumour cells will need to be developed [109]. The role of cytokines produced by HPV transformed keratinocytes in regulating immune responses in the cervix is unclear and will require analysis *in situ*. The potentially immunosuppressive effects of keratinocyte derived cytokines might be overcome either by local delivery of inflammatory cytokines [110] or simply through sheer numbers of CTL generated by vaccination or adoptive transfer.

PROSPECTS FOR OTHER VIRALLY ASSOCIATED CANCERS

Hepatitis viruses and primary liver cancer

It has been estimated that there are 300 million carriers of HBV worldwide. Up to 50% of the population in Southern Africa and South East Asia have been infected by Hepatitis B virus (HBV). Primary hepatomas (PH) are the most common form of cancer world-wide and their development is associated with chronic infection with HBV. While most liver tumour cells contain portions of the HBV, no common viral gene product is persistently expressed. This limits any direct attempts at immunotherapy of PH. However it could be argued that since primary hepatomas usually develop some 20-30 years after initial infection, there is plenty of scope for immune intervention. No viral gene product has been shown to have transforming activity and it is not known how HBV infected hepatocytes become transformed. As with other cancers it is the persistent infection of hepatocytes coupled with other host cell facts which leads to tumourigenesis. Thus eradicating or limiting the numbers of HBV infected hepatocyes may prevent subsequent development of PH. In this regard the CMI to HBV antigens has been well studied [111] and it is possible that CMI could be used prophylactically in patients considered at greatest risk of developing PH. This could also apply to Hepatitis C virus (HCV) which was characterised in 1989 and may also be involved in development of PH.

Human herpes virus 8 and Kaposi's sarcoma

Kaposi's sarcoma is a malignant skin tumour frequently found in HIV infected individuals and more rarely in men from Southern Europe. It is highly aggressive in AIDS patients spreading rapidly to gastrointestinal and respiratory tracts, causing severe internal bleeding. Recently a novel herpes virus (HHV8) has been isolated from the lesions of HIV positive patients with KS [112]. Epidemiologically there is strong evidence to link HHV8 infection with development of KS, as greater than 95% of KS lesions have HHV8 DNA as detected by PCR. Given the rapid spread of KS in HIV, combination adoptive immunotherapy using CTL against HIV and HHV8 would be a possible treatment option. However the actual expression of gene products in KS lesions is unknown and there has been no evidence that HHV8 has any transforming activity *in vitro*. What is known is that HHV8 encodes several proteins capable of down-regulating cell cycle control, inhibiting apoptosis and control of growth differentiation (chemokines). If such genes are overexpressed or sufficiently distinct from host genes, then these could be potential targets for CTL.

Human T lymphotropic virus and adult T cell leukaemia.

Human T lymphotropic virus (HTLV1) is human retrovirus associated with a number of diseases including malignancies and inflammatory conditions. Unlike the other viruses described in this review except HCV, HTLV1 is an RNA virus, replicating in cells via a DNA intermediate. This allows for rapid mutation by the virus in response to selective pressures as has been amply demonstrated for another human retrovirus, HIV. There is a strong epidemiological link between human T cell leukaemia virus (HTLV-1) which was the first human retrovirus isolated and adult T cell leukaemia (ATL) [113]. ATL predominates in the Southern Islands of Japan, and is characterised by the presence of leukaemic T cells, which express CD4 and CD25 (IL2 receptor). The genome of HTLV-1 has been mapped however no oncogene or transforming gene has been found [113]. Therefore the mechanism of leukaemic development is unknown.

HTLV-1 is thought to be transmitted in early life [114] thus the disease develops slowly but once acute disease has been diagnosed the mean survival time is 6-12 months. Besides the prospect of prophylactic vaccination of children with HTLV-1 positive mothers, this suggests that immunotherapy of ATL might be effective in seropositive individuals in early childhood. However it is unclear whether HTLV1 is expressed in vivo in ATL cells and similar to HBV there is no viral antigen that is consistently and persistently expressed in tumour cells. Another argument against the use of T cell responses against HTLV-1 is that about 1% of people infected with HTLV-I develop a disabling chronic inflammatory disease of the central nervous system known as HTLV-I-associated myelopathy/tropical spastic paraparesis (HAM/TSP) [113]. These patients have high frequencies of CTL specific for HTLV-1 proteins and it has been suggested that these CTL may be responsible for tissue damage. Therefore induction of HTLV-1 specific CTL may in some circumstances be harmful. Recently mathematical modeling studies combined with quantitation of viral load have questioned this view and suggest that CTL may have a beneficial effect in reducing the proviral load [115]. Thus vaccines aimed at developing strong CTL responses may reduce the risk of developing HAM or ATL. Recent studies using anti-retroviral vaccines in animal models suggest that this approach will be feasible [116, 117].

Emerging tumour viruses

Simian virus 40 (SV40) is a large DNA virus which infects primates. It was first isolated from macaques and due to its tumorigenicity in rodents has been a powerful model to study carcinogenesis . Furthermore murine CTL specific for large T antigen are able to protect against SV40 induced tumour challenge [118]. SV40 is not infectious to humans, however SV40 T antigen can transform human cells *in vitro*. SV40 was a contaminant of early poliovirus vaccines administered before 1964, leading to proposals that SV40 may be implicated in development of human cancers. Several laboratories have reported that SV40 specific sequences (T antigen) can be detected by PCR in patients with mesotheliomas and other tumours [119, 120]. This association remains controversial as a large epidemiological study in the US did not demonstrate any evidence that polio vaccination lead to a higher level of tumour development [121]. It remains to be seen whether environmental carcinogens such as asbestos or coal-dust act as co-factors in the development of mesothelioma. If this association is confirmed and large T antigen is shown to be consistently expressed in tumour cells, then immunotherapeutic appraoches could be considered.

JC virus is a human polyoma virus which is highly oncogenic in rodents but infects humans asymptomatically. In immunosuppressed individuals, JC virus is thought to cause the rare disease called progressive multifocal leukoencephalopathy (PML[122]. Interest in this virus as a tumour virus has been aroused by a recent report that used PCR techniques to show that ten times more JC viral DNA is present in malignant colorectal epithelial tissue than normal colonic tissue [123]. Since this virus was not considered a major pathogen, little is known about immune responses against it compared to other viruses such EBV. JC virus T antigen is a possible immunotherapeutic target as it is known to alter expression of cell cycle regulators and can induce tumours in the tissue in transgenic mice. It is possible that this could be targeted as a tumour specific antigen but as with SV40 larger scale human studies are required before it can unequivocally be linked with human cancer.

CONCLUDING REMARKS

Many immunological concepts established in the laboratory are now being tested in clinical trials. As usual for trials of this type using patients with advanced cancer, miracle cures are rare, however encouraging results have been obtained in a few patients. Sometimes it is impossible to detect CTL responses in these patients even if clinical responses have been obtained [124]. Too few patients have been tested to allow a consensus into the mechanisms of clinical responses. Do CTL have a direct or indirect benefit? The increased sensitivity of CTL detection made possible by new techniques [83] will allow these questions to be addressed. It will be possible to directly quantitate CTL in blood and sites of disease after vaccination [125], and isolate T cells with minimum *in vitro* manipulation to study function.

Finding the best formulation for a therapeutic vaccine is the holy grail for many tumour immunologists. Every research laboratory has convincing arguments for their particular approach. An example of the rapidly changing nature of the field is the diminishing optimism over the use of peptide vaccines. Recent research has revealed many theoretical problems with peptide vaccines which were not evident at the time vaccine trials were set up. As for the best formulation, the most likely scenario is that vaccine formulations will be tailored to be disease specific and perhaps even patient specific.

EBV and HPV have been the main targets for virus directed immunotherapy of cancer due to the obligate expression of viral genes in tumour cells. However many other virally associated tumours could be targeted using host cell proteins altered by viral gene products. For example mutated and overexpressed p53 is often found in tumours and could serve as a target [126], or inappropriately expressed hormone receptors [127] or differentiation specific markers [128]. Survival of adoptively transferred CTL *in vivo* is key for the success of immunotherapy. Recently a number of studies in HIV-infected patients have revealed some limitations of the adoptive therapy approach. For example transferred T cells transfected with a suicide gene (gangcyclovir) proved to be immunogenic to the recipient and they were rapidly eliminated [129]. Another potential mechanism for loss of CTL *in vivo* is apoptosis. Extended *in vitro* culturing of T cells prior to adoptive transfer could lead to expression of fas ligand and subsequent subsceptibility to apoptosis [130]. Survival of transferred CTL may also require growth promoting or apoptosis preventing cytokines produced by CD4$^+$ T cells [131]. There has been increasing research into defining CTL epitopes recognised by CD4 T cells with the hope of engineering vaccines able to stimulate both CD8 and CD4 responses simultaneously. In this regard NK cells, may also be attractive effectors.

Another problem is that transferred CTL may themselves cause inappropriate inflammatory or autoimmune reactions [97]. However this is a worthwhile risk when the trials involve patients with limited lifespan. The focus of this review has been the application of CTL recognising viral T cells to treatment of cancer but it is clear that the problem requires the understanding of both CTL and the tumour cell. It will be important to study the interactions between CTL and tumour cells, particularly *in situ*, to allow development of more efficient immunotherapies. Finally all the studies with CTL must be kept in context. Many of the approaches described can only be utilised in hospital settings in the developed world yet the global burden of virally associated cancers falls on the developing countries. These countries have insufficient resources for conventional treatments for cancer let alone adoptive immunotherapy. Thus the greatest impact upon the global burden of virally associated cancers will be made if immunotherapeutic approaches are combined with development of effective prophylactic vaccines.

ACKNOWLEDGEMENTS

Due to space constraints, I have only been able to reference a selection of the many excellent publications concerned with T cell recognition of virus associated tumours. I am grateful to the Royal Society, the Cancer Research Campaign and the Medical

Research Council for funding my research. Thanks go to Poling and Benjamin who tolerated my evening absences during the writing of this review.

REFERENCES

1. Old LJ, Immunotherapy for cancer. Sci Am, 1996; 275: 136-143.
2. Guidotti LG, Ishikawa T, Hobbs MV, Matzke B, Schreiber R, and Chisari FV, Intracellular inactivation of the hepatitis B virus by cytotoxic T lymphocytes. Immunity, 1996; 4: 25-36.
3. Townsend ARM, Gotch FM, and Davey J, Cyto-Toxic T-Cells Recognize Fragments of the Influenza Nucleoprotein. Cell, 1985; 42: 457-467.
4. Townsend ARM, Rothbard J, Gotch FM, Bahadur G, Wraith D, and McMichael AJ, The Epitopes of Influenza Nucleoprotein Recognized by Cytotoxic Lymphocytes-T Can Be Defined with Short Synthetic Peptides. Cell, 1986; 44: 959-968.
5. Pamer E and Cresswell P, Mechanisms of MHC class I - Restricted antigen processing. Annu Rev Immunol, 1998; 16: 323-358.
6. Pardoll D, Cancer vaccines. Nat Med, 1998; 4: 525-531.
7. Boon T, Cerottini JC, van den Eynde B, van der Bruggen P, and Vanpel A, Tumor antigens recognized by T lymphocytes. Annu Rev Immunol, 1994; 12: 337-365.
8. Mandelboim O, Vadai E, Fridkin M, Katzhillel A, Feldman M, Berke G, and Eisenbach L, Regression of Established Murine Carcinoma Metastases Following Vaccination with Tumor-Associated Antigen Peptides. Nat Med, 1995; 1: 1179-1183.
9. Mayordomo JI, Zorina T, Storkus WJ, Zitvogel L, Celluzzi C, Falo LD, Melief CJ, Ildstad ST, Kast WM, Deleo AB, and Lotze MT, Bone-Marrow-Derived Dendritic Cells Pulsed with Synthetic Tumor Peptides Elicit Protective and Therapeutic Antitumor Immunity. Nat Med, 1995; 1: 1297-1302.
10. Moss B, Carroll MW, Wyatt LS, Bennink JR, and Hirsch VM, Host range restricted non-replicating vaccina virus vectors as vaccine candidates. Adv Exp Med Biol, 1996; 397: 7-13.
11. Chen PW, Wang M, Bronte V, Zhai YF, Rosenberg SA, and Restifo NP, Therapeutic antitumor response after immunization with a recombinant adenovirus encoding a model tumor-associated antigen. J Immunol, 1996; 156: 224-231.
12. Liu MA, The immunologist's grail: Vaccines that generate cellular immunity. Proc Natl Acad Sci U S A, 1997; 94: 10496-10498.
13. Melief CJM, Offringa R, Toes REM, and Kast WM, Peptide-based cancer vaccines. Curr Opin Immunol, 1996; 8: 651-657.
14. Rickinson AB and Moss DJ, Human cytotoxic T lymphocyte responses to Epstein-Barr virus infection. Annu Rev Immunol, 1997; 15: 405-431.
15. de Campos-Lima PO, Gavioli R, Zhang QJ, Wallace LE, Dolcetti R, Rowe M, Rickinson AB, and Masucci MG, Hla-A11 Epitope Loss Isolates of Epstein-Barr-Virus from a Highly A11+ Population. Science, 1993; 260: 98-100.
16. Rooney CM, Smith CA, Ng CYC, Loftin SK, Sixbey JW, Gan YJ, Srivastava DK, Bowman LC, Krance RA, Brenner MK, and Heslop HE, Infusion of cytotoxic T cells for the prevention and treatment of Epstein-Barr virus-induced lymphoma in allogeneic transplant recipients. Blood, 1998; 92: 1549-1555.
17. Papadopoulos EB, Ladanyi M, Emanuel D, Mackinnon S, Boulad F, Carabasi MH, Castromalaspina H, Childs BH, Gillio AP, Small TN, Young JW, Kernan NA, and Oreilly RJ, Infusions of Donor Leukocytes to Treat Epstein-Barr Virus- Associated Lymphoproliferative Disorders after Allogeneic Bone- Marrow Transplantation. N Engl J Med, 1994; 330: 1185-1191.
18. Rooney CM, Smith CA, Ng CYC, Loftin S, Li CF, Krance RA, Brenner MK, and Heslop HE, Use of Gene-Modified Virus-Specific T-Lymphocytes to Control Epstein-Barr-Virus-Related Lymphoproliferation. Lancet, 1995; 345: 9-13.
19. Haque T, Amlot PL, Helling N, Thomas JA, Sweny P, Rolles K, Burroughs AK, Prentice HG, and Crawford DH, Reconstitution of EBV-specific T cell immunity in solid organ transplant recipients. J Immunol, 1998; 160: 6204-6209.
20. Khanna R, Bell S, Sherritt M, Galbraith A, Burrows SR, Rafter L, Clarke B, Slaughter R, Falk MC, Douglass J, Williams T, Elliott SL, and Moss DJ, Activation and adoptive transfer of Epstein-Barr

virus-specific cytotoxic T cells in solid organ transplant patients with posttransplant lymphoproliferative disease. Proc Natl Acad Sci U S A, 1999; 96: 10391-10396.

21. Rooney CM, Rowe M, Wallace LE, and Rickinson AB, Epstein-Barr Virus-Positive Burkitts-Lymphoma Cells Not Recognized by Virus-Specific T-Cell Surveillance. Nature, 1985; 317: 629-631.

22. Gregory CD, Murray RJ, Edwards CF, and Rickinson AB, Down-Regulation of Cell-Adhesion Molecules Lfa-3 and Icam-1 in Epstein-Barr Virus-Positive Burkitts-Lymphoma Underlies Tumor- Cell Escape from Virus-Specific T-Cell Surveillance. J Exp Med, 1988; 167: 1811-1824.

23. Levitskaya J, Coram M, Levitsky V, Imreh S, Steigerwaldmullen PM, Klein G, Kurilla MG, and Masucci MG, Inhibition of Antigen-Processing by the Internal Repeat Region of the Epstein-Barr-Virus Nuclear Antigen-1. Nature, 1995; 375: 685-688.

24. Rowe M, Khanna R, Jacob CA, Argaet V, Kelly A, Powis S, Belich M, Croomcarter D, Lee S, Burrows SR, Trowsdale J, Moss DJ, and Rickinson AB, Restoration of Endogenous Antigen-Processing in Burkitts- Lymphoma Cells by Epstein-Barr-Virus Latent Membrane Protein-1 - Coordinate up-Regulation of Peptide Transporters and Hla- Class-I Antigen Expression. Eur J Immunol, 1995; 25: 1374-1384.

25. Blake N, Lee S, Redchenko I, Thomas W, Steven N, Leese A, Steigerwald-Mullen P, Kurilla MG, Frappier L, and Rickinson A, Human CD8(+) T cell responses to EBV EBNA1: HLA class I presentation of the (Gly-Ala)-containing protein requires exogenous processing. Immunity, 1997; 7: 791-802.

26. Moss DJ, Chan SH, Burrows SR, Chew TS, Kane RG, Staples JA, and Kunaratnam N, Epstein-Barr Virus Specific T-Cell Response in Nasopharyngeal Carcinoma Patients. Int J Cancer, 1983; 32: 301-305.

27. Deacon EM, Pallesen G, Niedobitek G, Crocker J, Brooks L, Rickinson AB, and Young LS, Epstein-Barr-Virus and Hodgkins-Disease - Transcriptional Analysis of Virus Latency in the Malignant-Cells. J Exp Med, 1993; 177: 339-349.

28. Khanna R, Burrows SR, Kurilla MG, Jacob CA, Misko IS, Sculley TB, Kieff E, and Moss DJ, Localization of Epstein-Barr-Virus Cytotoxic T-Cell Epitopes Using Recombinant Vaccinia - Implications for Vaccine Development. J Exp Med, 1992; 176: 169-176.

29. Herbst H, Foss HD, Samol J, Araujo I, Klotzbach H, Krause H, Agathanggelou A, Niedobitek G, and Stein H, Frequent expression of interleukin-10 by Epstein-Barr virus- harboring tumor cells of Hodgkin's disease. Blood, 1996; 87: 2918-2929.

30. Frisan T, Sjoberg J, Dolcetti R, Boiocchi M, Dere V, Carbone A, Brautbar C, Battat S, Biberfeld P, Eckman M, Ost O, Christensson B, Sundstrom C, Bjorkholm M, Pisa P, and Masucci MG, Local Suppression of Epstein-Barr-Virus (Ebv)-Specific Cytotoxicity in Biopsies of Ebv-Positive Hodgkins-Disease. Blood, 1995; 86: 1493-1501.

31. Ranieri E, Herr W, Gambotto A, Olson W, Rowe D, Robbins PD, Kierstead LS, Watkins SC, Gesualdo L, and Storkus WJ, Dendritic cells transduced with an adenovirus vector encoding Epstein-Barr virus latent membrane protein 2B: A new modality for vaccination. J Virol, 1999; 73: 10416-10425.

32. Lee SP, Tierney RJ, Thomas WA, Brooks JM, and Rickinson AB, Conserved CTL epitopes within EBV latent membrane protein 2 - A potential target for CTL-based tumor therapy. J Immunol, 1997; 158: 3325-3334.

33. Roskrow MA, Suzuki N, Gan YJ, Sixbey JW, Ng CYC, Kimbrough S, Hudson M, Brenner MK, Heslop HE, and Rooney CM, Epstein-Barr virus (EBV)-specific cytotoxic T lymphocytes for the treatment of patients with EBV-positiye relapsed Hodgkin's disease. Blood, 1998; 91: 2925-2934.

34. Finerty S, Mackett M, Arrand JR, Watkins PE, Tarlton J, and Morgan AJ, Immunization of Cottontop Tamarins and Rabbits with a Candidate Vaccine against the Epstein-Barr-Virus Based on the Major Viral Envelope Glycoprotein Gp340 and Alum. Vaccine, 1994; 12: 1180-1184.

35. Gu SY, Huang TM, Ruan L, Miao H, and Lu H, First EBV vaccine trial in humans using recombinant vaccina virus expressing the major membrane antigen. Dev Biol Stand, 1995; 84: 171-177.

36. Thomson SA, Khanna R, Gardner J, Burrows SR, Coupar B, Moss DJ, and Suhrbier A, Minimal Epitopes Expressed in a Recombinant Polyepitope Protein Are Processed and Presented to Cd8(+) Cytotoxic T-Cells - Implications for Vaccine Design. Proc Natl Acad Sci U S A, 1995; 92: 5845-5849.

37. Mateo L, Gardner J, Chen QY, Schmidt C, Down M, Elliott SL, Pye SJ, Firat H, Lemonnier FA, Cebon J, and Suhrbier A, An HLA-A2 polyepitope vaccine for melanoma immunotherapy. J Immunol, 1999; 163: 4058-4063.

38. Walboomers JMM, Jacobs MV, Manos MM, Bosch FX, Kummer JA, Shah KV, Snijders PJF, Peto J, Meijer C, and Munoz N, Human papillomavirus is a necessary cause of invasive cervical cancer worldwide. J Pathol, 1999; 189: 12-19.

140

39. Stanley M, Genital human papillomaviruses - Prospects for vaccination. Curr Opin Infect Dis, 1997; 10: 55-61.
40. Stanley MA, Replication of Human Papillomaviruses in Cell-Culture. Antiviral Res, 1994; 24: 1-15.
41. Laimins LA, Human papillomaviruses target differentiating epithelia for virion production and malignant conversion. Semin Virol, 1996; 7: 305-313.
42. Hawley-Nelson P, Vousden KH, Hubbert NL, Lowy DR, and Schiller JT, Hpv16 E6-Proteins and E7-Proteins Cooperate to Immortalize Human Foreskin Keratinocytes. EMBO J, 1989; 8: 3905-3910.
43. Romanczuk H and Howley PM, Disruption of Either the E1-Regulatory or the E2-Regulatory Gene of Human Papillomavirus Type-16 Increases Viral Immortalization Capacity. Proc Natl Acad Sci U S A, 1992; 89: 3159-3163.
44. Daniel B, Rangarajan A, Mukherjee G, Vallikad E, and Krishna S, The link between integration and expression of human papillomavirus type 16 genomes and cellular changes in the evolution of cervical intraepithelial neoplastic lesions. J Gen Virol, 1997; 78: 1095-1101.
45. Vousden K, *Mechanisms of transformation by HPV*, in *Human papilloma viruses and cervical cancer - biology and immunology*, P.L. Stern and M. Stanley, Editors. 1994, Oxford Medical Publications: Oxford. p. 92-115.
46. Ho GYF, Bierman R, Beardsley L, Chang CJ, and Burk RD, Natural history of cervicovaginal papillomavirus infection in young women. N Engl J Med, 1998; 338: 423-428.
47. Forsmo S, Buhaug H, Skjeldestad FE, and Haugen OA, Treatment of pre-invasive conditions during opportunistic screening and its effectiveness on cervical cancer incidence in one Norwegian county. Int J Cancer, 1997; 71: 4-8.
48. McIndoe WA, McLean MR, Jones RW, and Mullins PR, The Invasive Potential of Carcinoma Insitu of the Cervix. Obstet Gynecol, 1984; 64: 451-458.
49. Soutter WP, Lopes AD, Fletcher A, Monaghan JM, Duncan ID, Paraskevaidis E, and Kitchener HC, Invasive cervical cancer after conservative therapy for cervical intraepithelial neoplasia. Lancet, 1997; 349: 978-980.
50. Schiller JT and Lowy DR, Papillomavirus-like particles and HPV vaccine development. Semin Cancer Biol, 1996; 7: 373-382.
51. Bal V, McIndoe A, Denton G, Hudson D, Lombardi G, Lamb J, and Lechler R, Antigen Presentation by Keratinocytes Induces Tolerance in Human T-Cells. Eur J Immunol, 1990; 20: 1893-1897.
52. Frazer IH, Thomas R, Zhou JA, Leggatt GR, Dunn L, McMillan N, Tindle RW, Filgueira L, Manders P, Barnard P, and Sharkey M, Potential strategies utilised by papillomavirus to evade host immunity. Immunol Rev, 1999; 168: 131-142.
53. Kundig TM, Bachmann MF, Dipaolo C, Simard JJL, Battegay M, Lother H, Gessner A, Kuhlcke K, Ohashi PS, Hengartner H, and Zinkernagel RM, Fibroblasts as Efficient Antigen-Presenting Cells in Lymphoid Organs. Science, 1995; 268: 1343-1347.
54. Beverley PCL, Sadovnikova E, Zhu X, Hickling J, Gao L, Chain B, Collins S, Crawford L, Vousden K, and Stauss HJ, *Strategies for Studying Mouse and Human Immune-Responses to Human Papillomavirus Type-16*, in *Vaccines against Virally Induced Cancers*. 1994. p. 78-96.
55. Halpert R, Fruchter RG, Sedlis A, Butt K, Boyce JG, and Sillman FH, Human Papillomavirus and Lower Genital Neoplasia in Renal- Transplant Patients. Obstet Gynecol, 1986; 68: 251-258.
56. Kiviat NB, Critchlow CW, Holmes KK, Kuypers J, Sayer J, Dunphy C, Surawicz C, Kirby P, Wood R, and Daling JR, Association of Anal Dysplasia and Human Papillomavirus with Immunosuppression and Hiv-Infection among Homosexual Men. AIDS, 1993; 7: 43-49.
57. Petry KU, Scheffel D, Bode U, Gabrysiak T, Kochel H, Kupsch E, Glaubitz M, Niesert S, Kuhnle H, and Schedel I, Cellular Immunodeficiency Enhances the Progression of Human Papillomavirus-Associated Cervical Lesions. Int J Cancer, 1994; 57: 836-840.
58. Shamanin V, zurHausen H, Lavergne D, Proby CM, Leigh IM, Neumann C, Hamm H, Goos M, Haustein UF, Jung EG, Plewig G, and deVilliers EM, Human papillomavirus infections in nonmelanoma skin cancers from renal transplant recipients and nonimmunosuppressed patients. J Natl Cancer Inst, 1996; 88: 802-811.
59. Coleman N, Birley HDL, Renton AM, Hanna NF, Ryait BK, Byrne M, Taylorrobinson D, and Stanley MA, Immunological Events in Regressing Genital Warts. Am J Clin Pathol, 1994; 102: 768-774.
60. Jarrett WFH, Smith KT, Oneil BW, Gaukroger JM, Chandrachud LM, Grindlay GJ, McGarvie GM, and Campo MS, Studies on Vaccination against Papillomaviruses - Prophylactic and Therapeutic Vaccination with Recombinant Structural Proteins. Virology, 1991; 184: 33-42.
61. Knowles G, Oneil BW, and Campo MS, Phenotypical characterization of lymphocytes infiltrating regressing papillomas. J Virol, 1996; 70: 8451-8458.

62. Selvakumar R, Schmitt A, Iftner T, Ahmed R, and Wettstein FO, Regression of papillomas induced by cottontail rabbit papillomavirus is associated with infiltration of CD8+ cells and persistence of viral DNA after regression. J Virol, 1997; 71: 5540-5548.
63. Tosi P, Cintorino M, Santopietro R, Lio R, Barbini P, Ji HX, Chang FJ, Kataja V, Syrjanen S, and Syrjanen K, Prognostic Factors in Invasive Cervical Carcinomas Associated with Human Papillomavirus (Hpv) - Quantitative Data and Cytokeratin Expression. Pathology Research and Practice, 1992; 188: 866-873.
64. Meneguzzi G, Cerni C, Kieny MP, and Lathe R, Immunization against Human Papillomavirus Type-16 Tumor-Cells with Recombinant Vaccinia Viruses Expressing E6 and E7. Virology, 1991; 181: 62-69.
65. Chen LP, Thomas EK, Hu SL, Hellstrom I, and Hellstrom KE, Human Papillomavirus Type-16 Nucleoprotein-E7 Is a Tumor Rejection Antigen. Proc Natl Acad Sci U S A, 1991; 88: 110-114.
66. Chen L, Mizuno MT, Singhal MC, Hu SL, Galloway DA, Hellstrom I, and Hellstrom KE, Induction of Cytotoxic Lymphocytes-T Specific for a Syngeneic Tumor Expressing the E6 Oncoprotein of Human Papillomavirus Type-16. J Immunol, 1992; 148: 2617-2621.
67. Tindle R and Frazer IH, Immune response to human papillomavirus and the prospects for human papilloma virus specific immunisation. Curr Top Microbiol Immunol, 1994; 186: 217-253.
68. Ressing ME, Sette A, Brandt RMP, Ruppert J, Wentworth PA, Hartman M, Oseroff C, Grey HM, Melief CJM, and Kast WM, Human Ctl Epitopes Encoded by Human Papillomavirus Type-16 E6 and E7 Identified through in-Vivo and in-Vitro Immunogenicity Studies of Hla-a-Asterisk-0201-Binding Peptides. J Immunol, 1995; 154: 5934-5943.
69. Ressing ME, vanDriel WJ, Celis E, Sette A, Brandt RMP, Hartman M, Anholts JDH, Schreuder GMT, terHarmsel WB, Fleuren GJ, Trimbos BJ, Kast WM, and Melief CJM, Occasional memory cytotoxic T-cell responses of patients with human papillomavirus type 16-positive cervical lesions against a human leukocyte antigen-A*0201-restricted E7-encoded epitope. Cancer Res, 1996; 56: 582-588.
70. Evans C, Bauer S, Grubert T, Brucker C, Baur S, Heeg K, Wagner H, and Lipford GB, HLA-A2-restricted peripheral blood cytolytic T lymphocyte response to HPV type 16 proteins E6 and E7 from patients with neoplastic cervical lesions. Cancer Immunology Immunotherapy, 1996; 42: 151-160.
71. Evans EML, Man S, Evans AS, and Borysiewicz LK, Infiltration of cervical cancer tissue with human papillomavirus-specific cytotoxic T-lymphocytes. Cancer Res, 1997; 57: 2943-2950.
72. Jochmus I, Osen W, Altmann A, Buck G, Hofmann B, Schneider A, Gissmann L, and Rammensee HG, Specificity of human cytotoxic T lymphocytes induced by a human papillomavirus type 16 E7-derived peptide. J Gen Virol, 1997; 78: 1689-1695.
73. Youde SJ, Dunbar PRR, Evans EML, Fiander AN, Borysiewicz LK, Cerundolo V, and Man S, Use of fluorogenic histocompatibility leukocyte antigen- A*0201/HPV 16 E7 peptide complexes to isolate rare human cytotoxic T-lymphocyte-recognizing endogenous human papillomavirus antigens. Cancer Res, 2000; 60: 365-371.
74. Tan LC, Gudgeon N, Annels NE, Hansasuta P, O'Callaghan CA, Rowland-Jones S, McMichael AJ, Rickinson AB, and Callan MFC, A re-evaluation of the frequency of CD8(+) T cells specific for EBV in healthy virus carriers. J Immunol, 1999; 162: 1827-1835.
75. Dunbar PR, Ogg GS, Chen J, Rust N, van der Bruggen P, and Cerundolo V, Direct isolation, phenotyping and cloning of low-frequency antigen- specific cytotoxic T lymphocytes from peripheral blood. Curr Biol, 1998; 8: 413-416.
76. Nimako M, Fiander AN, Wilkinson GWG, Borysiewicz LK, and Man S, Human papillomavirus-specific cytotoxic T lymphocytes in patients with cervical intraepithelial neoplasia grade III. Cancer Res, 1997; 57: 4855-4861.
77. Nakagawa M, Stites DP, Farhat S, Sisler JR, Moss B, Kong F, Moscicki AB, and Palefsky JM, Cytotoxic T lymphocyte responses to E6 and E7 proteins of human papillomavirus type 16: Relationship to cervical intraepithelial neoplasia. J Infect Dis, 1997; 175: 927-931.
78. Santin AD, Hermonat PL, Ravaggi A, Chiriva-Internati M, Zhan DJ, Pecorelli S, Parham GP, and Cannon MJ, Induction of human papillomavirus-specific CD4(+) and CD8(+) lymphocytes by E7-pulsed autologous dendritic cells in patients with human papillomavirus type 16-and 18-positive cervical cancer. J Virol, 1999; 73: 5402-5410.
79. Murakami M, Gurski KJ, Marincola FM, Ackland J, and Steller MA, Induction of specific CD8+ T-lymphocyte responses using a human papillomavirus-16 E6/E7 fusion protein and autologous dendritic cells. Cancer Res, 1999; 59: 1184-1187.
80. Jacobs N, Giannini SL, Al-Saleh W, Hubert P, Boniver J, and Delvenne P, Generation of T lymphocytes from the epithelium and stroma of squamous pre-neoplastic lesions of the uterine cervix. J Immunol Methods, 1999; 223: 123-129.

142

81. Bontkes HJ, deGruijl TD, Walboomers JMM, vandenMuysenberg AJC, Gunther AW, Scheper RJ, Meijer C, and Kummer JA, Assessment of cytotoxic T-lymphocyte phenotype using the specific markers granzyme B and TIA-1 in cervical neoplastic lesions. Br J Cancer, 1997; 76: 1353-1360.

82. Romero P, Dunbar PR, Valmori D, Pittet M, Ogg GS, Rimoldi D, Chen JL, Lienard D, Cerottini JC, and Cerundolo V, Ex vivo staining of metastatic lymph nodes by class I major histocompatibility complex tetramers reveals high numbers of antigen-experienced tumor-specific cytolytic T lymphocytes. J Exp Med, 1998; 188: 1641-1650.

83. McMichael AJ and O'Callaghan CA, A new look at T cells. J Exp Med, 1998; 187: 1367-1371.

84. Kono K, Ressing ME, Brandt RMP, Melief CJM, Potkul RK, Andersson B, Petersson M, Kast WM, and Kiessling R, Decreased expression of signal-transducing zeta chain in peripheral T cells and natural killer cells in patients with cervical cancer. Clin Cancer Res, 1996; 2: 1825-1828.

85. Boursnell MEG, Rutherford E, Hickling JK, Rollinson EA, Munro AJ, Rolley N, McLean CS, Borysiewicz LK, Vousden K, and Inglis SC, Construction and characterisation of a recombinant vaccinia was expressing human papillomavirus proteins for immunotherapy of cervical cancer. Vaccine, 1996; 14: 1485-1494.

86. Moss B, Vaccina virus: a tool for research and vaccine development. Science, 1991; 252: 1662-1667.

87. Restifo NP, The new vaccines: building viruses that elicit antitumor immunity. Curr Opin Immunol, 1996; 8: 658-663.

88. Borysiewicz LK, Fiander A, Nimako M, Man S, Wilkinson GWG, Westmoreland D, Evans AS, Adams M, Stacey SN, Boursnell MEG, Rutherford E, Hickling JK, and Inglis SC, A recombinant vaccinia virus encoding human papillomavirus types 16 and 18, E6 and E7 proteins as immunotherapy for cervical cancer. Lancet, 1996; 347: 1523-1527.

89. Fiander AN, Adams M, Evans AS, Bennett AJ, and Borysiewicz LK, Immunocompetent for Immunotherapy - a Study of the Immunocompetence of Cervical-Cancer Patients. Int J Gynecol Cancer, 1995; 5: 438-442.

90. Fiander A, Man S, Nimako M, Evans A, and Adams M, *Clinical HPV vaccination programme utilising recombinant vaccina virus encoding E6 and E7 p[roteins of HPV 16 and 18*, in *17th International Papilloma virus Conference*. 1999: Charleston, USA. p. 215.

91. Melief CJM and Kast WM, *Prospects for T-Cell Immunotherapy of Tumors by Vaccination with Immunodominant and Subdominant Peptides*, in *Vaccines against Virally Induced Cancers*. 1994. p. 97-112.

92. Feltkamp MCW, Vreugdenhil GR, Vierboom RPM, Ras E, Vanderburg SH, Terschegget J, Melief CJM, and Kast WM, Cytotoxic T-Lymphocytes Raised against a Subdominant Epitope Offered as a Synthetic Peptide Eradicate Human Papillomavirus Type 16-Induced Tumors. Eur J Immunol, 1995; 25: 2638-2642.

93. Alexander J, Sidney J, Southwood S, Ruppert J, Oseroff C, Maewal A, Snoke K, Serra HM, Kubo RT, Sette A, and Grey HM, Development of High Potency Universal Dr-Restricted Helper Epitopes by Modification of High-Affinity Dr-Blocking Peptides. Immunity, 1994; 1: 751-761.

94. Ressing ME, de Jong JH, Brandt RMP, Drijfhout JW, Benckhuijsen WE, Schreuder GMT, Offringa R, Kast WM, and Melief CJM, Differential binding of viral peptides to HLA-A2 alleles. Implications for human papillomavirus type 16 E7 peptide-based vaccination against cervical carcinoma. Eur J Immunol, 1999; 29: 1292-1303.

95. Ellis JRM, Keating PJ, Baird J, Hounsell EF, Renouf DV, Rowe M, Hopkins D, Duggankeen MF, Bartholomew JS, Young LS, and Stern PL, The Association of an Hpv16 Oncogene Variant with Hla-B7 Has Implications for Vaccine Design in Cervical-Cancer. Nat Med, 1995; 1: 464-470.

96. Toes REM, Offringa R, Blom RJJ, Melief CJM, and Kast WM, Peptide vaccination can lead to enhanced tumor growth through specific T-cell tolerance induction. Proc Natl Acad Sci U S A, 1996; 93: 7855-7860.

97. Toes REM, Blom RJJ, Offringa R, Kast WM, and Melief CJM, Enhanced tumor outgrowth after peptide vaccination - Functional deletion of tumor-specific CTL induced by peptide vaccination can lead to the inability to reject tumors. J Immunol, 1996; 156: 3911-3918.

98. Toes REM, van der Voort EIH, Schoenberger SP, Drijfhout JW, van Bloois L, Storm G, Kast WM, Offringa R, and Melief CJM, Enhancement of tumor outgrowth through CTL tolerization after peptide vaccination is avoided by peptide presentation on dendritic cells. J Immunol, 1998; 160: 4449-4456.

99. Toes REM, Hoeben RC, van der Voort EIH, Ressing ME, van der Eb AJ, Melief CJM, and Offringa R, Protective anti-tumor immunity induced by vaccination with recombinant adenoviruses encoding multiple tumor-associated cytotoxic T lymphocyte epitopes in a string-of-beads fashion. Proc Natl Acad Sci U S A, 1997; 94: 14660-14665.

100. Tindle RW, Human papillomavirus vaccines for cervical cancer. Curr Opin Immunol, 1996; 8: 643-650.
101. Chu Y, Hu HM, Winter H, Wood WJ, Doran T, Lashley D, Bashey J, Schuster J, Wood J, Lowe BA, Vetto JT, Weinberg AD, Puri R, Smith JW, Urba WJ, and Fox BA, Examining the immune response in sentinel lymph nodes of mice and men. Eur J Nucl Med, 1999; 26: S50-S53.
102. Connor ME and Stern PL, Loss of Mhc Class-I Expression in Cervical Carcinomas. Int J Cancer, 1990; 46: 1029-1034.
103. Chen LP, Ashe S, Brady WA, Hellstrom I, Hellstrom KE, Ledbetter JA, McGowan P, and Linsley PS, Costimulation of Antitumor Immunity by the B7 Counterreceptor for the Lymphocyte-T Molecules Cd28 and Ctla-4. Cell, 1992; 71: 1093-1102.
104. Chambers MA, Stacey SN, Arrand JR, and Stanley MA, Delayed-Type Hypersensitivity Response to Human Papillomavirus Type-16 E6 Protein in a Mouse Model. J Gen Virol, 1994; 75: 165-169.
105. Nickoloff BJ, Turka LA, Mitra RS, and Nestle FO, Direct and Indirect Control of T-Cell Activation by Keratinocytes. J Invest Dermatol, 1995; 105: S25-S29.
106. Doan T, Herd K, Street M, Bryson G, Fernando G, Lambert P, and Tindle R, Human papillomavirus type 16 E7 oncoprotein expressed in peripheral epithelium tolerizes E7-directed cytotoxic T-lymphocyte precursors restricted through human (and mouse) major histocompatibility complex class I alleles. J Virol, 1999; 73: 6166-6170.
107. Ikeda H, Lethe B, Lehmann F, VanBaren N, Baurain JF, DeSmet C, Chambost H, Vitale M, Moretta A, Boon T, and Coulie PG, Characterization of an antigen that is recognized on a melanoma showing partial HLA loss by CTL expressing an NK inhibitory receptor. Immunity, 1997; 6: 199-208.
108. Porgador A, Yewdell JW, Deng YP, Bennink JR, and Germain RN, Localization, quantitation, and in situ detection of specific peptide MHC class I complexes using a monoclonal antibody. Immunity, 1997; 6: 715-726.
109. AlexanderMiller MA, Leggatt GR, and Berzofsky JA, Selective expansion of high- or low-avidity cytotoxic T lymphocytes and efficacy for adoptive immunotherapy. Proc Natl Acad Sci U S A, 1996; 93: 4102-4107.
110. Dranoff G, Jaffee E, Lazenby A, Golumbek P, Levitsky H, Brose K, Jackson V, Hamada H, Pardoll D, and Mulligan RC, Vaccination with Irradiated Tumor-Cells Engineered to Secrete Murine Granulocyte-Macrophage Colony-Stimulating Factor Stimulates Potent, Specific, and Long-Lasting Antitumor Immunity. Proc Natl Acad Sci U S A, 1993; 90: 3539-3543.
111. Bertoletti A, Sette A, Chisari FV, Penna A, Levrero M, Decarli M, Fiaccadori F, and Ferrari C, Natural Variants of Cytotoxic Epitopes Are T-Cell Receptor Antagonists for Antiviral Cytotoxic T-Cells. Nature, 1994; 369: 407-410.
112. Chang Y, Cesarman E, Pessin MS, Lee F, Culpepper J, Knowles DM, and Moore PS, Identification of Herpesvirus-Like DNA-Sequences in Aids- Associated Kaposis-Sarcoma. Science, 1994; 266: 1865-1869.
113. Uchiyama T, Human T cell leukemia virus type I (HTLV-I) and human diseases. Annu Rev Immunol, 1997; 15: 15-37.
114. Murphy EL, Hanchard B, Figueroa JP, Gibbs WN, Lofters WS, Campbell M, Goedert JJ, and Blattner WA, Modeling the Risk of Adult T-Cell Leukemia Lymphoma in Persons Infected with Human T-Lymphotropic Virus Type-I. Int J Cancer, 1989; 43: 250-253.
115. Bangham CRM, Hall SE, Jeffery KJM, Vine AM, Witkover A, Nowak MA, Wodarz D, Usuku K, and Osame M, Genetic control and dynamics of the cellular immune response to the human T-cell leukaemia virus, HTLV-I. Philos Trans R Soc Lond Ser B-Biol Sci, 1999; 354: 691-700.
116. Hislop AD, Good MF, Mateo L, Gardner J, Gatei MH, Daniel RCW, Meyers BV, Lavin MF, and Suhrbier A, Vaccine-induced cytotoxic T lymphocytes protect against retroviral challenge. Nat Med, 1998; 4: 1193-1196.
117. Ohashi T, Hanabuchi S, Kato H, Koya Y, Takemura F, Hirokawa K, Yoshiki T, Tanaka Y, Fujii M, and Kannagi M, Induction of adult T-cell leukemia-like lymphoproliferative disease and its inhibition by adoptive immunotherapy in T-cell- deficient nude rats inoculated with syngeneic human T-cell leukemia virus type 1-immortalized cells. J Virol, 1999; 73: 6031-6040.
118. Newmaster RS, Mylin LM, Fu TM, and Tevethia SS, Role of a subdominant H-2K(d)-restricted SV40 tumor antigen cytotoxic T lymphocyte epitope in tumor rejection. Virology, 1998; 244: 427-441.
119. Pepper C, Jasani B, Navabi H, WynfordThomas D, and Gibbs AR, Simian virus 40 large T antigen (SV40LTAg) primer specific DNA amplification in human pleural mesothelioma tissue. Thorax, 1996; 51: 1074-1076.

120. Testa JR, Carbone M, Hirvonen A, Khalili K, Krynska B, Linnainmaa K, Pooley FD, Rizzo P, Rusch V, and Xiao GH, A multi-institutional study confirms the presence and expression of simian virus 40 in human malignant mesotheliomas. Cancer Res, 1998; 58: 4505-4509.

121. Strickler HD, Rosenberg PS, Devesa SS, Hertel J, Fraumeni JF, and Goedert JJ, Contamination of poliovirus vaccines with simian virus 40 (1955-1963) and subsequent cancer rates. JAMA-J Am Med Assoc, 1998; 279: 292-295.

122. Blaho JA and Aaronson SA, Convicting a human tumor virus: Guilt by association? Proc Natl Acad Sci U S A, 1999; 96: 7619-7621.

123. Laghi L, Randolph AE, Chauhan DP, Marra G, Major EO, Neel JV, and Boland CR, JC virus DNA is present in the mucosa of the human colon and in colorectal cancers. Proc Natl Acad Sci U S A, 1999; 96: 7484-7489.

124. Marchand M, van Baren N, Weynants P, Brichard V, Dreno B, Tessier MH, Rankin E, Parmiani G, Arienti F, Humblet Y, Bourlond A, Vanwijck R, Lienard D, Beauduin M, Dietrich PY, Russo V, Kerger J, Masucci G, Jager E, De Greve J, Atzpodien J, Brasseur F, Coulie PG, Van der Bruggen P, and Boon T, Tumor regressions observed in patients with metastatic melanoma treated with an antigenic peptide encoded by gene MAGE-3 and presented by HLA-A1. Int J Cancer, 1999; 80: 219-230.

125. Dhodapkar MV, Steinman RM, Sapp M, Desai H, Fossella C, Krasovsky J, Donahoe SM, Dunbar PR, Cerundolo V, Nixon DF, and Bhardwaj N, Rapid generation of broad T-cell immunity in humans after a single injection of mature dendritic cells. J Clin Invest, 1999; 104: 173-180.

126. Theobald M, Biggs J, Dittmer D, Levine AJ, and Sherman LA, Targeting p53 as a general tumor antigen. Proc Natl Acad Sci U S A, 1995; 92: 11993-11997.

127. Lustgarten J, Theobald M, Labadie C, LaFace D, Peterson P, Disis ML, Cheever MA, and Sherman LA, Identification of Her-2/Neu CTL epitopes using double transgenic mice expressing HLA-A2.1 and human CD.8. Hum Immunol, 1997; 52: 109-118.

128. Boon T and van der Bruggen P, Human Tumor-Antigens Recognized By T-Lymphocytes. J Exp Med, 1996; 183: 725-729.

129. Riddell SR, Elliott M, Lewinsohn DA, Gilbert MJ, Wilson L, Manley SA, Lupton SD, Overell RW, Reynolds TC, Corey L, and Greenberg PD, T-cell mediated rejection of gene-modified HIV-specific cytotoxic T lymphocytes in HIV-infected patients. Nat Med, 1996; 2: 216-223.

130. Tan RS, Xu XN, Ogg GS, Hansasuta P, Dong T, Rostron T, Luzzi G, Conlon CP, Screaton GR, McMichael AJ, and Rowland-Jones S, Rapid death of adoptively transferred T cells in acquired immunodeficiency syndrome. Blood, 1999; 93: 1506-1510.

131. Zajac AJ, Murali-Krishna K, Blattman JN, and Ahmed R, Therapeutic vaccination against chronic viral infection: the importance of cooperation between CD4(+) and CD8(+) T cells. Curr Opin Immunol, 1998; 10: 444-449.

8
The immune response to oncogenic fusion proteins

LORENA PASSONI & CARLO GAMBACORTI-PASSERINI

INTRODUCTION

Chromosomal translocations represent somatically acquired cytogenetic mutations. When chromosomal breaks occur within exons of two different genes, the consequence of chromosomal translocation is the creation of a new fusion gene encoding for a chimeric protein. It is well established that these proteins are necessary and sufficient for the malignant transformation of normal cells [1, 2]. Chromosomal translocations coding for oncogenic fusion proteins (OFP) have been described in a number of human cancers, including both leukemias [3] and solid tumours [4]. More than 30 different oncogenic fusion proteins have been identified since the first cloning of the 9; 22 translocation from leukaemia cells which yields the *BCR/ABL* fusion gene [5]. Table 8.1 lists several examples of these translocations.

TABLE 8.1   Chromosomal translocations which generate oncogenic fusion proteins in human cancer

DISEASE	TRANSLOCATION	INVOLVED GENES
CML/ALL	9;22	BCR/ABL
CML-BC	3;21	AML1/EAP
AML/M3 (APL)	15;17	PML/RARα
AML/M3 (APL)	11;17	PLZF/RARα
PRE-B ALL	1;19	E2A/PBX
ALL	17;19	E2A/HFL

R.A. Robins and R.C. Rees (eds.), Cancer Immunology, 147–156.
© 2001 *Kluwer Academic Publishers. Printed in the Netherlands.*

DISEASE	TRANSLOCATION	INVOLVED GENES
ALL	4;11	ALL-1/AF-4
ALL	11;19	ALL-1/ENL or ELL
ALL/AML	9;11	ALL-1/AF-9
AML	11;17	ALL-1/AF-17
AML	6;11	ALL-1/AF-6
T-NHL	4;16	IL2/BCM
NHL	INS 2;2	REL/NRG
AML/M2	8;21	AML1/MTG8
AML	6;9	DEK/CAN
AML	INV.16	CBF-ß/MYH11
AML	16;21	ERG/TLS-FUS
CMML	5;12	TEL/PDGFRβ
LARGE CELLS ANAPLASTIC LYMPHOMA	2;5	NPM/ALK
EWING'S SARCOMA	11;22	EWS/hFLI-1
CLEAR CELL SARCOMA	12;22	EWS/ATF-1
THYROID PAPILLARY CARCINOMA	INV 10, t 10;17 1	PTC-1,-2 or -3 (RET) TRP/TRK or TPM/TRK
MYXOID LIPOSARCOMA	12;16	FUS/CHOP
ALVEOLAR RABDOMYOSARCOMA	2;13 1;13	PAX3/FKHR PAX7/FKHR

Fusion proteins represent an attractive target for antitumor immune response. They are uniquely express in tumour cells and thus they can be considered as tumour specific markers. By joining the sequences of two different genes normally not related, an abnormal protein is created which reaches the maximal difference within its junctional region. Therefore, the intracellular processing of the junctional region product could generate novel peptides, which might result to be highly immunogenic and theoretically represent tumour specific antigens.

In this respect, the bcr/abl fusion region has been the object of intensive research aiming at demonstrating whether an immune response to fusion proteins occurs naturally or could be induced and/or enhanced through *in vitro* manipulations. The most significant studies and relevant achievements on the immune response to bcr/abl will be presented in a following section.

The first example of OFP immune recognition is represented by the chimeric protein pml/RARα. This OFP, generated by a t(15:17) chromosomal translocation, is present in 80%-90% cases of Acute Promyelocytic Leukaemia (APL). A peptide corresponding to the fusion region can be specifically recognised by healthy donor CD4 lymphocytes. This recognition seems to be restricted to HLA-DR11 molecules only. The absence of reactivity toward peptides from normal pml and RARα sequences flanking the fusion point demonstrates that the translocation directly generates the specific immune recognition [6].

Recently, two different groups reported that in pre-B Acute Lymphoblastic Leukaemia (ALL) the fusion protein etv6/aml1, which results from a t(12;21) chromosomal translocation , acts as a tumour specific antigen. CD4 [7] and CD8 [8] clones recognising peptides from the junctional region in a HLA restricted manner have been generated. CD8 clones can recognise tumour cells expressing endogenous etv6/aml1, and CTLs specific for the junction peptide were identified with high frequency in one ALL patient. CD4 clones were not tested for their ability to recognise tumour cells.

Interesting and different is the case of the chimeric protein npm/alk. The t(2;5) breakpoint found in approximately 10% of all non-Hodgkin lymphomas was first cloned by Morris et al. in 1994. This rearrangement was shown to fuse the amino terminal portion of the nucleolar phosphoprotein nucleophosmin (npm) to the catalytic domain of a novel anaplastic lymphoma kinase (alk) [9]. Low levels of expression of the native *ALK* gene are normally restricted to a limited number of neural cells. On the other hand, as a result of the t(2;5) translocation, the alk catalytic domain, driven by the strong npm promoter, is highly expressed in tumour cells [10, 11]. Therefore it is conceivable to hypothesise a possible break of tolerance and/or an activation of cryptic populations of T cells that have escaped tolerance by virtue of their low affinity for the alk protein. This may results in the increase of the potential immunogenicity of alk, thus inducing the immune system to react against the alk positive lymphoma cells. In this case, not only the junction region of npm/alk but also the entire portion of the alk protein can be good candidates for a specific tumour antigen.

Recently, the presence of anti-alk circulating antibodies in Anaplastic Large Cell Lymphoma patient's serum has been reported [12]. Studies are currently ongoing to verify alk kinase aptitude at inducing an anti-tumour immune response.

BCR/ABL

The so called "Philadelphia chromosome -positive" (Ph+) haematologic malignancies are characterised by the reciprocal translocation between the *BCR* gene on chromosome 22 (Philadelphia Chromosome) and the proto-oncogene *c-ABL* on chromosome 9 which encodes for a nonreceptor tyrosine kinase. The t(9;22) translocation generates two different types of fusion proteins, p210 and p190 bcr/abl. The enhanced tyrosine-kinase activity of bcr/abl is necessary and sufficient for the neoplastic transformation. The p210 bcr/abl protein is expressed in leukemic cells of Chronic Myeloid Leukaemia (CML) patients and in part of Acute Lymphoblastic Leukaemia's (ALL), where p190 is also found.

CML immunotherapy

Experimental and clinical evidences support the existence of a graft versus leukaemia (GVL) effect in CML patients after allogenic bone marrow transplantation (BMT) [13].

In the murine model it has been demonstrated that donor T cells are the critical component of GVL induction [14]. In humans, when T cells are depleted from the donor graft as graft versus host disease (GVHD) prophylaxis in clinical transplantation, GVL activity is severely compromised, especially in CML patients, and correlates to an increased risk of relapse [15].

Given the indirect evidence that donor T cells are likely to play a major role in the control or eradication of leukaemia after allografting, in 1990, Kolb et al. first reported that infusions of lymphocytes from the original marrow donor could restore remission in patients with relapsed CML after allogenic BMT [16]. The effectiveness of Donor Lymphocyte Infusion (DLI) in the treatment of relapsed CML has since then been confirmed and studied in greater detail, demonstrating that CML is very sensitive to immune recognition by donor lymphocytes [17]. Unfortunately, the use of DLI is not free of complications. In fact, the majority of patients experience either acute or chronic GVHD as toxic side effects [18, 19]

Despite the important role of donor T cells in the control and/or eradication of leukaemia after allografting, the target antigens on the tumour cells still remain poorly defined. The identification of these targets is of critical importance because it may help in designing a more specific immunotherapy strategy targeting only the leukaemia cells and avoiding the toxic GVHD effects.

Specific recognition of the bcr/abl protein

The fact that GVL induction exhibits disease specificity suggests that the target antigens may be tumour specific. It is intriguing to think that the novel bcr/abl peptide expressed in CML could be involved in tumour cell recognition. In fact, in addition to having aminoacid sequences not normally assembled within the same protein, the potential for immunogenicity of bcr/abl is enhanced by the presence at the fusion point of a codon for an aminoacid which does not derive from either the bcr or abl constituent proteins.

Peripheral blood mononuclear cells (PBMCs) from CML patients in complete cytogenetic remission after interferon treatment are stimulated to *in vitro* proliferate in response to extracts of p210 bcr/abl expressing COS-1 transfected cells, which suggests a specific cellular immune response against sequences of the oncoprotein p210 bcr/abl [20].

Two variants of p210 bcr/abl OFP can be generated depending on where breakpoint on chromosome 22 is located. Breakpoints between bcr exons b2 and b3 or exons b3 and b4 give rise to p210 b2a2 or p210 b3a2 proteins respectively.

p210 b2a2 and b3a2 junction regions have been the object of several studies intented at demonstrating their immunogenicity. It appears clear that these two proteins have a different potential in inducing an anti tumour activity. Although the b3a2 junction is able to induce an immune response, an anti-b2a2 response is very difficult to achieve. The reason for this apparent difference is still unclear.

The b3a2 fusion protein contains a novel lysine residue at the fusion point. Unlike b3a2, the b2a2 fusion region lacks a novel aminoacid carrying instead a glutamic acid encoded by the new b2a2 fusion triplet, which is also present in the original abl sequence. Therefore, the b2a2 fusion region shows more similarity to the physiologic abl counterpart when compared to the b3a2 fusion. This might contribute to the reduced immunogenicity of b2a2.

In vitro studies have confirmed that different synthetic peptides derived from the b3a2 fusion region can bind class I HLA molecules such as A2 [21], A3 [22, 23], A11 and B8 [22], A24 [24] and class II DRB1 0402, DRB1 0301, and DR11 [25] molecules with high affinity. Interestingly, some of these peptides lack the typical major anchor motifs of HLA-binding molecules.

The immunogenicity of the resulting HLA-peptide complex has been confirmed as the ability to provoke an *in vitro* peptide-specific primary CTL response from Peripheral Blood Lymphocytes (PBLs) of HLA-matched healthy donor. The approach undertaken allowed the generation of anti bcr/abl-specific CD4 [25, 26] and CD8 [24, 26] T cell lines and/or clones. In some cases these clones were able to react against *BCR-ABL* positive tumour cells endogenously expressing the chimeric molecule. These results indicate that bcr/abl is intracellularly processed and that natural peptides from the b3a2 junction region are presented by HLA molecules [21, 24, 26]. The ability of these peptides to elicit an *in vivo* immune response needs to be verified in CML patients.

Up to date, there are only two reports of induction of a b3a2 junction peptide-specific CTL HLA-restricted immune response. Specific lysis was obtained in HLA-A3, HLA-B8 and HLA-A2.1 patients [21, 23]. In addition, by using a Limiting Dilution Analysis to determine the frequency of specific CTL precursors, an higher frequency of bcr/abl b3a2 specific CTLs were found in 5 out of 21 CML patients when compared to healthy donors [21]. On the other hand, no T-cells recognising b3a2 junction peptides in a HLA class II restricted fashion could be detected in CML patients [27, 28].

Taken together these data document the likely presence of a T cell-mediated antitumor immunity in leukaemia patients. It is worthy of note that the immune response seems to be limited to the p210b3a2 junction antigens presented by HLA Class I molecules. As CML cells express both HLA Class I and Class II molecules [29], the reason for a lack of Class II restricted response should not be attributed to a loss of expression of HLA molecules which is typical of many tumours.

Several groups as mentioned above have demonstrated the immunogenicity of fusion region-derived peptides of p210b3a2. On the other hand, an immune response against fusion peptides from the b2a2 junctional region seems difficult to elicit. Binding studies on HLA class I molecules report that all the possible peptides spanning the b2a2 junction region failed to bind to any alleles [30, 31].

HLA Class II binding assays revealed that b2a2 synthetic peptides are unable to bind strongly to any of the HLA-DR alleles, with the possible exception of HLA-DR3 [32] and HLA-DR2a [33].

CML vaccination

The identification of tumour antigens that are recognised by T-cells has led to the development of vaccination strategies aimed at generating an antigen-specific immune response capable of mediating tumour regression in cancer patients.

A therapeutic approach to CML based on T cell immunity is particularly attractive. Bcr/abl derived fusion proteins represent a reasonable target for an immunologic approach to the treatment of CML. The *in vitro* data mentioned before provided the rationale for developing a peptide-based vaccine for CML.

A Phase 1 clinical trial was conducted in 12 patients with chronic-phase CML. Patients were vaccinated with a combination of 5 peptides (4 CML class I peptides and a single class II peptide) spanning the p210b3a2 junction region. Patients were subdivided in four groups. Each group received different doses of vaccine starting from a dose of 10μg up to 300μg of single peptide per vaccination. Peptides were injected subcutaneosly together with an immunological adjuvant. After vaccination, specific proliferative response was detected in 3 patients and two of them generated a DTH positive response against the administrated peptides. No autologous killing of CML cells was tested [34].

This represents the first reported clinical trial of vaccination with peptides derived from tumour-specific OFP. Unfortunately, the interpretation of the outcome of immunisation is unclear. A limited number of patients have been tested and some of them received low doses of single peptide, which might enhance tolerance rather than immunity. Moreover. no selection based on the peptides HLA binding restriction elements was applied. Infact, all patients, regardless of HLA type, were eligible for this trial.

On the basis of this report it is difficult to draw conclusions on the effectiveness of a peptide-based vaccine strategy in controlling CML. Clearly more work is needed to understand the feasibility of this approach applied to CML.

FUSION PROTEINS AND TUMOUR ESCAPE

Despite the increasing evidences that cellular immune response to tumour antigens can be elicited both *in vitro* and *in vivo*, effective endogenous immunity against human cancer is rarely observed.

While a generalised suppression of the cellular immunity, due to the poor health condition of the patients, is usually present in the late stage of the disease, at an earlier time cancer patients are immunologically competent [28].

Among the reasons proposed to explain the failure of developing an effective immune response lies the ability of tumour cells to evade the immune attack. The main mechanisms of tumour escape are the loss of MHC expression and the production of immunosuppressive molecules such as Prostaglandin E_2, Transforming Growth Factor-β, Fas ligand and Interleukin-10 (IL-10) [35].

The absence of relevant restriction element HLA-DR molecules in APL cells can be considered as an example of tumour escape in OFP neoplastic cells.

pml/RARα is recognised by T lymphocytes only when presented by the restriction element HLA-DR11 [6]. A specific CD4 T cell clone recognising a peptide encompassing the pml/RARα fusion region has been generated from HLA-DR11 healthy donor lymphocytes. This clone exerts a specific cytotoxic activity upon stimulation with pml/RARα expressing LCLs derived from HLA-DR11 APL patients. No specific lysis is observed against APL blasts coming from the same patients [36] as expected, due to the lack of expression of any HLA-DR element in promyelocytes. The unsuccessful attempts in generating anti pml/RARα T cell clones in four HLA-DR11 APL patients confirms the APL blasts inability of inducing an immune response [36].

The loss of HLA-DR molecules is of particular relevance for the design of any pml/RAR-α specific immunotherapeutic strategy. In fact, considering the lack of HLA class I binding motif in the pml/RARα junction region, the suppression of the expression of HLA-DR molecules in APL cells severely compromises any kind of immunological approach.

Another example of escape is the spontaneous secretion of IL-10 by PBMC from chronic phase CML. IL-10 is detectable in the serum of CML patients. It has been widely demonstrated that IL-10 suppresses both Antigen Presenting Cells (APCs) and responding T cells [37]. T-cells of patients producing high levels of IL-10 are unable to respond with proliferation to autologous tumour cells. Proliferation is, instead, observed in cells from patients producing low amount of IL-10 [27]. *In vitro* spontaneous secretion of IL-10 by CML cells is depressed by the addition of Interferon-α to the culture medium [38]. It remains to demonstrate whether the reduction in IL-10 release observed *in vitro* is also present in CML patients receiving Interferon-α treatment and whether it correlates with a higher T cell reactivity.

The presence of high levels of IL-10 in the serum of some CML patients could also influence the antigen-presenting capacities of the APCs. It is possible to generate Dendritic Cells by *in vitro* differentiation of peripheral blood cells from CML patients. More than 70% of the leukemic Dendritic Cells were shown to be *BCR/ABL* positive by FISH analysis. *In vitro* stimulation of T cells with leukemic DCs significantly increases lymphocyte cytotoxicity against CML autologous cells [39].

The possibility to *in vitro* mature competent DC cells from CML precursors suggests that, potentially, there is no impaired antigen processing and presentation in CML patients. However, it could be speculated that these processes are negatively influenced *in vivo* by the production of IL-10 observed in CML patients.

CONCLUDING REMARKS

The identification of specific tumour-antigen epitopes has opened new perspectives for the immunotherapy of cancer. This finding led to the possibility to exploit minimal peptide sequences as cancer vaccines with the purpose of inducing or enhancing *in vivo* a systemic anti-tumour specific T-cell response. Clinical trials have been attempted using peptide-based vaccines in metastatic melanoma [40], HER2/neu positive breast and ovarian cancer [41] and HPV16 positive cervical carcinoma [42] patients. Successful immunisation has been achived in the majority of the patients vaccinated.

The conspicuous amount of data generated *in vitro* on OFP immune recognition indicates that peptides from the junction region can be processed and presented to the immune system in a HLA restricted way. In some cases, this gives rise to a specific T-cell response able to target tumour cells. Thus, it is conceivable to think that synthetic peptides derived from OFP can be utilise in peptide-based cancer vaccines similarly to what have been done for other tumour antigens.

Up to date, only one clinical trial has been reported involving the chimeric protein bcr/abl. Despite no evidence of successful clinical outcome, repeated vaccinations with bcr/abl-derived peptides is feasible, no toxic, and capable of eliciting specific immune response to the fusion peptides [34].

This should encourage to extend this approach to other OFP which immunogenicity has been previous established *in vitro*.

The challenge for the next few years will be to define the most appropriate mode of immunisation to generate CTL responses strong enough to mediate tumour rejection.

REFERENCES

1. Rabbitts TH, Chromosomal Translocations in Human Cancer. Nature, 1994; 372: 143-149.
2. Rabbitts TH, Perspective: Chromosomal translocations can affect genes controlling gene expression and differentiation - Why are these functions targeted? J Pathol, 1999; 187: 39-42.
3. Drexler HG, Macleod RAF, Borkhardt A, and Janssen JWG, Recurrent Chromosomal Translocations and Fusion Genes in Leukemia-Lymphoma Cell-Lines. Leukemia, 1995; 9: 480-500.
4. Aman P, Fusion genes in solid tumors. Semin Cancer Biol, 1999; 9: 303-318.
5. de Klein A, Vankessel AG, Grosveld G, Bartram CR, Hagemeijer A, Bootsma D, Spurr NK, Heisterkamp N, Groffen J, and Stephenson JR, A Cellular Oncogene Is Translocated to the Philadelphia- Chromosome in Chronic Myelocytic-Leukemia. Nature, 1982; 300: 764-767.
6. Gambacorti-Passerini C, Grignani F, Arienti F, Pandolfi PP, Pelicci PG, and Parmiani G, Human Cd4 Lymphocytes Specifically Recognize a Peptide Representing the Fusion Region of the Hybrid Protein Pml Rar- Alpha Present in Acute Promyelocytic Leukemia-Cells. Blood, 1993; 81: 1369-1375.
7. Yun C, Senju S, Fujita H, Tsuji Y, Irie A, Matsushita S, and Nishimura Y, Augmentation of immune response by altered peptide ligands of the antigenic peptide in a human CD4(+) T-cell clone reacting to TEL/AML1 fusion protein. Tissue Antigens, 1999; 54: 153-161.
8. Yotnda P, Garcia F, Peuchmaur M, Grandchamp B, Duval M, Lemonnier F, Vilmer E, and Langlade-Demoyen P, Cytotoxic T cell response against the chimeric ETV6-AML1 protein in childhood acute lymphoblastic leukemia. J Clin Invest, 1998; 102: 455-462.
9. Morris SW, Kirstein MN, Valentine MB, Dittmer KG, Shapiro DN, Saltman DL, and Look AT, Fusion of a Kinase Gene, Alk, to a Nucleolar Protein Gene, Npm, in Non-Hodgkins-Lymphoma. Science, 1994; 263: 1281-1284.

IMMUNE RESPONSES TO FUSION PROTEINS

10. Pulford K, Lamant L, Morris SW, Butler LH, Wood KM, Stroud D, Delsol G, and Mason DY, Detection of anaplastic lymphoma kinase (ALK) and nucleolar protein nucleophosmin (NPM)-ALK proteins in normal and neoplastic cells with the monoclonal antibody ALK1. Blood, 1997; 89: 1394-1404.
11. Falini B, Bigerna B, Fizzotti M, Pulford K, Pileri SA, Delsol G, Carbone A, Paulli M, Magrini U, Menestrina F, Giardini R, Pilotti S, Mezzelani A, Ugolini B, Billi M, Pucciarini A, Pacini R, Pelicci PG, and Flenghi L, ALK expression defines a distinct group of T/null lymphomas ("ALK lymphomas") with a wide morphological spectrum. Am J Pathol, 1998; 153: 875-886.
12. Pulford K, Falini B, Banham AH, Codrington D, Hatten CSR, and Mason DY, Immune response to the ALK oncogenic tyrosine kinase in patients with anaplastic large cell lymphoma. Blood, 1999; 94: 373.
13. Porter DL and Antin JH, The graft-versus-leukemia effects of allogeneic cell therapy. Annu Rev Med, 1999; 50: 369-386.
14. Truitt RL and Atasoylu AA, Contribution of Cd4+ and Cd8+ T-Cells to Graft-Versus-Host Disease and Graft-Versus-Leukemia Reactivity after Transplantation of Mhc-Compatible Bone-Marrow. Bone Marrow Transplant, 1991; 8: 51-58.
15. Goldman JM, Gale RP, Horowitz MM, Biggs JC, Champlin RE, Gluckman E, Hoffmann RG, Jacobsen SJ, Marmont AM, McGlave PB, Messner HA, Rimm AA, Rozman C, Speck B, Tura S, Weiner RS, and Bortin MM, Bone-Marrow Transplantation for Chronic Myelogenous Leukemia in Chronic Phase - Increased Risk for Relapse Associated with T- Cell Depletion. Ann Intern Med, 1988; 108: 806-814.
16. Kolb HJ, Mittermuller J, Clemm C, Holler E, Ledderose G, Brehm G, Heim M, and Wilmanns W, Donor Leukocyte Transfusions for Treatment of Recurrent Chronic Myelogenous Leukemia in Marrow Transplant Patients. Blood, 1990; 76: 2462-2465.
17. Dazzi F, Szydlo RM, and Goldman JM, Donor lymphocyte infusions for relapse of chronic myeloid leukemia after allogeneic stem cell transplant: Where we now stand. Exp Hematol, 1999; 27: 1477-1486.
18. Kolb HJ, Schattenberg A, Goldman JM, Hertenstein B, Jacobsen N, Arcese W, Ljungman P, Ferrant A, Verdonck L, Niederwieser D, Vanrhee F, Mittermueller J, Dewitte T, Holler E, and Ansari H, Graft-Versus-Leukemia Effect of Donor Lymphocyte Transfusions in Marrow Grafted Patients. Blood, 1995; 86: 2041-2050.
19. Collins RH, Shpilberg O, Drobyski WR, Porter DL, Giralt S, Champlin R, Goodman SA, Wolff SN, Hu W, Verfaillie C, List A, Dalton W, Ognoskie N, Chetrit A, Antin JH, and Nemunaitis J, Donor leukocyte infusions in 140 patients with relapsed malignancy after allogeneic bone marrow transplantation. J Clin Oncol, 1997; 15: 433-444.
20. Oka T, Sastry KJ, Nehete P, Schapiro SJ, Guo JQ, Talpaz M, and Arlinghaus RB, Evidence for specific immune response against P210 BCR-ABL in long-term remission CML patients treated with interferon. Leukemia, 1998; 12: 155-163.
21. Yotnda P, Firat H, Garcia-Pons F, Garcia Z, Gourru G, Vernant JP, Lemonnier FA, Leblond V, and Langlade-Demoyen P, Cytotoxic T cell response against the chimeric p210 BCR-ABL protein in patients with chronic myelogenous leukemia. J Clin Invest, 1998; 101: 2290-2296.
22. Bocchia M, Korontsvit T, Xu Q, Mackinnon S, Yang SY, Sette A, and Scheinberg DA, Specific human cellular immunity to bcr-abl oncogene-derived peptides. Blood, 1996; 87: 3587-3592.
23. Greco G, Fruci D, Accapezzato D, Barnaba V, Nisini R, Alimena G, Montefusco E, Vigneti E, Butler R, Tanigaki N, and Tosi R, Two bcr-abl junction peptides bind HLA-A3 molecules and allow specific induction of human cytotoxic T lymphocytes. Leukemia, 1996; 10: 693-699.
24. Nieda M, Nicol A, Kikuchi A, Kashiwase K, Taylor K, Suzuki K, Tadokoro K, and Juji T, Dendritic cells stimulate the expansion of bcr-abl specific CD8(+) T cells with cytotoxic activity against leukemic cells from patients with chronic myeloid leukemia. Blood, 1998; 91: 977-983.
25. Mannering SI, McKenzie JL, Fearnley DB, and Hart DNJ, HLA-DR1-restricted bcr-abl (b3a2)-specific CD4(+) T lymphocytes respond to dendritic cells pulsed with b3a2 peptide and antigen-presenting cells exposed to b3a2 containing cell lysates. Blood, 1997; 90: 290-297.
26. Osman Y, Takahashi M, Zheng Z, Koike T, Toba K, Liu A, Furukawa T, Aoki S, and Aizawa Y, Generation of bcr-abl specific cytotoxic T-lymphocytes by using dendritic cells pulsed with bcr-abl (b3a2) peptide: its applicability for donor leukocyte transfusions in marrow grafted CML patients. Leukemia, 1999; 13: 166-174.
27. Pawelec G, Rehbein A, Schlotz E, and daSilva P, Cellular immune responses to autologous chronic myelogenous leukaemia cells in vitro. Cancer Immunology Immunotherapy, 1996; 42: 193-199.

28. Bertazzoli C, Marchesi E, Passoni L, Barni R, Ravagnani F, Lombardo C, Corneo GM, Pioltelli P, Pogliani E, and Gambacorti-Passerini C, Differential recognition of a BCR/ABL peptide by lymphocytes from normal donors and chronic myeloid leukemia patients. Clin Cancer Res, 2000; 6: 1931-1935.

29. Valiron O, Clemanceymarcille G, Troesch A, Schweitzer A, Prenant M, Hollard D, and Berthier R, Immunophenotype of Blast Cells in Chronic Myeloid-Leukemia. Leuk Res, 1988; 12: 861-&.

30. Cullis JO, Barrett AJ, Goldman JM, and Lechler RI, Binding of Bcr/Abl Junctional Peptides to Major Histocompatibility Complex (Mhc) Class-I Molecules - Studies in Antigen-Processing Defective Cell-Lines. Leukemia, 1994; 8: 165-170.

31. Bocchia M, Wentworth PA, Southwood S, Sidney J, McGraw K, Scheinberg DA, and Sette A, Specific Binding of Leukemia Oncogene Fusion Protein-Peptides to Hla Class-I Molecules. Blood, 1995; 85: 2680-2684.

32. Pawelec G, Max H, Halder T, Bruserud O, Merl A, daSilva P, and Kalbacher H, BCR/ABL leukemia oncogene fusion peptides selectively bind to certain HLA-DR alleles and can be recognized by T cells found at low frequency in the repertoire of normal donors. Blood, 1996; 88: 2118-2124.

33. ten Bosch GJA, Kessler JH, Joosten AM, Bres-Vloemans AA, Geluk A, Godthelp BC, van Bergen J, Melief CJM, and Leeksma OC, A BCR-ABL oncoprotein p210b2a2 fusion region sequence is recognized by HLA-DR2a restricted cytotoxic T lymphocytes and presented by HLA-DR matched cells transfected with an Ii(b2a2) construct. Blood, 1999; 94: 1038-1045.

34. Pinilla-Ibarz J, Cathcart K, Korontsvit T, Soignet S, Bocchia M, Caggiano J, Lai L, Jimenez J, Kolitz J, and Scheinberg DA, Vaccination of patients with chronic myelogenous leukemia with bcr-abl oncogene breakpoint fusion peptides generates specific immune responses. Blood, 2000; 95: 1781-1787.

35. Marincola F, Jaffee E, Hicklin DJ, and Ferrone S, Escape of human solid tumours from T cell recognition: molecular mechanisms and functional significance. Adv Immunol, 2000; 74: 181-273.

36. Dermime S, Bertazzoli C, Marchesi E, Ravagnani F, Blaser K, Corneo GM, Pogliani E, Parmiani G, and GambacortiPasserini C, Lack of T-cell-mediated recognition of the fusion region of the pml RAR-alpha hybrid protein by lymphocytes of acute promyelocytic leukemia patients. Clin Cancer Res, 1996; 2: 593-600.

37. Salazar-Onfray F, Interleukin-10: a cytokine used by tumors to escape immunosurveillance. Med Oncol, 1999; 16: 86-94.

38. Pawelec G, Schlotz E, and Rehbein A, IFN-alpha regulates IL 10 production by CML cells in vitro. Cancer Immunology Immunotherapy, 1999; 48: 430-434.

39. Choudhury A, Gajewski JL, Liang JC, Popat U, Claxton DF, Kliche KO, Andreeff M, and Champlin RE, Use of leukemic dendritic cells for the generation of antileukemic cellular cytotoxicity against Philadelphia chromosome-positive chronic myelogenous leukemia. Blood, 1997; 89: 1133-1142.

40. Rosenberg SA, Yang JC, Schwartzentruber DJ, Hwu P, Marincola FM, Topalian SL, Restifo NP, Dudley ME, Schwarz SL, Spiess PJ, Wunderlich JR, Parkhurst MR, Kawakami Y, Seipp CA, Einhorn JH, and White DE, Immunologic and therapeutic evaluation of a synthetic peptide vaccine for the treatment of patients with metastatic melanoma. Nat Med, 1998; 4: 321-327.

41. Disis ML, Grabstein KH, Sleath PR, and Cheever MA, Generation of immunity to the HER-2/neu oncogenic protein in patients with breast and ovarian cancer using a peptide-based vaccine. Clin Cancer Res, 1999; 5: 1289-1297.

42. van Driel WJ, Ressing ME, Kenter GG, Brandt RMP, Krul EJT, van Rossum AB, Schuuring E, Offringa R, Bauknecht T, Tamm-Hermelink A, van Dam PA, Fleuren GJ, Kast WM, Melief CJM, and Trimbos JB, Vaccination with HPV16 peptides of patients with advanced cervical carcinoma: Clinical evaluation of a phase I-II trial. Eur J Cancer, 1999; 35: 946-952.

9
Immunological significance of hsp70 in tumor rejection

ANTOINE MÉNORET

INTRODUCTION.

The immune system whose function is to protect the host against the infectious agents of endless antigenic diversity has been shaped during evolution under the selective pressure of infectious agents. To the contrary, tumors that arise generally after the age of reproduction should have no major influence on the evolution of the immune system. Nevertheless, animal and human tumors can sometimes be rejected spontaneously by the immune system of the host [1-3]. On one hand, the previous years have been marked by significant advances in understanding the molecular mechanisms of tumor rejection in the context of immunotherapy of cancer [4]. On the other hand, little is known about the circumstances and mechanisms by which spontaneous tumor rejection happens and its immunological significance [5, 6]. In this chapter I have considered the hypothesis that the stress inducible Heat Shock Proteins (HSP) in general and the inducible hsp70 in particular, may play a determining role in tumor immunogenicity and might be responsible for the spontaneous rejection of tumors by the immune system.

PROGRESSOR AND REGRESSOR TUMORS.

The spontaneous regression of tumors of the brain, bone, skin, liver, kidney, lungs and other organs has consistently been reported in humans as a rare, heterogeneous but well established event [6]. The circumstances of the regression of tumors have not provided the opportunity for insight into the patho-physiologic mechanism or into causality. Although it seems likely that an immunological mechanism is involved in these circumstances, no direct observation can sustain this thesis or disprove it. One of the most compelling study on this topic has been performed on progressive and regressive human melanomas [7]. The regressive melanomas present lymphocytic infiltrates that penetrates and disrupts the tumor cells, *in vivo* degeneration of the tumor, extension of

157

R.A. Robins and R.C. Rees (eds.), Cancer Immunology, 157–169.
© 2001 *Kluwer Academic Publishers. Printed in the Netherlands.*

angiogenesis and fibroblast proliferation, whereas the progressive melanoma were not showing these characteristics. Interestingly the regressive melanomas were infiltrated with a larger number of CD4+ T cells and associated with production of Th1 type cytokines more than that in progressive melanomas. Although the authors were not able to demonstrate that these cytokines were responsible for the rejection of the melanomas, these observations support the concept that the tumor can regress under the pressure of the immune system. Regressing tumors are difficult to study in humans since they have to be isolated before eradication and cannot, for obvious reasons, be inoculated in patients to test their *in vivo* immunogenicity. The experimental animal tumor models that have been established to study this topic have provided only partial answers, yet they have opened novel avenues of tumor immunology.

One of these models, the mouse mastocytoma p815, has been extensively studied for its immune rejection in syngeneic host and its ability to generate immune escape variants. A P815 variant, collected from the peritoneal cavity after partial rejection has been shown to be much less sensitive to specific Cytotolytic T Lymphocytes (CTL) than the parental P815 cells [8] due to the loss of an MHC-I epitope [9]. This phenomenon was exploited by Boon and collaborators to clone by "reverse immunology", P1A, the first molecularly defined MHC-I tumor epitope [10]. The same strategy has been used for the molecular characterization of the human equivalent of the mouse P1A antigen in melanoma, and other type of cancers [11]. However, the recent finding that P1A T cell-transgenic mice do not reject a P1A expressing tumor (J558), but reject the same tumor transfected with the co-stimulatory molecule B7-1 suggests that the effector function of P1A-specific CD8+ T lymphocytes is restrained in vivo [12].

Analysis of another type of model, the mouse UV-induced skin tumors had permitted the establishment of highly immunogenic tumors, which are most often regressors [1]. The results from systematic immunological analysis of a large number of these UV-induced tumors and their progressor and regressor variants have led to identification of tumor antigens presented by the MHC-I of the tumor cells and to provocative conclusions. (a) Regressor tumors expressed a seemingly infinite diversity of antigens, as no cross reactivity could be detected when a CTL clone raised against one tumor was tested against as many as 25 other syngeneic UV-induced tumor targets [13]. The concept that clonal T cells cannot recognize all the cells of a tumor has obvious consequences for immunotherapy against cancer. (b) The level of expression of MHC class I antigen shows no correlation with the *in vivo* tumor immunogenicity [13]. Identical observations have been seen in chemically induced tumors of varying immunogenicities [14]. (c) Finally, loss of a CTL-defined antigen does not always lead to progressive growth of the tumor *in vivo* [15]. These conclusions do not conflict with the key role of CD8+ T lymphocytes and MHC-I epitopes during the rejection of tumors, yet they suggest that other complementary mechanisms need to be considered for the understanding of the spontaneous rejection of tumors.

CO-SEGREGATION OF EXPRESSION OF THE INDUCIBLE HSP70, BUT NOT OF THE CONSTITUTIVE HSC70, WITH A REGRESSIVE PHENOTYPE.

Progressor and regressor tumors have also been isolated in rats. A transplantable colon carcinoma tumor has been fractionated to derive clones of various immunogencicities [16]. Several clones (named PRO for progressor) gave rise to tumors that, like the primary tumor, grew progressively, produced distant metastasis and killed the host. On the contrary, other clones (named REG for regressor) gave rise to tumors that first progressed for 2 or 3 weeks, regressed and completely disappeared. The regression of REG clones can be reverted by depletion of $\alpha\beta$-TCR positive lymphocytes, underlying the key role of the immune system in this rejection [17]. Interestingly, the PRO and REG tumors are cross-reactive suggesting that antigenic variation among these clones cannot explain by itself the difference of immunogenicity [17]. Surprisingly, classical immunological markers like MHC-I, MHC-II, I-CAM and cytokine expression were not associated with this difference of *in vivo* behavior of the different clones [18]. One important finding was that all the clones having the ability to synthesize the strictly inducible hsp70, and other inducible HSPs, were rejected by the immune system. Conversely, the clones that grew progressively do not synthesize the inducible hsp70 (see fig. 9.1).

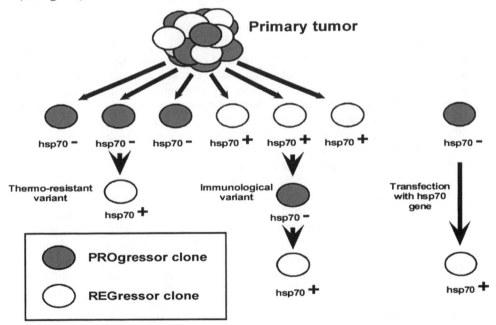

Figure 9.1. Co-segregation of tumor immunogenicity with expression of inducible hsp70. (From [18, 19] and unpublished data).

159

This observation was quite surprising since the inducible hsp70 has not been described as a classical stimulator of the specific immune system. In fact, HSP are classically considered as natural protector of stressed cells, in that they chaperone and refold proteins damaged by stress. Another study made in the same animal model has shown that the expression of hsp27 enhances the tumorigenicity of these rat colon carcinomas [20].

Altogether these observation suggest that some HSPs like the hsp27 and hsc70 have mainly a protector function, whereas other HSPs, like the inducible hsp70 have a functional duality of protector and immune stimulator. This idea is consistent with the clinical finding that high expression of constitutively expressed HSPs in human tumors correlate with poor clinical prognosis [21-23]. The co-segregation of tumor immunogenicity and expression of the inducible hsp70 in rat has been further confirmed through several selection cycles and transfection. An immunological variant of a REG clone has been generated by passaging in immuno-supressed animals. This clone had lost the ability to synthesis the inducible hsp70 after stress, and was able to form large progressively growing tumors in syngenic hosts (Fig 9.1). Further selection of this variant showed that the progressor phenotype is unstable, in that passage of this variant tumor in syngenic host indicate a regressor phenotype. Interestingly, this revertant had regained the ability to synthesize the inducible hsp70. Co-segregation of immunogenicity with induction of hsp70 was also tested in a thermo-resistant variant (Ph8) of a Progressor clone. From a non-immunologic selection process at 45^0C a clone that gained the ability to synthesize the inducible hsp70 was isolated (Fig.9.1). This thermoresistant variant was significantly more immunogenic than the parental PRO clone in syngenic animal but not in animal depleted of T lymphocytes. Importantly, the expression of classical immunological markers of the variants remained comparable to the parental clones and was not accountable for the increase or decrease of immunogenicity of the variants [18]. Another key observation is that the constitutively expressed hsc70 remain stable in these clones, suggesting that despite a high structural identity with the inducible hsp70, these two HSP of 70 kDa have profound different immunological properties. We have since confirmed the immunological importance of the inducible hsp70 by showing an increase in immunogenicity of the inducible hsp70-transfected fibrosarcoma MethA over the mock-transfected tumor (unpublished results).

Recently, Melcher et al. [19] have used a suicide gene transfer to generate non-apoptotic cell death in vivo and observed that non-apoptotic cell death increases tumor immunogenicity and induces hsp70 expression. Furthermore, stable transfection of colorectal tumors and melanomas with a plasmid encoding for cDNA of the inducible mouse hsp70 under the control of a constitutive promotor enhanced tumor immunogencity. Interestingly, inducible hsp70-transfected cells promoted more infiltration of T cells and antigen presenting cells (APC) and secretion of intra-tumoral Th1 type cytokines. Once again, the expression of the constitutive hsc70 remain stable in the transfected cells and cannot be accounted for the change of immunogenicity. These observations could be partially explained by the release and APC uptake of inducible hsp70, (additionally to other HSPs) from non-apoptotic dying cells [24]. These authors also reported that hsp induction occurs in vivo, but not in vitro, in clones of B16 transfected with IL-2 or GM-CSF genes, both of which are more immunogenic in vivo than the parental cell line. It seems, even if the reason for this increase is unclear, that hsp induction may play a broad role in the immune response against tumor. The recent association of the notion of cell death with the concept of danger signal is central in the understanding of physiological immunity and may be directly applicable to immunotherapy of cancer [25, 26]. The debate that is centered today on the balance between apoptotic and necrotic cell death might find its solution in the concept that dying cells that do not release HSPs should be poorly immunogenic [27].

Independently of this work Wells et al. [28] have reported that transfection of B16 melanoma variant deficient for presentation of antigen by the MHC-I with the gene encoding the human inducible hsp70 restore endogenous antigen presentation to specific CD8$^+$ T cells. The hsp70 transfection significantly increased MHC-I expression, measured by conformation-dependent antibodies suggesting that hsp70 participates in the processing of intracellular peptides. This idea was reinforced by the observation that transfection of hsp70 in cells lacking the activity of the transporter associated with antigen presentation (TAP) did not improve antigen presentation to specific CD8$^+$ T cells. These results are consistent with the proposed idea that HSPs participate in the processing of immunogenic peptides to the MHC I pathway [29], yet the respective role of the inducible hsp70 and constitutive hsc70 in this pathway remains unclear. Interestingly, similar observations have been obtained using cells transfected with the mycobacterial hsp65 suggesting that the chaperoning function of these proteins is conserved across distant forms of life [30].

Altogether these findings promote the idea, that we are currently exploring, that the inducible hsp70 can participate in the stimulation of the immune system differently than the constitutive hsc70.

IMMUNIZATION WITH TUMOR-DERIVED HEAT SHOCK PROTEIN OF 70 KDA (HSP70/HSC70), NATURALLY OR ARTIFICIALLY COMPLEXED WITH ANTIGENIC PEPTIDES.

In order to understand the immunological properties and the putative differences between the inducible hsp70 and the constitutive hsc70 we considered their ability to generate specific immunity after isolation from tumor cells. One key property of the hsp70/hsc70, which explains their specific immunogenicity, is related to their ability to chaperone peptides. Udono and Srivastava [31] first showed that tumor-derived hsp70/hsc70-peptide complexes, immunized specifically against tumor from which the HSP was isolated. Remarkably, the hsp70/hsc70 purified from tumor lose their immunogenicity after elution of the peptides they chaperone, demonstrating that the hsp70/hsc70 are not immunogenic per se whereas the hsp70/hsc70-peptide complexes are. Induction of a powerful specific anti-tumor immunity is not restricted to the hsp70/hsc70. Tumor rejection assays, induction of cytotoxic T lymphocytes (CTL) and anti-viral responses have been carried out successfully not only with hsp70/hsc70 immunization but also with various HSPs: gp96, hsp90, and calreticulin (see review by Ménoret and Chandawarkar [32]). Immunization with other HSPs, (grp170 and hsp110) that physiologically accept peptides in the cytosol and the ER ([33], Subjeck, personal communication) are under investigation and may increase the number of HSP-based vaccines. Since tumors are not always available in large quantity, a major challenge remaines the development of a procedure to simultaneously isolate these HSPs from the same sample. We have recently reported that hsp40, hsp60, hsc70, hsp70, hsp84, hsp86, and gp96 (grp94) but not BiP (grp78) and calreticulin can be separated from a single tumor sample in one step using heparin-agarose chromatography [34]. Individual HSP can then be further isolated to homogeneity and used alone or in combination with other HSPs.

It is worth noting that the immunogenicity of HSPs has been discovered, without pre-established view, by trying to isolate the immunological active principal of tumors among the multitude of molecules in the cell. The vaccination against cancer, using tumor-derived HSP-PCs was generalizable not only across different species, but also across tumor types, irrespective of their histology, or means of generation. This strategy was shown to be successful in rats, mice, even in *Xenopus*; against chemically-induced tumors, UV-induced tumors and spontaneous tumors of different histological origins (fibrosarcomas, thymomas, prostate cancers, lung carcinomas, melanomas, colonic cancers), under prophylactic and therapeutic strategies (see reviews by Ménoret and Chandawarkar [32], and by Srivastava et al. [27]). The possibility to immunize with *in vitro* reconstituted HSP-immunogenic peptide complexes has also been demonstrated [35]. Remarkably, immunogenic peptides complexed with another carrier, the mouse serum albumin, was not able to induce immunogenic peptide-specific CD8+ T lymphocytes *in vivo*, suggesting that HSPs can be considered as chaperone molecules with adjuvant properties. The mechanism by which the HSP-PC immunization primes CD8+ T lymphocytes has been proposed [29, 36], tested [37] and described in detail elsewhere [27, 32]. The current view is that the antigenic peptides chaperoned by the HSPs can be endocytosed by a putative receptor expressed on professional APC and represented by their MHC-I in a proteasome and TAP-dependent manner. The APC then home to the lymphatic organ where they prime specifically the CD8+ T lymphocytes responsible for the rejection of the tumor.

Independently of the ability to immunize against tumor and virus infected cells it has been reported that an HSP of 70 kDa is a putative NK target on the surface of tumor cells [38]. The characterization of the surface protein revealed that this protein is recognized by an inducible-hsp70 specific antibody, however, the expression of this HSP of 70 kDa is not inducible under stress suggesting that either its regulation is compromised or that a new member of this family of protein is being implicated in NK recognition.

Collectively these findings have promoted the thesis that HSPs might be *"the"*, or one of the physiological agents of priming [27, 37] We believe that the individual purification and the exploration of the structural differences between the inducible hsp70 and constitutive hsc70 will reveal new insights into the physiological ways by which these two HSPs respectively influence the priming and expansion of the immune response.

DIFFERENCE OF PEPTIDE BINDING DOMAINS BETWEEN THE INDUCIBLE HSP70 AND CONSTITUTIVE HSC70.

The peptide-binding domains of most HSP have been identified. Recently, crystallization of hsp70 and hsp90 revealed a 3-dimensional domain capable of binding peptide[39, 40]. Li and Srivastava [41], and Udono and Srivastava [31] showed for the first time that peptides bound under physiological conditions inside the cell can be separated from the chaperone itself by trifluoroacetic acid treatment (gp96) or by ATP treatment (hsc70/hsp70). Conversely, hsc70/hsp70, gp96 [35] and calreticulin [42] can be conjugated *in vitro* via a non-covalent bond with synthetic peptides. Re-constituted HSP-peptide complexes could also elicit significant anti-tumor immunity when tested *in vivo*. A possible reason for the immunological differences between the hsp70 and the hsc70 might be related to a structural variation in their ability to chaperone peptides.

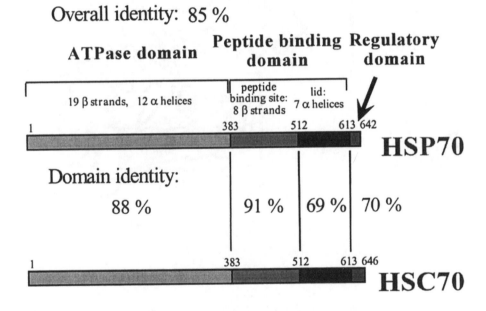

Figure 9.2. amino-acid identity between the inducible hsp70 and the constitutive hsc70. Amino acid percent identity between the inducible mouse hsp70 (NCBI accession NB: M35021) and the constitutive mouse hsc70 (NCBI accession NB: U73744) was produced by LALIGN (GENESTREAM Network Service, Montpellier, France). The ATPase domain and the peptide binding domain were respectively defined according to the 3 dimensional structure of the amino-terminal region of the bovine hsc70 [43] and to the 3 dimensional structure of the carboxyl-terminal region of the E. Coli hsp70, DnaK [39].

The genetic identity between the constitutive hsc70 and inducible hsp70 is high (85% identity). The amino-terminal ATPase domain is conserved (88%) as well as the peptide-binding pocket of the peptide binding site (91%) (Fig.9.2).On the contrary, the lid (amino acid 512 to 615) of the peptide-binding domain shows 69% identity between the hsp70 and the hsc70 (Fig.9.2). The carboxyl extremity of these 2 proteins is also poorly conserved (70%). The function of this last domain (amino acid 615 to 642) is not yet defined neither was it crystallized, it could be a part of the lid and/or an important sequence related to the stability of the protein [44]. The importance of the Lid of the peptide-binding site of the HSP70 is illustrated on figure 9.3.

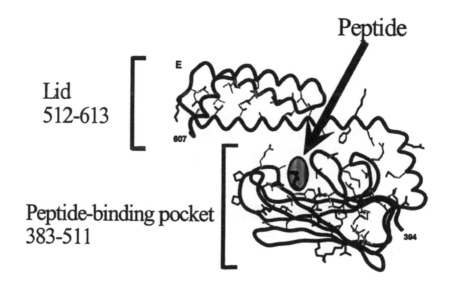

Figure 9.3. Interaction of hsp70 (DnaK) with peptide.The crystal of the *E. Coli* hsp70, DnaK, was obtained from a recombinant fragment missing the ATPase domain and the extreme carboxyl-fragment (amino acid 608-638) of the protein [39]. DnaK was crystallized in presence of a synthetic peptide (NRLLLTG) which interact with this chaperone through numerous van der Waals contacts from its side chains and seven main-chain hydrogen bounds, as well as additional main-chain van der Waals interactions

The crystal structure of the *E Coli* hsp70, DnaK, shows that the peptide is bound in an extended conformation through a channel defined by loops from a β sandwich. An α-helical domain (lid) stabilizes the complex, but does not contact the peptide directly.

This domain is rotated in the molecule of a second crystal lattice, which suggest a model of conformation-dependent substrate binding that features a latch mechanism for maintaining long life complexes. The fact that the main structural heterogeneity between the inducible hsp70 and the constitutive hsc70 resides in the lid of the peptide-binding site suggests that the quality and/or the quantity of peptides chaperoned by the proteins is different.

This concept is consistent with the observation that the chaperoning activity of hsp70 was enhanced after heat shock treatment, whereas no differences were observed for the hsc70 [45]. The differences in the lid of the peptide-binding domain of the hsp70 and the hsc70 may play a crucial function in the stability of the hsp70-peptide interaction inside the cell and outside the cell after cell lysis. It may also participate in the endogenous selection of immunogenic peptides, promoting an intracellular self/non-self discrimination by interacting differently with intracellular immunogenic peptides derived from unfolded, aggregated, mutated, or pathogen-derived proteins.

IMPLICATION FOR IMMUNOTHERAPY OF CANCER AND BEYOND.

It would be of interest here to imagine that the physiological conditions promoting the expression of the inducible HSPs, like systemic fever, metabolic starvation, chemical stress and intracellular protein aggregation might be implicated in spontaneous rejection of tumor. We have previously discussed that the micro-environmental conditions of the tumor, i.e. hypoxia, variable pH, low nutriment have a profound influence on the immune response against cancer [46]. The new development of hyperthermia of cancer at a "fever-like temperature" (38^0C -39.5^0C) promotes the idea that the immune system might be extremely sensitive to conditions that enhance expression of inducible HSPs [47]. Such parameters are clearly difficult to control and evaluate in humans, yet they can be more easily evaluated in animal models. The molecular regulation of the hsp70 and hsc70 genes has been studied in detail (see reviews by Morimoto [48] and Wu [49]). It remains that the *in vivo* expression of hsp70 in tumors is extremely heterogeneous (Ménoret *et al.* unpublished results, [50, 51]), it differs from tissue to tissue even in absence of external stress [52] and may even vary at a single cell level in non-transformed lymphocytes [51]. The basis for these variations in expression is still unclear, yet it may influence considerably the immune system. One may also propose that human tumors expressing inducible hsp70 should be of good prognostic for immunotherapeutical interventions and that inducible hsp70-derived human tumor should constitute a more immunogenic anti-cancer vaccine than the constitutive hsc70-derived tumors.

An interesting approach has been to vaccinate mice with hsp70 genetically fused with a known antigen circumventing the chaperoning function of these proteins [53]. Immunization with both the mycobacterial and mouse hsp70 gene fused with the ovalbumin gene elicited a specific CD8[+] T cell response. Recently the region of the hsp70 required for the CTL priming has been mapped in a 200 amino acid segment of its ATPase domain [54]. The ability of the hsp70 fusion protein to elicit CD8+ response

165

in absence of CD4+ T cells has been shown in CD4 knock-out transgenic mice suggesting that this strategy might be useful for development of HIV therapy.

The use of hsp70/hsc70 based vaccine against cancer and infectious diseases is currently entering into a development phase for the treatment of lymphomas and breast cancers. Currently, the immunological difference between the inducible and constitutive hsp of 70 kDa is under intense examination. It will participate in both the fundamental understanding of the immune system and the new generation of HSP-based anti-cancer vaccines that might be of enormous benefit for public health.

It is worth noting that the inducible mouse hsp70 is encoded on Chromosome 17, in the H-2 histocompatibility locus whereas the constitutive hsc70 is on the Chromosome 9 ([55], Hunt personal communication). By analogy with the localization of other immunologically important genes in the H-2 locus, (TAP1, TAP, LMP2, LMP7, TNFα, TNFβ, MHC-I, MHC-II and MHC-III) it is tantalizing to suggest that the inducible hsp70 gene cosegregates with immunological functions. This hypothesis has been tested in the *Botryllus schlosseri* [56], a colonial protochordate that can generate an allo-recognition mediated by blood cells after contact with another colony and controlled by a single Mendelian locus that might be homologous to the vertebrate MHC. The authors have cloned two inducible hsp70 genes exhibiting the characteristics of MHC-linked hsp70 genes of the vertebrates [57] and found that the segregation patterns of hsp70 genes is not linked to the historecognition locus of *B. schlosseri*. On the contrary an inducible MHC-encoded hsp70 in the ascidian *Ciona intestinalis* has been shown to participate to a self / non-self discrimination during the regulation of gamete auto-fecondation [58].

These observations and the other studies presented here argue that the heat shock proteins in general and the inducible hsp70 in particular should be considered as the classical components of the immune system. The integration of these highly conserved proteins into the immune system during evolution remains unclear. Nevertheless, the hypothesis that the HSPs were an important part of the primitive immunological backbone [59] may have direct consequences for the understanding and for the immunological treatment of cancers and infectious diseases.

ACKNOWLEDGMENTS

The author is grateful to Dr. Zihai Li and Dr. Pramod K. Srivastava for their beneficial comments and criticisms and to Gillian Bell for her critical reading of the manuscript. The author is supported by a startup grant from the University of Connecticut, a grant from the American Cancer Society (ACSIN 152-O-169) and a grant from the National Institue of Health (RO1CA/AI84042-01).

REFERENCES

1. Ward PL and Schreiber H, MHC I restricted T cells and immune surveillance against ultraviolet light-induced tumors. Semin Cancer Biol, 1991; 2: 321-328.

2. Lokich J, Spontaneous regression of metastatic renal cancer - Case report and literature review. Am J Clin Oncol-Cancer Clin Trials, 1997; 20: 416-418.
3. Zorn E and Hercend T, A natural cytotoxic T cell response in a spontaneously regressing human melanoma targets a neoantigen resulting from a somatic point mutation. Eur J Immunol, 1999; 29: 592-601.
4. Berd D, Cancer vaccines: Reborn or just recycled? Semin Oncol, 1998; 25: 605-610.
5. Woodruff MFA, Cellular Heterogeneity in Tumors. Br J Cancer, 1983; 47: 589-594.
6. Papac RJ, Spontaneous regression of cancer: Possible mechanisms. In Vivo, 1998; 12: 571-578.
7. Lowes MA, Bishop GA, Crotty K, Barnetson RS, and Halliday GM, T helper 1 cytokine mRNA is increased in spontaneously regressing primary melanomas. J Invest Dermatol, 1997; 108: 914-919.
8. Biddison WE and Palmer JC, Development of tumor cell resistance to syngeneic cell-mediated cytotoxicity during growth of ascitic mastocytoma P815Y. Proc Natl Acad Sci U S A, 1977; 74: 329-333.
9. Uyttenhove C, Maryanski J, and Boon T, Escape of Mouse Mastocytoma P815 after Nearly Complete Rejection Is Due to Antigen-Loss Variants Rather Than Immunosuppression. J Exp Med, 1983; 157: 1040-1052.
10. van den Eynde B, Lethe B, Vanpel A, Deplaen E, and Boon T, The Gene Coding for a Major Tumor Rejection Antigen of Tumor P815 Is Identical to the Normal Gene of Syngeneic Dba-2 Mice. J Exp Med, 1991; 173: 1373-1384.
11. Boon T and van der Bruggen P, Human Tumor-Antigens Recognized By T-Lymphocytes. J Exp Med, 1996; 183: 725-729.
12. Sarma S, Guo Y, Guilloux Y, Lee C, Bai XF, and Liu Y, Cytotoxic T lymphocytes to an unmutated tumor rejection antigen P1A: Normal development but restrained effector function in vivo. J Exp Med, 1999; 189: 811-820.
13. Ward PL, Koeppen HK, Hurteau T, Rowley DA, and Schreiber H, Major Histocompatibility Complex Class-I and Unique Antigen Expression by Murine Tumors That Escaped from Cd8+ T-Cell- Dependent Surveillance. Cancer Res, 1990; 50: 3851-3858.
14. Zennadi R, Garrigue L, Ringeard S, Menoret A, Blanchardie P, and Lependu J, Analysis of Factors Associated with the Tumorigenic Potential of 12 Tumor Clones Derived from a Single-Rat Colon Adenocarcinoma. Int J Cancer, 1992; 52: 934-940.
15. Haywood GR and McKhann CF, Antigenic specificities on murine sarcoma cells. Reciprocal relationship between normal transplantation antigens (H2) and tumour specific immunogenicity. J Exp Med, 1971; 133: 1171-1187.
16. Martin F, Caignard A, Jeannin JF, Leclerc A, and Martin M, Selection by Trypsin of 2-Sublines of Rat Colon Cancer-Cells Forming Progressive or Regressive Tumors. Int J Cancer, 1983; 32: 623-627.
17. Caignard A, Martin MS, Michel MF, and Martin F, Interaction between 2 Cellular Subpopulations of a Rat Colonic- Carcinoma When Inoculated to the Syngeneic Host. Int J Cancer, 1985; 36: 273-279.
18. Menoret A, Patry Y, Burg C, and Lependu J, Co-Segregation of Tumor Immunogenicity with Expression of Inducible but Not Constitutive Hsp70 in Rat Colon Carcinomas. J Immunol, 1995; 155: 740-747.
19. Melcher A, Todryk S, Hardwick N, Ford M, Jacobson M, and Vile RG, Tumor immunogenicity is determined by the mechanism of cell death via induction of heat shock protein expression. Nat Med, 1998; 4: 581-587.
20. Garrido C, Fromentin A, Bonnotte B, Favre N, Moutet M, Arrigo AP, Mehlen P, and Solary E, Heat shock protein 27 enhances the tumorigenicity of immunogenic rat colon carcinoma cell clones. Cancer Res, 1998; 58: 5495-5499.
21. Ciocca DR, Clark GM, Tandon AK, Fuqua SAW, Welch WJ, and McGuire WL, Heat-Shock Protein-Hsp70 in Patients with Axillary Lymph Node- Negative Breast-Cancer - Prognostic Implications. J Natl Cancer Inst, 1993; 85: 570-574.
22. Kimura E, Enns RE, Alcaraz JE, Arboleda J, Slamon DJ, and Howell SB, Correlation of the Survival of Ovarian-Cancer Patients with Messenger-Rna Expression of the 60-Kd Heat-Shock Protein Hsp-60. J Clin Oncol, 1993; 11: 891-898.
23. Jameel A, Law M, Coombes RC, and Luqmani YA, Significance of Heat-Shock Protein-90 as a Prognostic Indicator in Breast-Cancer. Int J Oncol, 1993; 2: 1075-1080.
24. Todryk S, Melcher AA, Hardwick N, Linardakis E, Bateman A, Colombo MP, Stoppacciaro A, and Vile RG, Heat shock protein 70 induced during tumor cell killing induces Th1 cytokines and targets immature dendritic cell precursors to enhance antigen uptake. J Immunol, 1999; 163: 1398-1408.
25. Matzinger P, Tolerance, danger, and the extended family. Annu Rev Immunol, 1994; 12: 991-1045.

26. Langman RE and Cohn M, Terra Firma: A retreat from "danger". J Immunol, 1996; 157: 4273-4276.
27. Srivastava PK, Menoret A, Basu S, Binder RJ, and McQuade KL, Heat shock proteins come of age: Primitive functions acquire new roles in an adaptive world. Immunity, 1998; 8: 657-665.
28. Wells AD, Rai SK, Salvato MS, Band H, and Malkovsky M, Hsp72-mediated augmentation of MHC class I surface expression and endogenous antigen presentation. Int Immunol, 1998; 10: 609-617.
29. Srivastava PK, Udono H, Blachere NE, and Li ZH, Heat-Shock Proteins Transfer Peptides During Antigen-Processing and Ctl Priming. Immunogenetics, 1994; 39: 93-98.
30. Wells AD, Rai SK, Salvato MS, Band H, and Malkovsky M, Restoration of MHC class I surface expression and endogenous antigen presentation by a molecular chaperone. Scand J Immunol, 1997; 45: 605-612.
31. Udono H and Srivastava PK, Heat-Shock Protein-70 Associated Peptides Elicit Specific Cancer Immunity. J Exp Med, 1993; 178: 1391-1396.
32. Menoret A and Chandawarkar R, Heat-shock protein-based anticancer immunotherapy: An idea whose time has come. Semin Oncol, 1998; 25: 654-660.
33. Spee P, Subjeck J, and Neefjes J, Identification of novel peptide binding proteins in the endoplasmic reticulum: ERp72, calnexin, and grp170. Biochemistry (Mosc), 1999; 38: 10559-10566.
34. Menoret A and Bell G, Purification of multiple heat shock proteins from a single tumor sample. J Immunol Methods, 2000; 237: 119-130.
35. Blachere NE, Li ZH, Chandawarkar RY, Suto R, Jaikaria NS, Basu S, Udono H, and Srivastava PK, Heat shock protein-peptide complexes, reconstituted in vitro, elicit peptide-specific cytotoxic T lymphocyte response and tumor immunity. J Exp Med, 1997; 186: 1315-1322.
36. Udono H, Levey DL, and Srivastava PK, Cellular-Requirements for Tumor-Specific Immunity Elicited by Heat-Shock Proteins - Tumor Rejection Antigen-Gp96 Primes Cd8+ T-Cells in-Vivo. Proc Natl Acad Sci U S A, 1994; 91: 3077-3081.
37. Suto R and Srivastava PK, A Mechanism for the Specific Immunogenicity of Heat-Shock Protein-Chaperoned Peptides. Science, 1995; 269: 1585-1588.
38. Multhoff G, Botzler C, Jennen L, Schmidt J, Ellwart J, and Issels R, Heat shock protein 72 on tumor cells - A recognition structure for natural killer cells. J Immunol, 1997; 158: 4341-4350.
39. Zhu XT, Zhao X, Burkholder WF, Gragerov A, Ogata CM, Gottesman ME, and Hendrickson WA, Structural analysis of substrate binding by the molecular chaperone DnaK. Science, 1996; 272: 1606-1614.
40. Stebbins CE, Russo AA, Schneider C, Rosen N, Hartl FU, and Pavletich NP, Crystal structure of an Hsp90-geldanamycin complex: Targeting of a protein chaperone by an antitumor agent. Cell, 1997; 89: 239-250.
41. Li ZH and Srivastava PK, Tumor Rejection Antigen Gp96/Grp94 Is an Atpase - Implications for Protein-Folding and Antigen Presentation. EMBO J, 1993; 12: 3143-3151.
42. Basu S and Srivastava PK, Calreticulin, a peptide-binding chaperone of the endoplasmic reticulum, elicits tumor- and peptide-specific immunity. J Exp Med, 1999; 189: 797-802.
43. Flaherty KM, Delucaflaherty C, and McKay DB, 3-Dimensional Structure of the Atpase Fragment of a 70k Heat- Shock Cognate Protein. Nature, 1990; 346: 623-628.
44. Boice JA and Hightower LE, A mutational study of the peptide-binding domain of Hsc70 guided by secondary structure prediction. J Biol Chem, 1997; 272: 24825-24831.
45. Angelidis CE, Lazaridis I, and Pagoulatos GN, Aggregation of hsp70 and hsc70 in vivo is distinct and temperature-dependent and their chaperone function is directly related to non-aggregated forms. Eur J Biochem, 1999; 259: 505-512.
46. Menoret A and Srivastava DK, *The cancer microenvironment and its impact on immune response to cancer.*, in *Molecular approaches to tumor immunotherapy*, L. Yang, Editor. 1998, World Scientific. p. 109-221.
47. Repasky EA, Tims E, Pritchard M, and Burd R, Characterisation of mild whole body hyperthermia protocols using human breast, ovarian and colon tumours grown in severe combinded immunodeficient mice. Infect Dis Obstet Gynecol, 1999; 7: 91-97.
48. Morimoto RI, Cells in Stress - Transcriptional Activation of Heat-Shock Genes. Science, 1993; 259: 1409-1410.
49. Wu C, Heat shock transcription factors: structure and regulation. Annu Rev Cell Dev Biol, 1995; 11: 441-469.
50. Dressel R, Johnson JP, and Gunther E, Heterogeneous patterns of constitutive and heat shock induced expression of HLA-linked HSP70-1 and HSP70-2 heat shock genes in human melanoma cell lines. Melanoma Res, 1998; 8: 482-492.

51. Dressel R and Gunther E, Heat-induced expression of MHC-linked HSP70 genes in lymphocytes varies at the single-cell level. J Cell Biochem, 1999; 72: 558-569.
52. Tanguay RM, Wu Y, and Khandjian EW, Tissue-Specific Expression of Heat-Shock Proteins of the Mouse in the Absence of Stress. Dev Genet, 1993; 14: 112-118.
53. Suzue K, Zhou XZ, Eisen HN, and Young RA, Heat shock fusion proteins as vehicles for antigen delivery into the major histocompatibility complex class I presentation pathway. Proc Natl Acad Sci U S A, 1997; 94: 13146-13151.
54. Huang Q, Richmond JFL, Suzue K, Eisen HN, and Young RA, In vivo cytotoxic T lymphocyte elicitation by mycobacterial heat shock protein 70 fusion proteins maps to a discrete domain and is CD4(+) T cell independent. J Exp Med, 2000; 191: 403-408.
55. Hunt CR, Gasser DL, Chaplin DD, Pierce JC, and Kozak CA, Chromosomal Localization of 5 Murine Hsp70 Gene Family Members - Hsp70-1, Hsp70-2, Hsp70-3, Hsc70t, and Grp78. Genomics, 1993; 16: 193-198.
56. Fagan MB and Weissman IL, Linkage analysis of HSP70 genes and historecognition locus in Botryllus schlosseri. Immunogenetics, 1998; 47: 468-476.
57. Fagan MB and Weissman IL, Sequence and characterization of two HSP70 genes in the colonial protochordate Botryllus schlosseri. Immunogenetics, 1996; 44: 134-142.
58. Marino R, Pinto MR, Cotelli F, Lamia CL, and De Santis R, The hsp70 protein is involved in the acquisition of gamete self-sterility in the ascidian Ciona intestinalis. Development, 1998; 125: 899-907.
59. Srivastava PK and Heike M, Tumour specific immunogenicity of stress induced proteins: convergence of two evolutionary pathways of antigen presentation? Semin Immunol, 1991; 3: 57-64.

10
Anti-idiotypic vaccination

LG DURRANT, I SPENDLOVE AND RA ROBINS

INTRODUCTION

An effective cancer vaccine should stimulate cytotoxic T cells (CTL), helper T cells and antibodies. The CTLs will efficiently kill all tumour cells expressing target antigen and class I MHC. Helper T cells responding to MHC class II presented epitopes will help in the production of CTLs but will also migrate to tissues expressing locally presented target antigen. Once they have localised within the tissues they will release the cytotoxic cytokines (TNFα, TNFβ, IFNγ) and recruit non specific effector cells such as macrophages; there is also evidence that the products of CD4 T cells can damage the vasculature of tumours[1]. All of these effects will result in tumour cell death of antigen positive or negative cells. They are therefore synergistic with CTL killing. T helper cells can also recruit natural killer (NK) cells that will kill any tumour cells that have lost MHC expression[2]. As this is a common mechanism for tumours to evade CTL killing it is an important component of any immune response induced by a cancer vaccine. The potential of antibody responses to contribute to anti-tumour effects is less clear. The 'type 1' T cells that help in the activation of CTLs can help in the production of specific subclasses of antibodies (IgG2a in mice and IgG1in humans). These antibodies will kill any tumour cell expressing target antigen by antibody dependent cellular cytotoxicity that is mediated by Fc receptor expressing leucocytes, including NK cells. T helper cell recruitment of NK cells into tumour tissues is therefore also essential for antibody mediated tumour killing. Complement fixation could also play a role, either as a lytic effector mechanism, or as a trigger for activating local immune responses. The remainder of this chapter will now consider how an anti-idiotypic antibody can fulfil these requirements for this effective cancer vaccine.

ANTI-IDIOTYPIC ANTIBODIES

Anti-idiotypic antibodies are produced by in response to unique features of the binding site of an antibody, and anti-idiotypic antibodies can themselves stimulate immune

R.A. Robins and R.C. Rees (eds.), Cancer Immunology, 171–180.

responses; this sequence of relationships is described as an anti-idiotypic network[3]. In the terminology of these networks, an antibody which recognises an antigen is described as an Ab1. Antibodies recognise antigens via the interaction of hypervariable loops (complementarity determining regions, CDRs). These loops are constrained by the framework regions of the antibody. The consequence of these features is the positioning of the CDRs in prominent surface locations that allow them to interact with specific antigens. This overall conformation, termed the idiotype, is itself immunogenic and can result in the generation of anti-idiotypic antibodies or Ab2s. Anti-idiotypic antibodies can also induce a third antibody (Ab3). Since Ab1 binds to both antigen and Ab2 these molecules may show sequence of structural similarity. Hence Ab3 that is stimulated by Ab2 might also recognise the original antigen. Thus anti-idiotypic antibodies can mimic antigenic epitopes and be used as surrogate antigens. The ease of production of anti-idiotypic antibodies makes them attractive candidates for cancer vaccines.

Can anti-idiotypic antibodies stimulate anti-tumour T cell responses?

Naïve T cells can only be activated by antigen that has been processed and presented on MHC molecules of antigen presenting cells in the appropriate stage of differentiation/activation, including expression of the costimulatory molecules CD80 and CD86. These costimulatory molecules provide a vital second signal via CD28 on the T cells. In contrast T cells encountering signal 1 (peptide/MHC) on a cell that does not express the appropriate costimulatory environment, receives a negative signal and is anergised. As discussed in Chapter 1, the only cells thought to stimulate naïve T cells are dendritic cells that constantly survey tissues then migrate to lymph nodes. If they have been activated they express costimulatory molecules and activate naïve T cells. In contrast if they have not been activated they fail to provide costimulation and anergise naïve T cells[4]. An effective cancer vaccine must therefore target activated dendritic cells. The signal that activates dendritic cells is poorly defined although bacterial products such as LPS or cytokines such as TNFα can elicit the response. More recently Matzinger has proposed her danger hypothesis that states that antigen presenting cells are activated by "danger"[5]. This could be unprogrammed cell death or necrosis that results in the release of intracellular molecules such as mitochondria or heat shock proteins.

Human anti-idiotypic antibodies may be particularly effective at targeting activated antigen presenting cells. Dendritic cells constantly survey tissues where they can either endocytose antigen by fluid phase macropinocytosis or by receptor mediated endocytosis. The latter process is more efficient and can result in a 1,000 fold greater accumulation of antigen than pinocytosis. Receptor mediated uptake is also reported to favour processing into the class I pathway[6]. Antigen presenting cells express both the high (CD64) and low affinity (CD32) Fc receptor for internalisation of either monomeric of complexed human IgG respectively, and studies with fusion proteins have demonstrated efficient antigen presentation using constructs containing intact Fc [7]. A human monoclonal antibody can therefore be rapidly internalised by antigen presenting cells by Fc mediated endocytosis. Interestingly resting dendritic cells do not express the high affinity receptor but can be induced to express it by inflammatory cytokines. Thus monomeric human anti-idiotypic antibodies can target activated dendritic cells. Mouse Fc binds poorly to CD64 and therefore mouse anti-idiotypes are very poor at stimulating unprimed human T cells. A mouse anti-idiotypic antibody that mimics CEA could stimulate T cell responses *in vitro* with lymphocytes from cancer patients but could not stimulate unprimed T cells from healthy donors. However when this anti-idiotypic antibody was chimerised to a human IgG1 antibody it stimulated strong proliferative responses in unprimed T cells [8].

The various types of antigens that can be targeted on tumour cells by T cells are discussed in detail in the early chapters of this volume: a major subdivision is between tumour specific and tumour associated antigens. Tumour specific antigens are novel proteins only expressed in tumours as a result of mutations. They include the products of both oncogenes and tumour supressor genes. T cells recognising these antigens have the advantage that they will only attack tumour cells and normal cells will be unaffected. Evidence that anti-idiotypic networks may be stimulated by products of tumour supressor genes was provided by the elegant studies of Ruiz et al. Resistance to tumour challenge was induced by induction of an anti-idiotypic network by immunisation of mice with a monoclonal antibody that was specific for mutated p53. The immunised mice produced IgG antibodies to p53 (Ab3) and mounted a cytotoxic reaction to a tumour line bearing mutated p53[9].

Tumour associated antigens are differentiation antigens that are highly over-expressed on tumour cells as compared to normal tissues. Many peptides can be selected from these antigens that can bind to a wide range of MHC antigens and stimulate effective T cell responses. The main disadvantage of this approach is that T cells that recognise these antigens may also attack normal cells. The solution may be to select epitopes from these antigens that bind with moderate affinity to MHC. These epitopes will be expressed at a lower frequency on MHC compared to higher affinity epitopes. The affinity of the T-cell receptor interaction with peptide-MHC must also be considered. High affinity T cells capable of responding to low levels of peptide expression may be deleted from the repertoire. This will have several consequences: firstly, T cells recognising moderate affinity epitopes may avoid negative selection in the thymus. Secondly that the level of expression of these epitopes on normal cells will be below the threshold for T cell recognition. This will mean that dendritic cells surveying normal tissues will express low levels of these epitopes. As there is also no danger signal these dendritic cells will fail to provide either signal 1 or 2 to the T cells specific for moderate affinity epitopes. The result will be that these T cells will be neither anergised or activated by normal tissues. However if a cancer vaccine presents large amounts of the moderate affinity epitope in the context of danger, then the dendritic cells will present both signal one and signal two and activate T cells. These activated T cells will leave the lymph node and migrate to tissues expressing antigen and MHC. This will include both normal and tumour tissues. The normal tissues will still only present moderate affinity epitopes that would be below the threshold for T cell killing. However tumour cells over-expressing tumour associated antigens would result in increased expression of even the moderate affinity epitopes to above the threshold for T cell killing. In experimental systems, conditions for driving T cell responses to tumour associated antigen to cause tumour rejection without auto-immune damage have been demonstrated[10].

A cancer vaccine targeting a tumour associated antigen must therefore efficiently present the moderate affinity epitope in the context of "danger". This can be achieved by immunising with the moderate affinity epitope alone to prevent competition for MHC occupancy with higher affinity epitopes. One approach is to use peptides but these are rapidly degraded in vivo and are poorly taken up by antigen presenting cells. In contrast a human anti-idiotypic antibody is very stable *in vivo*, is efficiently internalised by antigen presenting cells by receptor mediated endocytosis and is unlikely to contain any competing high affinity T cell epitopes. Therefore a human antibody can be used to effectively present a selected moderate affinity epitope from a tumour associated antigen. This can be achieved by either cloning a human anti-idiotypic antibody from a cancer patient [11] or by directly inserting a T cell epitope into the CDR region of a human antibody [12]. It is interesting that anti-idiotypic antibody immunisation appears to be effective in the context of aluminium hydroxide (traditionally viewed as a mild adjuvant) [13, 14].

The human anti-idiotypic monoclonal antibody 105AD7 was isolated from a cancer patient receiving the anti-CD55 monoclonal antibody, 791T/36[15] for diagnostic imaging. He made a very strong anti-idiotypic response that was cloned and characterised[11]. 105AD7 bound specifically to the binding site of 791T/36 and could induce antibodies in mice that bound to CD55 and could prime DTH responses in mice and rats to human tumour cells expressing the CD55 antigen[16]. Over 200 patients have now received this human anti-idiotypic vaccine with no associated toxicity. Inflammatory T cell responses were measured both in the blood and at the tumour site of immunised patients[17-20].

For an anti-idiotypic antibody to stimulate T cells that also recognise antigen, a similar T cell epitope must be processed and presented on MHC from both anti-idiotype and antigen. An anti-idiotypic antibody that mimics hepatitis B surface antigen showed significant amino acid homology between antigen and its CDRH3[21]. The minimal B and T cell epitope was defined as a 6 amino acid peptide expressed by both the anti-idiotypic antibody and the antigen. Similarly a mouse anti-idiotypic antibody which mimics CEA (3H1) showed significant homology between its CDRL1 region and the N terminus of CEA. Peptide based upon either of these regions could stimulate T cell from patients who had been immunised with the 3H1 anti-idiotype[22].

A conceptual difficulty arises with the presence of T cell epitopes in the variable region of anti-idiotypes, because the T cell essentially recognises short peptide sequences, whereas antibodies recognise the topography of the native antigen. Thus, how can sequence information be transferred from the antigen to the anti-idiotype through the medium of the Ab1? In some cases this could be because the anti-idiotype uses a similar amino acid sequence to mimic the antigen; there are remarkable examples of this type in the literature[23]. Another possibility is that helper T cells restricted by antigen specific peptide sequence would preferentially favour the expansion of anti-idiotypic B cell clones whose antibody contained the same sequences, because these would be presented by the B cell and allow its interaction with the helper T cell[24].

The human anti-idiotype 105AD7 is unusual in that it shows three areas of homology between 3 of its CDR regions and 3 regions of CD55. All three regions on both anti-idiotype and antigen define the binding site for the Ab1, 791T/36. However only the CDRH3 region stimulates T cell responses. T cell epitope analysis of the

CDRH3 region identifies peptides that could bind to HLAA1,A3 and A24 and HLA DR1,3,7. Ninety six percent of all patients who show a T cell response to 105AD7 vaccination are of the predicted phenotype[14]. Interestingly the epitopes in 105AD7 have a lower predicted dissociation rate than the homologous epitopes in CD55. The epitopes in CD55 are of moderate to low affinity binding to MHC, and therefore should not be expressed sufficiently on normal cells for T cell recognition. This is important as CD55 is a complement regulatory protein that is expressed by a wide range of normal cells. However it is over-expressed 10-1,000 fold on tumour cells [25]. If the T cell epitope presented from 105AD7 is of higher affinity than the homologous epitope presented from antigen then this would make 105AD7 a more effective immunogen than antigen. Rosenberg et al demonstrated this principle using T cell epitopes within melanoma antigens. When the anchor residues of these epitopes were mutated they bound with higher affinity to MHC but still stimulated T cells that recognised the unmutated epitope. A clinical trial with these mutated peptides resulted in tumour responses in melanoma patients[26]. Similarly, a recent study from the group of J Schlom showed that mutated amino acids within a T cell epitope of CEA and found a peptide that did not bind better to MHC but was more effective at stimulating T cells[27]; see also chapter 5. These T cells could also still recognise the unmutated epitope on target cells. This approach could easily be extended to anti-idiotypic immunisation as antibodies can be cloned and residues mutated by site directed mutagenesis. Anti-idiotypic antibodies could be genetically engineered to express any T cell epitope of choice. Bona et al compared the immunogenicity of an influenza T cell epitope when presented as either antigen, a peptide or an anti-idiotypic antibody engineered to express the T cell epitope within its CDRH3. Anti-idiotypic antibody was the most effective immunogen stimulating stronger proliferative responses than either peptide or antigen[28].

There are two potential limitations in using anti-idiotypic antibodies as immunogens. The first is the limited number of T cell epitopes that anti-idiotypic antibodies can present. Like peptides they usually only present one or two epitopes. However recent results have suggested that the immune response to viruses which contain hundreds of potential epitopes is usually restricted to one or two immunodominant epitopes[29]. Furthermore, in acute viral infections, up to 44% of CD8 cells can be selectively activated by a single epitope[30]. Therefore the number of epitopes presented is unlikely to be a limitation for an effective vaccine. An important caveat is the possibility of the tumour losing expression of the target antigen. This is less likely in a vaccine that stimulates all arms of the immune response as recruitment of non specific effector cells or secretion of cytokines would also kill antigen negative cells.

Their second limitation is as to whether anti-idiotypic antibodies can stimulate CTL responses. Two recent pieces of evidence suggest that anti-idiotypes can indeed induce cytotoxic T cell responses. The chimeric but not the mouse anti-idiotype, 708 that mimics CEA stimulated primary *in vitro* CTL responses that showed MHC restricted CEA specific tumour cell killing[31, and unpublished findings]. This implies that Fc uptake by dendritic cells may allow cross priming of CTL responses by exogenous antigen. The second piece of evidence was provided by the study that stimulated an anti-idiotypic network to p53. Lymphocytes were induced that specifically killed a tumour cell line expressing mutated p53[9].

Can anti-idiotypic antibodies stimulate anti-tumour antibody responses ?

In contrast to T cells which recognise linear peptides antibodies predominantly recognise conformational determinants. If an anti-idiotypic antibody is therefore going to mimic a B cell epitope on antigen it will have to share some structural similarity with antigen. One excellent example of conformational mimicry between and anti-idiotypic antibody and antigen was provided by the elegant study of Bentley et al. They compared the crystal structure of an Ab1-anti-idiotypic antibody complex with the crystal structure of Ab1 complexed to antigen[32]. Although there was no evidence of sequence homology in this case, both complexes showed similar interactions. Thus anti-idiotype can differ greatly from antigen in structure and still be recognised as similar by the same antibody. Indeed anti-idiotypic antibodies can effectively mimic non protein antigens such as carbohydrates and lipids[33]. An anti-idiotypic antibody mimicking the ganglioside GD2 has been shown to induce anti-tumour antibodies in melanoma patients[34].

105AD7 not only displays amino acid homology between three of its CDRs and 3 separate regions of CD55, but also shows structural similarity. Analysis of molecular models of 105AD7 and CD55 highlights this similarity. The model of 105AD7 shows that the three CDRs that show homology with CD55 brought into close proximity with each other. Molecular modelling of CD55, based on the NMR solved structure of factor H complement control protein, shows that the regions homologous to 105AD7 are arranged in similar positions within the antigen as the homologous CDRs are within the antibody. This concept is supported by the results showing that 105AD7 Ab3s shows identical binding specificities against CD55, 105AD7 and its peptides as 791T/36. As conformation is very important in the mimicry of CD55 by 105AD7 it is unlikely that any linear peptide would be as effective an immunogen as the human anti-idiotype. In contrast it is possible for B cell to recognise linear peptides as was clearly demonstrated with an anti-idiotypic antibody which mimics the type 3 reovirus receptor. An area of homology was observed between antigen and the CDR2 of both heavy and light chains. When the sequences were linked together VL/VH peptide could induce virus neutralising antibodies[35].

Numerous other anti-idiotypic antibodies have been shown to recognise tumour associated antigens although the precise molecular mimicry has not been elucidated. Unfortunately however even with anti-idiotypic antibodies which show good molecular mimicry and induce antibodies which recognise antigen this is only a small component of a polyclonal response; in many cases most of the antibodies recognise components of the anti-idiotype that does not mimic antigen. Mouse serum raised against the human anti-idiotype 105AD7 shows titres of 1/100 against CD55, 1/1000 against the 105AD7 binding site and 1/10,000 against whole 105AD7 antibody (includes mouse anti-human antibodies). If only an antibody response is required (virus neutralisation) it will be more effective to immunise with antigen than anti-idiotypic antibody. However as previously discussed to effectively treat cancer it will be necessary to stimulate both B and T cell responses. As human anti-idiotypic antibodies can effectively stimulate all arms of the immune system they may indeed be viable alternative vaccine.

Clinical trials

Several clinical trials with anti-idiotypic antibodies have been reported. The earliest was immunisation of colorectal cancer patients with a goat anti-idiotypic polyclonal antiserum that mimicked the tumour associated antigen 17-IA[36, 37]. Anti-tumour antibody responses were induced in 15/18 patients. The survival of these patients was difficult to assess as half of them had also received chemotherapy. Further trials using a similar approach also gave encouraging results as all 9 patients are still well 7 years later. More recently, encouraging responses have been observed with human monoclonal antibody in this system[38]. A mouse monoclonal anti-idiotypic antibody mimicking a high molecular weight (HMW) melanoma associated antigen also induced anti-tumour antibody responses. Patients who produced these antibodies survived significantly longer than patients who failed to respond[39]. Although these results were encouraging neither of these anti-idiotypic vaccines were shown to produce antigen specific helper or cytotoxic T cell responses. Recent studies have shown that if mice with a tumour expressing the mouse 17-1A antigen are immunised with either anti-idiotype, antigen or antigen presented in vaccinia virus. Only the viral expression construct induced CTL responses and gave protective immunity[40].

A mouse anti-idiotypic antibody (3H1) that mimics CEA has also been administered to colorectal cancer patients. 18/25 patients showed an anti-CEA antibody response and 15/25 showed a CEA specific T cell proliferation response[34]. However there was no detectable clinical benefit. This was attributed to the extensive disease of these immunised patients. A randomised adjuvant trial with this anti-idiotypic antibody is now in progress. Following resection of their tumours colorectal cancer patients are randomised to receive chemotherapy with or without anti-idiotypic vaccination.

Two human anti-idiotypic antibodies have been administered to colorectal cancer patients. A human anti-idiotypic antibody which mimics 17-1A[38] and the human monoclonal anti-idotypic antibody (105AD7) that mimics CD55[41]. The human anti-idiotypic antibody mimicking 17-1A induced both antibody and helper T cell responses in 7/10 patients. 105AD7 anti-idiotype induces both helper and cytotoxic T cell responses in cancer patients. In advanced colorectal cancer patients this was not associated with any survival benefit. However in an neoadjuvant trial there was increased infiltration of activated lymphocytes[20] and a highly significant increase in apoptosis of tumour cells in 105AD7 immunised as compared to control patients[42]. Four year survival for these patients is 71% which is better than contemporary controls but is difficult to interpret in a non randomised trial.

One of the main problems in evaluating not only anti-idiotypic immunisation but all vaccine approaches is the clinical evaluation of the tumour and immune response. Tumour apoptosis as exemplified by the 105AD7 studies may be a way of measuring tumour response. However current in vitro cell culture assays such as T cell blastogenesis or chromium release cytotoxicity assays are at best insensitive and at worst difficult to interpret. Recent developments in methods to enumerate antigen specific T cells by tetramer[43, 44] or intracellular cytokine staining[45, 46] could be the solution to this problem.

Apart from providing an accurate assessment of the number and phenotype (CD4 or CD8) of cells responding to vaccination it may allow optimisation of immunisation protocols. Thus it may be possible to compare antigen and anti-idiotype vaccines or to compare a range of immune adjuvants. It may also be possible to determine the frequency and number of immunisations that are necessary for successful treatment. These measurements could also address perhaps the most important questions of all. Is there synergy between vaccines which target different antigens? Is there synergy between vaccines and chemotherapy ?

CONCLUSION

Cancer vaccines are still in their infancy, developments in the understanding of the molecular basis of immune responses have enabled design of many new approaches. A similar development in our ability to measure both tumour and immune responses in patients will allow selection of the most effective vaccines. Human monoclonal anti-idiotypic antibodies offer a real possibility of fulfilling the role of the "ideal cancer vaccine".

REFERENCES

1. Qin Z and Blankenstein T, CD4+ T cell mediated tumour rejection involves inhibition of angiogenesis that is dependent on IFNgamma receptor expression by nonhematopoietic cells. Immunity, 2000; 12: 677-686.
2. Karre K, How to recognize a foreign submarine. Immunological Reviews, 1997; 155: 5-9.
3. Jerne NK, Idiotypic networks and other preconceived ideas. Immunological Reviews, 1984; 79: 5-24.
4. Kurts C, Kosaka H, Carbone FR, Miller J, and Heath WR, Class I-restricted cross-presentation of exogenous self- antigens leads to deletion of autoreactive CD8(+) T cells. J Exp Med, 1997; 186: 239-245.
5. Matzinger P, An innate sense of danger. 1044-5323, 1998; 10: 399-415.
6. Ke Y and Kapp JA, Exogenous antigens gain access to the major histocompatibility complex class I processing pathway in B cells by receptor- mediated uptake. J Exp Med, 1996; 184: 1179-1184.
7. Liu CL, Goldstein J, Graziano RF, He J, Oshea JK, Deo Y, and Guyre PM, Fc gamma RI-targeted fusion proteins result in efficient presentation by human monocytes of antigenic and antagonist T cell epitopes. J Clin Invest, 1996; 98: 2001-2007.
8. Irvine K and Schlom J, Induction Of Delayed-Type Hypersensitivity Responses By Monoclonal Antiidiotypic Antibodies to Tumor-Cells Expressing Carcinoembryonic Antigen and Tumor-Associated Glycoprotein-72. Cancer Immunol Immunother, 1993; 36: 281-292.
9. Ruiz PJ, Wolkowicz R, Waisman A, Hirschberg DL, Carmi P, Erez N, Garren H, Herkel J, Karpuj M, Steinman L, Rotter V, and Cohen IR, Idiotypic immunization induces immunity to mutated p53 and tumor rejection. Nature Medicine, 1998; 4: 710-712.
10. Bronte V, Apolloni E, Ronca R, Zamboni P, Overwijk WW, Surman DR, Restifo NP, and Zanovello P, Genetic vaccination with "self" tyrosinase-related protein 2 causes melanoma eradication but not vitiligo. Cancer Res, 2000; 60: 253-258.
11. Austin EB, Robins RA, Durrant LG, Price MR, and Baldwin RW, Human Monoclonal Anti-Idiotypic Antibody to the Tumor-Associated Antibody 791T/36. Immunol, 1989; 67: 525-530.
12. Zaghouani H, Kuzu Y, Kuzu H, Brumeanu TD, Swiggard WJ, Steinman RM, and Bona CA, Contrasting efficacy of presentation by major histocompatibility complex class-I and class-II products

ANTI-IDIOTYPIC ANTIBODY AS IMMUNOGEN

when peptides are administered within a common protein carrier, self immunoglobulin. Euop J Immunol, 1993; 23: 2746-2750.

13. Foon KA, John WJ, Chakraborty M, Das R, Teitelbaum A, Garrison J, Kashala O, Chatterjee SK, and Bhattacharya-Chatterjee M, Clinical and immune responses in resected colon cancer patients treated with anti-idiotype monoclonal antibody vaccine that mimics the carcinoembryonic antigen. J Clin Oncol, 1999; 17: 2889-2895.

14. Durrant LG, Buckley DJ, Robins RA, and Spendlove I, 105AD7 cancer vaccine stimulates anti-tumour helper and cytotoxic T- cell responses in colorectal cancer patients but repeated immunisations are required to maintain these responses. Int J Cancer, 2000; 85: 87-92.

15. Spendlove I, Li L, Carmichael J, and Durrant LG, Decay accelerating factor (CD55): A target for cancer vaccines? Cancer Res, 1999; 59: 2282-2286.

16. Austin EB, Robins RA, Baldwin RW, and Durrant LG, Induction Of Delayed-Hypersensitivity to Human Tumor-Cells With a Human Monoclonal Antiidiotypic Antibody. J natl Cancer Inst, 1991; 83: 1245-1248.

17. Robins RA, Denton GWL, Hardcastle JD, Austin EB, Baldwin RW, and Durrant LG, Antitumor Immune-Response and Interleukin-2 Production Induced In Colorectal-Cancer Patients By Immunization With Human Monoclonal Antiidiotypic Antibody. Cancer Res, 1991; 51: 5425-5429.

18. Denton GWL, Durrant LG, Hardcastle JD, Austin EB, Sewell HF, and Robins RA, Clinical Outcome Of Colorectal-Cancer Patients Treated With Human Monoclonal Antiidiotypic Antibody. Int J Cancer, 1994; 57: 10-14.

19. Durrant LG, Buckley TJD, Denton GWL, Hardcastle JD, Sewell HF, and Robins RA, Enhanced Cell-Mediated Tumor Killing In Patients Immunized With Human Monoclonal Antiidiotypic Antibody 105AD7. Cancer Res, 1994; 54: 4837-4840.

20. Maxwell-Armstrong CA, Durrant LG, Robins RA, Galvin AM, Scholefield JH, and Hardcastle JD, Increased activation of lymphocytes infiltrating primary colorectal cancers following immunisation with the anti-idiotypic monoclonal antibody 105AD7. Gut, 1999; 45: 593-598.

21. Pride MW, Shi H, Anchin JM, Linthicum DS, Loverde PT, Thakur A, and Thanavala Y, Molecular Mimicry Of Hepatitis-B Surface-Antigen By an Antiidiotype- Derived Synthetic Peptide. Proc Natl Acad Sci USA, 1992; 89: 11900-11904.

22. Chatterjee SK, Tripathi PK, Chakraborty M, Yannelli J, Wang HT, Foon KA, Maier CC, Blalock JE, and Bhattacharya-Chatterjee M, Molecular mimicry of carcinoembryonic antigen by peptides derived from the structure of an anti-idiotype antibody. Cancer Res, 1998; 58: 1217-1224.

23. Ban N, Escobar C, Garcia R, Hasel K, Day J, Greenwood A, and McPherson A, Crystal-Structure Of an Idiotype Antiidiotype Fab Complex. Proc Natl Acad Sci USA, 1994; 91: 1604-1608.

24. Williams WV, London SD, Weiner DB, Wadsworth S, Berzofsky JA, Robey F, Rubin DH, and Greene MI, Immune response to a molecularly defined internal image anti-idiotype. J Immunol, 1989; 142: 4392-4400.

25. Durrant LG, Robins RA, and Baldwin RW, Flow Cytometric Screening Of Monoclonal-Antibodies For Drug or Toxin Targeting to Human Cancer. J natl Cancer Inst, 1989; 81: 688-696.

26. Rosenberg SA, Yang JC, Schwartzentruber DJ, Hwu P, Marincola FM, Topalian SL, Restifo NP, Dudley ME, Schwarz SL, Spiess PJ, Wunderlich JR, Parkhurst MR, Kawakami Y, Seipp CA, Einhorn JH, and White DE, Immunologic and therapeutic evaluation of a synthetic peptide vaccine for the treatment of patients with metastatic melanoma. Nature Medicine, 1998; 4: 321-327.

27. Salazar E, Zaremba S, Arlen PM, Tsang KY, and Schlom J, Agonist peptide from a cytotoxic T-lymphocyte epitope of human carcinoembryonic antigen stimulates production of TC1-type cytokines and increases tyrosine phosphorylation more efficiently than cognate peptide. Int J Cancer, 2000; 85: 829-838.

28. Bona C, Brumeanu TD, and Zaghouani H, Immunogenicity of Microbial Peptides Grafted in Self Immunoglobulin Molecules. Cell Mol Biol, 1994; 40: 21-30.

29. Altman JD, Moss PAH, Goulder PJR, Barouch DH, McHeyzer-Williams MG, Bell JI, McMichael AJ, and Davis MM, Phenotypic Analysis of Antigen-Specific T-Lymphocytes. Science, 1996; 274: 94-96.

30. Callan MFC, Tan L, Annels N, Ogg GS, Wilson JDK, Ocallaghan CA, Steven N, McMichael AJ, and Rickinson AB, Direct visualization of antigen-specific CD8(+) T cells during the primary immune response to Epstein-Barr virus in vivo. J Exp Med, 1998; 187: 1395-1402.

31. Durrant LG, Denton GWL, Jacobs E, Mee M, Moss R, Austin EB, Baldwin RW, Hardcastle JD, and Robins RA, An Idiotypic Replica Of Carcinoembryonic Antigen Inducing Cellular and Humoral Responses Directed Against Human Colorectal Tumors. Int J Cancer, 1992; 50: 811-816.

179

32. Bentley GA, Bhat TN, Boulot G, Fischmann T, Navaza J, Poljak RJ, Riottot MM, and Tello D, Immunochemical and Crystallographic Studies of Antibody D1.3 in Its Free, Antigen-Liganded, and Idiotope-Bound States. Cold Spring Harbor Symp Quant Biol, 1989; 54: 239-245.

33. Kirch RD, Beale D, He M, Corper AL, Krawinkel-Brenig U, and Taussig MJ, Anti-anti-idiotypic (Ab3) antibodies that bind progesterone 11alpha-bovine serum albumin differ in their combining sites from antibodies raised directly against the antigen. Immunol, 2000; 100: 152-164.

34. Foon KA, Lutzky J, Baral RN, Yannelli JR, Hutchins L, Teitelbaum A, Kashala OL, Das R, Garrison J, Reisfeld RA, and Bhattacharya-Chatterjee M, Clinical and immune responses in advanced melanoma patients immunized with an anti-idiotype antibody mimicking disialoganglioside GD2. J Clin Oncol, 2000; 18: 376-384.

35. Sharpe AH, Gaulton GN, McDade KK, Fields BN, and Greene MI, Syngeneic monoclonal anti-idiotype can induce cellular immunity to Reovirus. J Exp Med, 1984; 160: 1195-1205.

36. Herlyn D, Wettendorff M, Schmoll E, Iliopoulos D, Schedel I, Dreikhausen U, Raab R, Ross AH, Jaksche H, Scriba M, and Koprowski H, Anti-Idiotype Immunization Of Cancer-Patients - Modulation Of the Immune-Response. Proc Natl Acad Sci USA, 1987; 84: 8055-8059.

37. Herlyn D, Ross AH, Iliopoulos D, and Koprowski H, Induction Of Specific Immunity to Human-Colon Carcinoma By Anti- Idiotypic Antibodies to Monoclonal-Antibody Co17-1a. Euop J Immunol, 1987; 17: 1649-1652.

38. Fagerberg J, Steinitz M, Wigzell H, Askelof P, and Mellstedt H, Human Antiidiotypic Antibodies Induced a Humoral and Cellular Immune- Response Against a Colorectal Carcinoma-Associated Antigen In Patients. Proc Natl Acad Sci USA, 1995; 92: 4773-4777.

39. Mittelman A, Chen ZJ, Yang H, Wong GY, and Ferrone S, Human High-Molecular-Weight Melanoma-Associated Antigen (Hmw-Maa) Mimicry By Mouse Antiidiotypic Monoclonal-Antibody Mk2-23 - Induction Of Humoral Anti-Hmw-Maa Immunity and Prolongation Of Survival In Patients With Stage-Iv Melanoma. Proc Natl Acad Sci USA, 1992; 89: 466-470.

40. Herlyn D, Somasundaram R, Zaloudik J, Li W, Jacob L, Harris D, Kieny MP, Ricciardi R, Gonczol E, Sears H, and Mastrangelo M, Cloned Antigens and Antiidiotypes. Hybridoma, 1995; 14: 159-166.

41. Durrant LG, MaxwellArmstrong C, Buckley D, Amin S, Robins RA, Carmichael J, and Scholefield JH, A neoadjuvant clinical trial in colorectal cancer patients of the human anti-idiotypic antibody 105AD7, which mimics CD55. 1078-0432, 2000; 6: 422-430.

42. Amin S, Robins RA, Maxwell-Armstrong CA, Scholefield JH, and Durrant LG, Vaccine-induced apoptosis: A novel clinical trial end point? Cancer Res, 2000; 60: 3132-3136.

43. McMichael AJ and O'Callaghan CA, A new look at T cells. J Exp Med, 1998; 187: 1367-1371.

44. Dunbar PR, Ogg GS, Chen J, Rust N, vanderBruggen P, and Cerundolo V, Direct isolation, phenotyping and cloning of low-frequency antigen- specific cytotoxic T lymphocytes from peripheral blood. Current Biology, 1998; 8: 413-416.

45. Waldrop SL, Pitcher CJ, Peterson DM, Maino VC, and Picker LJ, Determination of antigen-specific: Memory/effector CD4+ T cell frequencies by flow cytometry - Evidence for a novel, antigen- specific homeostatic mechanism in HIV-associated immunodeficiency. J Clin Invest, 1997; 99: 1739-1750.

46. Kern F, Surel IP, Brock C, Freistedt B, Radtke H, Scheffold A, Blasczyk R, Reinke P, Schneider-Mergener J, Radbruch A, Walden P, and Volk H-D, T-cell epitope mapping by flow cytometry. Nature Medicine, 1998; 4: 975-978.

11
Genetically modified tumour cells for cancer immunization

STEPHEN TODRYK, SELMAN ALI, ANGUS DALGLEISH and
ROBERT REES

ABSTRACT

Whole tumour cells are a logical basis for generating immunity against the cancers they
comprise or represent. In order to alert the immune system to respond to the tumour
antigens intervention is required. This can be achieved by transfection of the tumour
cells with genes encoding a variety of immunostimulatory molecules. The most obvious
approach is the transduction of tumour cells taken from the body with genes that encode
molecules (such as cytokines and costimulatory molecules) that enhance T cell or
antigen presenting cell function. Irradiated cells are then re-injected as a cancer vaccine
and an anti-tumour immune response is generated that can destroy tumour cells.
Molecules that effect antigen presenting cell function, such as Granulocyte-Macrophage
Colony-Stimulating Factor (GM-CSF), appear to hold the most promise as
demonstrated in preclinical and early clinical studies. The direct delivery of
immunostimulatory molecule genes to tumours *in vivo* also shows some efficacy,
especially the suicide gene Herpes Simplex Virus thymidine kinase. Future clinical
trials in earlier stage patients will provide the clearest indication of the efficacy of
immunization with transduced tumour cells since tumour burdens will be lower and
immunocompetence will be better than in present phase I/II trials.

INTRODUCTION

Although evidence is mounting to show that cancers can naturally elicit immune
responses, immune-mediated tumour regression seems to be the exception rather than
the rule. Nevertheless, a number of tumour antigens have been identified for a range of
tumour types and immune responses to some of these antigens are associated with
tumour regression [1]. This is particularly evident in the case of melanoma. The

R.A. Robins and R.C. Rees (eds.), Cancer Immunology, 181–194.

prevalence of tumours however suggests that they are not generally recognised by the immune system such that they are rejected. The aim of cancer immunisation using genetically modified tumour cells is to "persuade" the immune system to respond to antigens that are not perceived as being foreign or a threat to survival of the host. This approach is usually envisaged as being vaccination with the patients' own (autologous) tumour cells. These cells are obtained following tumour surgery or biopsy, or from the circulation in the case of leukaemias. The *ex-vivo* cells are transduced *in vitro* using one of a number of potential vectors, and there is a wide variety immunostimulatory molecules that can be transferred. Irradiated cells are then reinjected into the patient as a vaccine. A less obvious but nevertheless important approach is the direct transduction of tumours *in situ*, *in vivo*, with immunostimulatory molecules. Expression of these molecules may have a direct effect on the growth of the transduced tumour and could be especially relevant for treating non-resectable tumours. Importantly, systemic immune responses can be generated that feed back and kill the primary tumour and that can kill metastases. The latter process, a bystander effect, is crucial since only a limited proportion of tumour cells can be transduced *in vivo* using the currently available technology. Since whole tumour cells are the source of tumour antigens in both the above approaches, the exact nature of the antigens is not necessarily required. In addition, since histologically-related tumours often express common antigens, it is possible to use selected cell lines as candidate vaccines.

The aim of this article is to review cancer immunotherapy using gene-modified tumour cells both in the preclinical and clinical settings, and to relate this approach to cancer immunology generally. The choice from a large number of molecules to transfer, and from a number of vectors used to achieve transduction, will depend to some extent on the histological type of the tumour in addition to its location and other phenotypic properties. Overall, this approach appears to be one of the most promising for achieving successful cancer immunotherapy.

Table 11.1 Aims of cancer immunization using genetic modification of tumour cells

Induce an immunostimulatory environment in the vicinity of the vaccine / tumour
Induce direct or cross-priming of CTL and Th cells against tumour antigens
Overcome immunosuppression and/or T cell anergy
Generate immune memory against primary tumour regrowth and metastasis

CANCER IMMUNOLOGY AS THE BACKDROP FOR IMMUNIZATION

It has become clear that, in general, T cells are required to kill cancer cells. There is a great deal of evidence that they are not only the main effector cells (cytotoxic T lymphocytes, CTL) that kill tumours but are required, as T helper (Th) cells, in controlling the priming and activation of CTL. CTL recognise antigens synthesised within the tumour cell that are presented on the cell surface in combination with MHC class I molecules. Tumour antigen-specific Th (and also possibly CD8$^+$) cells also orchestrate non-specific immune effector mechanisms in tumour destruction by secreting appropriate cytokines such as IFNγ in the vicinity of the tumour [2]. In comparison to infectious diseases tumours are thus more akin to virally infected cells in regard to their therapeutic requirements. Therapy is the operative word with tumours in that immunization usually follows detection of a malignancy. Not only will the tumour have had the opportunity to firmly establish itself physically, with large numbers of tumour cells, but the immune system will have been exposed to tumour antigens in a non-stimulatory setting. This means that the immune system, and in particular T cells, will perceive the tumour as being self or "non-dangerous" to the host, and tolerance to tumour antigens may well result. Immunotherapy aims to change this by associating tumour antigens with molecules that are directly immunostimulatory or with molecular signals that are usually flagged up during tissue damage or infection ; "dangerous" situations that need immunological action to maintain the health of the host. The exact nature of such molecules will be described later, but notably have been mimicked non-genetically by administering tumour cell vaccines with immunological adjuvants such as bacillus Calmette-Guerin [3, 4]. In addition to breaking T cell immune tolerance to tumour antigens there is also the issue of appropriate T cell homing that may confound an effective immune response. The generation of immunity against antigens expressed by both tumour and normal tissue may occur but may not be too problematic as in the case of vitiligo associated with melanoma immunotherapy [5].

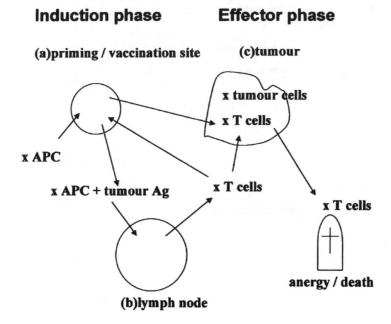

Figure 11.1 Anti-tumour immunization scheme

Unfortunately for cancer immunotherapy, tumours are moving targets in many respects, not only because they physically metastasise. They often express molecules that inhibit immune responses locally including Transforming Growth Factor (TGF)-β, Interleukin (IL)-10, Vascular Endothelial Growth Factor (VEGF) and Fas ligand [6]. Tumour cells can also potentially be poor targets for CTL by their loss or reduction of MHC molecules, reduction in antigen processing and presentation and loss or variation of tumour antigens. In addition, the possession of a tumour burden often results in a generalised immunosuppression of the host due the above and other mechanisms. Molecules involved in T cell receptor signalling, for instance, may be reduced, causing T cell dysfunction [7]. Immunization strategies need to keep occurrences such as these in mind in order to be effective and may only work effectively if the tumour burden is low e.g. following surgical resection.

The scheme described in Fig.11.1 illustrates the various checkpoints in tumour immunotherapy based on modulating APC function, which is emerging as one of the most important mechanisms in cancer immunotherapy. The processes at each stage are depicted in more detail in Fig.11.2. The immunomodulatory and immunoevasive mechanisms mentioned above are able to influence the outcome of immunotherapy at many of these checkpoints. In particular TGF-β and VEGF can reduce APC function during priming and IL-10 and TGF-β can influence T cell function during their effector phase.

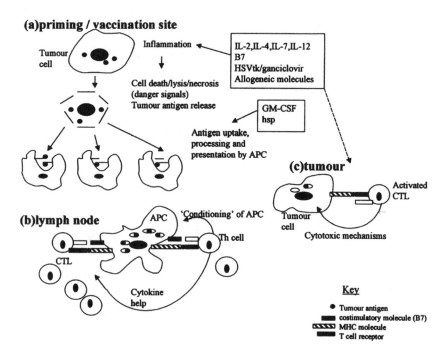

Figure 11.2 Detail of processes occurring during tumour immunization. Boxes contain genes that can be transfected to intervene at various points (vaccine and/or tumour site).

Also, Fas ligand expression on the surface of tumours may cause the death of Fas-bearing T cells, although this is a complex issue[8]. Thus tumours themselves are often not good APC and are certainly very poor if not totally ineffective at priming T cells that have never responded to the tumour antigens before (naïve T cells). Fig.11.1 emphasises the importance of numbers (x) of cells in the generation of effective anti-tumour immunity. Initially, appropriate numbers of APC (particularly dendritic cells, DC) must enter the vaccination site, take up tumour antigens, and exit and traffic to the local lymph nodes (Fig.11.2a). DC are known to be the most potent APC at priming naïve T cells [9]. This process requires the correct co-ordination of DC phagocytosis, maturation and migration. Once in the lymph nodes the DC must present tumour antigens in the context of MHC class II, and with appropriate B7 costimulatory molecules, to Th cells (Fig.11.2b). CD40 ligand (CD154) on these antigen-specific Th cells ligates CD40 on the DC and conditions them to go on to present tumour antigens on MHC class I together with upregulated costimulatory molecules and cytokines. The DC are thus able to prime and activate tumour-specific CTL. The presentation of tumour-derived antigens on MHC class I of host bone marrow-derived APC such as DC [10] is known as "cross-priming". Both these T cell types, though predominantly CTL, must exit the lymph nodes in sufficient numbers to be able to seek out tumour cells either at metastatic sites or at the priming site. Efficient homing requires that the tumours are vascularised and that the vasculature is adhered to by the T cells. Often, however, the tumours will not present themselves as any more attractive to T cells than normal tissues of the body. In this situation the sheer number of tumour-reactive T cells is vital. Once a small number of T cells do arrive and recognise the tumour (Fig.11.2c), in addition to direct tumour killing, they secrete molecules that will attract further cells into the tumour including further T cells and non-specific effector cells. These non-specific effectors include Natural Killer (NK) cells, macrophages and neutrophils. Whether the tumour is eradicated is dependant upon the size and speed of growth (aggression) of the tumour, i.e. the number of tumour cells present. Finally, T cells will be "consumed" during the effector process and will require replenishment by further priming. Modifying the nature of the priming process will be a major topic described in the following sections.

There now exists a large and perhaps daunting volume of literature on the use of gene transduction for cancer immunotherapy. In the animal models there are a number of variables that can exist and that must be clarified here (Fig.11.3). As mentioned earlier the tumours may be transduced *in vivo*, or *ex-vivo* prior to administration. The latter cells can be given live and changes in tumorigenicity due to the transfection can be observed. Such cells can also be irradiated before injection in the more traditional vaccination mode, so that they do not grow. Immune responses generated by either of these approaches can be tested on established tumours (therapy experiments) or on a new tumour challenge (prophylaxis experiment), though growing transduced tumours must first have been surgically removed. *In vitro*, immunological responses are measured as CTL which lyse tumour cells or tumour-specific T cell cytokine secretion. Therapy experiments clearly represent the human clinical situation more closely, but proof of principle for immunotherapy can be obtained from all these models. In addition, tumour cell lines used in these experiments and even clones from the same lines may vary in their intrinsic immunogenicity (possession of immunogenic antigens) and their rate of growth (aggression).

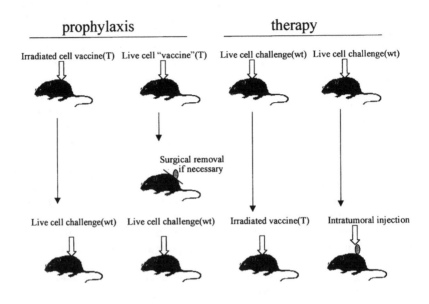

Figure 11.3 Approaches to studying transduced tumour cell immunization in animal models
T = transduced, wt = wild-type

TUMOUR CELL TRANSFECTION WITH CYTOKINE-ENCODING GENES

Interest in the use of cytokines for therapy of cancer goes back some two decades when IL-2 was administered systemically in human trials in order to boost T cell and NK cell-like anti-tumour activity [11]. Some efficacy was observed and systemic administration continued with cytokines such as IL-2 and IL-12. However, the associated toxicity forced many such trials to cease. The transduction of tumour cells with cytokine genes so that they secrete the cytokines locally, in a paracrine fashion, avoids much of the systemic toxicity. This sustained secretion also allows physical targeting of immune responses to the tumour cells in part by causing local inflammation in a manner similar to a bacterial adjuvant.

As with systemic cytokine administration, the first cytokine transfections were with molecules such as IL-2 in an attempt to boost anti-tumour T cell activity. One theory was that CTL, with their receptors engaged with tumour peptide on MHC on the tumour cell surface, would be activated by IL-2 to kill the tumour cell perhaps as though they had received cytokine help from Th cells. In mouse models this did appear to be the case and elimination of the transduced tumours was observed that was dependant on CD8[+] T cells [12]. Immune protection from subsequent challenge with wild type tumour was also found with IL-2-secreting vaccines [13]. Later studies, however, suggested that the inflammation generated by IL-2 was enhancing tumour antigen processing and presentation by APC and indirect T cell priming [14]. Similar findings were reported for a number of other cytokines [15]. When various cytokines were compared for irradiated tumour cell vaccines (including IL-2,4,6,IFNγ,TNFα) all were superseded in the generation of protection by Granulocyte-Macrophage Colony-Stimulating Factor (GM-CSF) [16]. This cytokine controls the local differentiation of DC, enhancing their ability to prime T cells to tumour antgens. This result was important because it used the poorly immunogenic B16 melanoma model. These findings with GM-CSF also extended to other tumour models. Like IL-2, IL-12 also activates T cells and NK cells. Other properties include induction of IFNγ secretion (which upregulates MHC) and the biasing a Th1 (cell mediated) immune response. IL-12 both inhibited tumorigenicity and elicited immunity in a colon cancer model [17]. Indeed, transfection with IFNγ itself also elicited immunity in some studies [18]. IL-7, possibly through its T cell-conditioning properties, has also shown immune-enhancing activity [19] as has IL-6, an inflammatory cytokine [20]. Since cytokines can often have numerous effects (pleiotropic) it was not entirely surprising that IL-4 [21] and IL-10 [22], which are known to be involved more with Th2 (antibody-generating) responses, also generated cell-mediated protective immunity. Cell vaccines comprising MHC non-matched (allogeneic) but histologically-related melanoma cells were able to treat tumours when the vaccines were transfected with GM-CSF [23]. More recently-identified cytokines that activate APC, Lag3 [24] and Flt3-ligand [25] have also elicited protective anti-tumour immunity when genetically transduced. It must be noted that different research groups will obtain varying levels of cytokine production from their transduced tumour cells and results may not be entirely comparable.

TUMOUR CELLS TRANSFECTED WITH GENES ENCODING COSTIMULATORY MOLECULES

The aim of transducing tumour cells with costimulatory molecules is to enhance the cells' ability to present their antigens to T cells. This is to some extent similar to transduction with T cell-activating cytokines. Specifically, CD8[+] CTL would be activated directly, possibly without the need for Th cells. Normally, B7 molecules on the surface of activated APC ligate CD28 molecules on the surface of T cells that are already recognising antigen on MHC molecules. The B7:CD28 interaction provides costimulation for full activation of T cells. Generally, B7.1 (CD80) transfection caused slowing of tumour growth or total regression [26]. However, systemic immunity was generated in some experiments but not others [27]. Where immunity was generated,

CD8[+] T cells were shown to be involved. A similar pattern of results was seen with B7.2 (CD86) transfection. The additional transfection with adhesion molecules such as ICAM-1 and LFA-3 has enhanced immunization with B7-expressing tumours in some studies. Certain findings called into question solely the direct presentation role of B7 molecules in such studies. This is because B7-induced regression was often associated with NK cell and neutrophil action. B7 may actually stimulate NK cells directly. A proposal that the induced inflammation and associated tumour-killing may give rise to increased tumour antigen cross-priming was backed up by the finding that bone marrow-derived APC were needed to generate immune protection [28]. Thus, as with many of the cytokine transductions, indirect antigen presentation appears to be a major mechanism for the generation of immunity. It may be beneficial to combine cytokine expression with costimulatory molecules as synergy, e.g between IL-12 and B7 [29]. Recently, tranduction of tumour cells genes for CD40 ligand and GM-CSF has given rise to enhanced CTL generation and immune protection above that for either molecule alone [30].

Table 11.2 Molecules to transfer for cancer immunotherapy

MOLECULES	NATURAL SOURCE	FUNCTION
Cytokines		
IL-2	Th cells	Proliferation/activation of CTL, Th and NK cells
IL-4	Th cells	Antibody responses, APC differentiation
IL-6	T cells, stromal cells	Inflammatory cytokine
IL-7	stromal cells	T cell maturation/survival
IL-10	T cells	Antibody responses
IL-12	APC	Activates Th1 cells, NK cells
IFNγ	T cells	Activates NK cells and macrophages
GM-CSF	T cells	APC differentiation/ maturation
Costimulatory molecules		
B7.1, B7.2	Activated APC	Stimulate T cells directly
Suicide genes		
HSVtk	Viral	Tumour cell killing
CD	Bacterial	Tumour cell killing
Other molecules		
Autologous MHC molecules	APC	Improve antigen presenting capacity
Heat shock proteins	Stressed cells	Enhance APC function
Immunogenic proteins	e.g. bacterial	Provide Th cell epitopes
Allogeneic MHC molecules	Transplants	Increase T cell-mediated tumour destruction

TRANSFECTION WITH GENES ENCODING SUICIDE GENES

Two suicide genes most commonly used in cancer therapy encode enzymes that can convert non-toxic prodrugs into toxic compounds, thus killing the transduced tumour cell. The first is Herpes Simplex Virus thymidine kinase (HSVtk) which converts ganciclovir into toxic metabolites that inhibit DNA replication [31]. The second is bacterial Cytosine Deaminase (CD) which converts non-toxic 5-fluorocytosine into toxic 5-fluoracil [32]. Since the current vector technology only allows a small proportion of a tumour to be transduced *in vivo*, the fact that non-transduced tumour cells in the vicinity also died was very useful. This "bystander effect" was thought to occur by the transfer of toxic metabolites from transduced to non-transduced cells via gap junctions or by apoptotic vesicle uptake. Direct *in vivo* administration of these genes using various vectors (see below) has resulted in the reduction in growth or often complete regression of tumour. An immune component in the action of these systems was implicated when the effect was seen to be reduced in nude mice that are deficient in T cells [33]. It was demonstrated that the cell killing causes an inflammatory response and secretion of cytokines that bias a Th1 (cell mediated) immune response [34, 35]. More recently it was shown that HSVtk/ganciclovir tumour killing was more immunogenic when the cells died by a necrotic mechanism than by an apoptotic mechanism. A proposed "danger signal" that was upregulated and that alerted the immune system during necrosis was hsp70 [36]. Thus suicide gene therapy of tumours can be considered as cancer immunotherapy.

OTHER TRANSFECTIONS

Apart from genes encoding cytokines and costimulatory molecules, genes for other molecules have also been transferred to tumour cells to increase their immunogenicity. Leading on from the last section, the transfer of genes encoding the proposed danger signal hsp70 enhanced the immune responses to wild-type tumours [36] and this enhancement may be due to the ability of hsp to modulate APC function [37]. Immune protection has also been elicited when mycobacterial hsp65 was transferred to tumour cells [38]. The transfer of genes encoding allogeneic MHC class I molecules (HLA-B7) has caused tumour regression and the generation of immunity [39]. Allogeneic MHC molecules resemble self MHC plus foreign peptide and are recognised by a relatively high frequency of peripheral T cells even without prior contact with the allo-MHC. The transfer of genes encoding highly immunogenic antigens such as mycobacterial proteins [40, 41] may also serve to provide additional epitopes for T cell help during anti-tumour CTL priming. It is argued that immunogenicity of the transferred molecules (including the vectors used) may contribute to some of the immune-enhancing effects for some transfections. Finally, the transduction of tumour cells with syngeneic MHC class II molecules has been performed to allow the cells to present antigens to CD4$^+$ Th cells [42] with some success in generating protective CTL-mediated immunity against MHC class II$^-$ tumours.

METHODS OF TRANSDUCTION

Modes of gene transduction of whole tumour cells continue to be developed in order to improve on targeting, efficiency and safety. The transduction method used (Table 11.3) depends very much on the application. *Ex-vivo* transduction does not particularly require targeting as the cells are isolated already, but needs good transduction efficiency. However, if autologous tumour cells are being used then rapid transduction is useful.

Table 11.3 Modes of transfection

Naked DNA	Viral Vectors
Calcium phosphate precipitation	Retoviruses
Cationic liposomes	Adenoviruses
Particle bombardment (gene gun)	Herpes simplex viruses
Electroporation	Vaccinia viruses
	Adeno-associated viruses

This can be achieved by replication-incompetent viral vectors such as those based on retroviruses, adenoviruses or herpes viruses. Adeno- and herpes viruses do not require the target cells to be in a proliferating phase and transduction occurs in a matter of hours. Full gene and protein expression, which is transient but probably of sufficient duration with these vectors, is usually evident within 24 hours and the tumour cells can be returned to the patient as a vaccine. There is no need for extended culture of the tumour cells, which could lead to alterations in antigen profile. Such viral vectors are a clear improvement over the relatively inefficient transduction approaches using naked DNA with precipitated salts or lipids. Retroviral vectors are excellent for making reliable, stable transfectants but require the cells to be dividing for gene integration. Considerable time is needed for selection since the transduction rate is relatively low, especially compared to adeno- and herpes viruses. The properties of the latter viruses, including their ability to infect a wide range of tumour cells, also make them useful for direct intratumoral delivery of genes and adenovirus for instance has been effective in delivering IL-12 to tumours *in vivo* and causing their regression [43]. A herpes vector encoding GM-CSF has also caused tumor regression by this approach [44], and when used in 'whole' cell vaccines [45]. Intratumoral injection of adenovirus encoding suicide genes such as HSVtk has effected tumour regression [46]. The use of viral vectors systemically to treat tumours depends on being able to effectively target them either at the level of surface molecules or at the transcriptional level (e.g. tyrosinase promotors in melanoma) [47]. Such approaches sound exciting but remain elusive clinically [48].

CLINICAL TRIALS

A plethora of clinical trials have been initiated using a number of the approaches described in this article. Such studies are essential as results from animal models may not necessarily extrapolate to humans with cancer. However, since these approaches are still in their infancy in relation to other protocols (e.g. whole cells + BCG [3, 4]) the main trials must be phase I/II toxicity studies, with the possibility of seeing some clinical benefit. But since such studies are carried out on very advanced cancer patients the chances of seeing clinical effects are small. Nevertheless, some effects on clinical and immunological parameters have been observed. In autologous, *ex-vivo*-transfected tumour cell vaccine approaches GM-CSF has been used for renal cancer [49] melanoma [50] and prostate cancer [51] and has given rise to immunological responses. Transduction of autologous tumour cells with T cell-stimulating cytokines IL-2 [52] and IL-7 [53] as vaccines have shown some efficacy in melanoma trials. In addition, allogeneic tumour cells secreting cytokines have also entered clinical trials for melanoma ([54]. All these vaccines comprised irradiated cells given intradermally. Certainly, safety and toxicity profiles associated with the above trials appear to be good even though clinical responses were limited. Trials with patients of earlier stage disease will really provide the most valuable evidence for the best approaches in terms of transduction methods and genes to transduce because the patients will have lower tumour burden and more competent immune systems.

CONCLUSIONS

Primary tumours are usually only treated successfully by surgery or radiotherapy. The role of cancer immunotherapy by gene transduction is to try and combat metastatic spread of the disease more effectively and with less toxic side-effects than chemotherapy. However, this is only realistic when the metastases are of small size and low number i.e.during minimal residual disease. Although there are a number of imunomodulatory genes that show pre-clinical efficacy, ones that promote tumour antigen processing and presentation by APC (cross-priming) such as GM-CSF have performed consistently and appear to hold the most promise clinically, especially in the whole-cell cancer vaccine approach. Whole cells for use as vaccines remains logical as they contain numerous tumour antigens which the growing tumours are unlikely to deviate from. Sufficient commonality of antigens between histologically-related tumours makes tumour cell lines of non-autologous origin (allogeneic vaccines) a feasible option. Indeed, such tumour lines are already established in culture and could be produced in very large numbers and to a high and reproducible standard [55]. *In vivo* delivery of some of the above-mentioned genes could also be beneficial but present trials of direct intratumoral injection using e.g. adenovirus vectors with HSVtk [56] are probably aimed more at direct killing of the tumour rather than immunization. Systemic administration of vectors awaits the development of better vector systems with regard to their targeting, transduction efficiency and safety.

REFERENCES

1.   Rosenberg SA, Cancer vaccines based on the identification of genes encoding cancer regression antigens. Immunol Today, 1997; 18: 175-182.
2.   Pardoll DM and Topalian SL, The role of CD4(+) T cell responses in antitumor immunity. Curr Opin Immunol, 1998; 10: 588-594.
3.   Morton DL, Foshag LJ, Hoon DSB, Nizze JA, Wanek LA, Chang C, Davtyan DG, Gupta RK, Elashoff R, and Irie RF, Prolongation of Survival in Metastatic Melanoma after Active Specific Immunotherapy with a New Polyvalent Melanoma Vaccine. Ann Surg, 1992; 216: 463-482.

4. Hoover HC, Brandhorst JS, Peters LC, Surdyke MG, Takeshita Y, Madariaga J, Muenz LR, and Hanna MG, Adjuvant Active Specific Immunotherapy for Human Colorectal- Cancer - 6.5-Year Median Follow-up of a Phase-Iii Prospectively Randomized Trial. J Clin Oncol, 1993; 11: 390-399.

5. Pardoll DM, Inducing autoimmune disease to treat cancer. Proc Natl Acad Sci U S A, 1999; 96: 5340-5342.

6. Chouaib S, AsselinPaturel C, MamiChouaib F, Caignard A, and Blay JY, The host-tumor immune conflict: from immunosuppression to resistance and destruction. Immunol Today, 1997; 18: 493-497.

7. Whiteside TL, Signaling defects in T lymphocytes of patients with malignancy. Cancer Immunology Immunotherapy, 1999; 48: 346-352.

8. Restifo NP, Not so Fas: Re-evaluating the mechanisms of immune privilege and tumor escape. Nat Med, 2000; 6: 493-495.

9. Banchereau J and Steinman RM, Dendritic cells and the control of immunity. Nature, 1998; 392: 245-252.

10. Huang AYC, Golumbek P, Ahmadzadeh M, Jaffee E, Pardoll D, and Levitsky H, Role Of Bone-Marrow-Derived Cells In Presenting Mhc Class I- Restricted Tumor-Antigens. Science, 1994; 264: 961-965.

11. Gore ME and Riches PG, Immunotherapy of Cancer. 1996: Wiley, UK.

12. Fearon ER, Pardoll DM, Itaya T, Golumbek P, Levitsky HI, Simons JW, Karasuyama H, Vogelstein B, and Frost P, Interleukin-2 Production by Tumor-Cells Bypasses T-Helper Function in the Generation of an Antitumor Response. Cell, 1990; 60: 397-403.

13. Cavallo F, Dipierro F, Giovarelli M, Gulino A, Vacca A, Stoppacciaro A, Forni M, Modesti A, and Forni G, Protective and Curative Potential of Vaccination with Interleukin-2-Gene-Transfected Cells from a Spontaneous Mouse Mammary Adenocarcinoma. Cancer Res, 1993; 53: 5067-5070.

14. Bannerji R, Arroyo CD, Cordoncardo C, and Gilboa E, The Role of Il-2 Secreted from Genetically-Modified Tumor-Cells in the Establishment of Antitumor Immunity. J Immunol, 1994; 152: 2324-2332.

15. Musiani P, Modesti A, Giovarelli M, Cavallo F, Colombo MP, Lollini PL, and Forni G, Cytokines, tumour-cell death and immunogenicity: A question of choice. Immunol Today, 1997; 18: 32-36.

16. Dranoff G, Jaffee E, Lazenby A, Golumbek P, Levitsky H, Brose K, Jackson V, Hamada H, Pardoll D, and Mulligan RC, Vaccination with Irradiated Tumor-Cells Engineered to Secrete Murine Granulocyte-Macrophage Colony-Stimulating Factor Stimulates Potent, Specific, and Long-Lasting Antitumor Immunity. Proc Natl Acad Sci U S A, 1993; 90: 3539-3543.

17. Brunda MJ, Luistro L, Warrier RR, Wright RB, Hubbard BR, Murphy M, Wolf SF, and Gately MK, Antitumor and Antimetastatic Activity Of Interleukin-12 Against Murine Tumors. J Exp Med, 1993; 178: 1223-1230.

18. Gansbacher B, Bannerji R, Daniels B, Zier K, Cronin K, and Gilboa E, Retroviral Vector-Mediated Gamma-Interferon Gene-Transfer into Tumor-Cells Generates Potent and Long Lasting Antitumor Immunity. Cancer Res, 1990; 50: 7820-7825.

19. Allione A, Consalvo M, Nanni P, Lollini PL, Cavallo F, Giovarelli M, Forni M, Gulino A, Colombo MP, Dellabona P, Hock H, Blankenstein T, Rosenthal FM, Gansbacher B, Bosco MC, Musso T, Gusella L, and Forni G, Immunizing and Curative Potential Of Replicating and Nonreplicating Murine Mammary Adenocarcinoma Cells Engineered With Interleukin (Il)- 2, Il-4, Il-6, Il-7, Il-10, Tumor-Necrosis-Factor-Alpha, Granulocyte- Macrophage Colony-Stimulating Factor, and Gamma-Interferon Gene or Admixed With Conventional Adjuvants. Cancer Res, 1994; 54: 6022-6026.

20. Porgador A, Tzehoval E, Katz A, Vadai E, Revel M, Feldman M, and Eisenbach L, Interleukin-6 Gene Transfection into Lewis Lung-Carcinoma Tumor-Cells Suppresses the Malignant Phenotype and Confers Immunotherapeutic Competence against Parental Metastatic Cells. Cancer Res, 1992; 52: 3679-3686.

21. Golumbek PT, Lazenby AJ, Levitsky HI, Jaffee LM, Karasuyama H, Baker M, and Pardoll DM, Treatment of Established Renal-Cancer by Tumor-Cells Engineered to Secrete Interleukin-4. Science, 1991; 254: 713-716.

22. Gerard CM, Bruyns C, Delvaux A, Baudson N, Dargent JL, Goldman M, and Velu T, Loss of tumorigenicity and increased immunogenicity induced by interleukin-10 gene transfer in B16 melanoma cells. Hum Gene Ther, 1996; 7: 23-31.

23. Kayaga J, Souberbielle BE, Sheikh N, Morrow WJW, Scott-Taylor T, Vile R, and Dalgleish AG, Anti-tumour activity against B16-F10 melanoma with a GM-CSF secreting allogeneic tumour cell vaccine. Gene Ther, 1999; 6: 1475-1481.

24. Prigent P, El mir S, Dreano M, and Triebel F, Lymphocyte activation gene-3 induces tumor regression and antitumor immune responses. Eur J Immunol, 1999; 29: 3867-3876.
25. Chen KY, Braun S, Lyman S, Fan Y, Traycoff CM, Wiebke EA, Gaddy J, Sledge G, Broxmeyer HE, and Cornetta K, Antitumor activity and immunotherapeutic properties of Flt3- Ligand in a murine breast cancer model. Cancer Res, 1997; 57: 3511-3516.
26. Townsend SE and Allison JP, Tumor Rejection after Direct Costimulation of Cd8+ T-Cells by B7-Transfected Melanoma-Cells. Science, 1993; 259: 368-370.
27. Chong H, Hutchinson G, Hart IR, and Vile RG, Expression of co-stimulatory molecules by tumor cells decreases tumorigenicity but may also reduce systemic antitumor immunity. Hum Gene Ther, 1996; 7: 1771-1779.
28. Huang AYC, Bruce AT, Pardoll DM, and Levitsky HI, Does B7-1 Expression Confer Antigen-Presenting Cell Capacity to Tumors In-Vivo. J Exp Med, 1996; 183: 769-776.
29. Zitvogel L, Robbins PD, Storkus WJ, Clarke MR, Maeurer MJ, Campbell RL, Davis CG, Tahara H, Schreiber RD, and Lotze MT, Interleukin-12 and B7.1 co-stimulation cooperate in the induction of effective antitumor immunity and therapy of established tumors. Eur J Immunol, 1996; 26: 1335-1341.
30. Chiodoni C, Paglia P, Stoppacciaro A, Rodolfo M, Parenza M, and Colombo MP, Dendritic cells infiltrating tumors cotransduced with granulocyte macrophage colony-stimulating factor (GM-CSF) and CD40 ligand genes take up and present endogenous tumor- associated antigens, and prime naive mice for a cytotoxic T lymphocyte response. J Exp Med, 1999; 190: 125-133.
31. Moolten FL, Tumor Chemosensitivity Conferred by Inserted Herpes Thymidine Kinase Genes - Paradigm for a Prospective Cancer Control Strategy. Cancer Res, 1986; 46: 5276-5281.
32. Mullen CA, Kilstrup M, and Blaese RM, Transfer of the Bacterial Gene for Cytosine Deaminase to Mammalian-Cells Confers Lethal Sensitivity to 5-Fluorocytosine - a Negative Selection System. Proc Natl Acad Sci U S A, 1992; 89: 33-37.
33. Vile RG, Nelson JA, Castleden S, Chong H, and Hart IR, Systemic Gene-Therapy Of Murine Melanoma Using Tissue-Specific Expression Of the Hsvtk Gene Involves an Immune Component. Cancer Res, 1994; 54: 6228-6234.
34. Ramesh R, Marrogi AJ, Munshi A, Abboud CN, and Freeman SM, In vivo analysis of the 'bystander effect': A cytokine cascade. Exp Hematol, 1996; 24: 829-838.
35. Vile RG, Castleden S, Marshall J, Camplejohn R, Upton C, and Chong H, Generation of an anti-tumour immune response in a non- immunogenic tumour: HSVtk killing in vivo stimulates a mononuclear cell infiltrate and a Th1-like profile of intratumoural cytokine expression. Int J Cancer, 1997; 71: 267-274.
36. Melcher A, Todryk S, Hardwick N, Ford M, Jacobson M, and Vile RG, Tumor immunogenicity is determined by the mechanism of cell death via induction of heat shock protein expression. Nat Med, 1998; 4: 581-587.
37. Todryk S, Melcher AA, Hardwick N, Linardakis E, Bateman A, Colombo MP, Stoppacciaro A, and Vile RG, Heat shock protein 70 induced during tumor cell killing induces Th1 cytokines and targets immature dendritic cell precursors to enhance antigen uptake. J Immunol, 1999; 163: 1398-1408.
38. Lukacs KV, Lowrie DB, Stokes RW, and Colston MJ, Tumor-Cells Transfected with a Bacterial Heat-Shock Gene Lose Tumorigenicity and Induce Protection against Tumors. J Exp Med, 1993; 178: 343-348.
39. Plautz GE, Yang ZY, Wu BY, Gao X, Huang L, and Nabel GJ, Immunotherapy of Malignancy by Invivo Gene-Transfer into Tumors. Proc Natl Acad Sci U S A, 1993; 90: 4645-4649.
40. Sfondrini L, Morelli D, Menard S, Maier JAM, Singh M, Melani C, Terrazzini N, Colombo MP, Colnaghi MI, and Balsari A, Anti-tumor immunity induced by murine melanoma cells transduced with the Mycobacterium tuberculosis gene encoding the 38-kDa antigen. Gene Ther, 1998; 5: 247-252.
41. Schweighoffer T, Tumor cells expressing a recall antigen are powerful cancer vaccines. Eur J Immunol, 1996; 26: 2559-2564.
42. Ostrand-Rosenberg S, Pulaski BA, Clements VK, Qi L, Pipeling MR, and Hanyok LA, Cell-based vaccines for the stimulation of immunity to metastatic cancers. Immunol Rev, 1999; 170: 101-114.
43. Caruso M, PhamNguyen K, Kwong YL, Xu BS, Kosai KI, Finegold M, Woo SLC, and Chen SH, Adenovirus-mediated interleukin-12 gene therapy for metastatic colon carcinoma. Proc Natl Acad Sci U S A, 1996; 93: 11302-11306.
44. Todryk S, McLean C, Ali S, Entwistle C, Boursnell M, Rees R, and Vile R, Disabled infectious single-cycle herpes simplex virus as an oncolytic vector for immunotherapy of colorectal cancer. Hum Gene Ther, 1999; 10: 2757-2768.
45. Ali SA, McLean CS, Boursnell MEG, Martin G, Holmes CL, Reeder S, Entwisle C, Blakeley DM, Shields JG, Todryk S, Vile R, Robins RA, and Rees RC, Preclinical evaluation of "whole" cell vaccines

for prophylaxis and therapy using a disabled infectious single cycle-herpes simplex virus vector to transduce cytokine genes. Cancer Res, 2000; 60: 1663-1670.

46. Chen SH, Shine HD, Goodman JC, Grossman RG, and Woo SLC, Gene-Therapy for Brain-Tumors - Regression of Experimental Gliomas by Adenovirus-Mediated Gene-Transfer in-Vivo. Proc Natl Acad Sci U S A, 1994; 91: 3054-3057.

47. Vile R, Miller N, Chernajovsky Y, and Hart I, A Comparison of the Properties of Different Retroviral Vectors Containing the Murine Tyrosinase Promoter to Achieve Transcriptionally Targeted Expression of the Hsvtk or Il-2 Genes. Gene Ther, 1994; 1: 307-316.

48. Vile RG, Gene therapy for cancer, the course ahead. Cancer Metastasis Rev, 1996; 15: 403-410.

49. Simons JW, Jaffee EM, Weber CE, Levitsky HI, Nelson WG, Carducci MA, Lazenby AJ, Cohen LK, Finn CC, Clift SM, Hauda KM, Beck LA, Leiferman KM, Owens AH, Piantadosi S, Dranoff G, Mulligan RC, Pardoll DM, and Marshall FF, Bioactivity of autologous irradiated renal cell carcinoma vaccines generated by ex vivo granulocyte-macrophage colony- stimulating factor gene transfer. Cancer Res, 1997; 57: 1537-1546.

50. Soiffer R, Lynch T, Mihm M, Jung K, Rhuda C, Schmollinger JC, Hodi FS, Liebster L, Lam P, Mentzer S, Singer S, Tanabe KK, Cosimi AB, Duda R, Sober A, Bhan A, Daley J, Neuberg D, Parry G, Rokovich J, Richards L, Drayer J, Berns A, Clift S, Cohen LK, Mulligan RC, and Dranoff G, Vaccination with irradiated autologous melanoma cells engineered to secrete human granulocyte- macrophage colony- stimulating factor generates potent antitumor immunity in patients with metastatic melanoma. Proc Natl Acad Sci U S A, 1998; 95: 13141-13146.

51. Simons JW, Mikhak B, Chang JF, DeMarzo AM, Carducci MA, Lim M, Weber CE, Baccala AA, Goemann MA, Clift SM, Ando DG, Levitsky HI, Cohen LK, Sanda MG, Mulligan RC, Partin AW, Carter HB, Piantadosi S, Marshall FF, and Nelson WG, Induction of immunity to prostate cancer antigens: Results of a clinical trial of vaccination with irradiated autologous prostate tumor cells engineered to secrete granulocyte- macrophage colony-stimulating factor using ex vivo gene transfer. Cancer Res, 1999; 59: 5160-5168.

52. Palmer K, Moore J, Everard M, Harris JD, Rodgers S, Rees RC, Murray AK, Mascari R, Kirkwood J, Riches PG, Fisher C, Thomas JM, Harries M, Johnston SRD, Collins MKL, and Gore ME, Gene therapy with autologous, interleukin 2-secreting tumor cells in patients with malignant melanoma. Hum Gene Ther, 1999; 10: 1261-1268.

53. Moller P, Sun Y, Dorbic T, Alijagic S, Makki A, Jurgovsky K, Schroff M, Henz BM, Wittig B, and Schadendorf D, Vaccination with IL-7 gene-modified autologous melanoma cells can enhance the anti-melanoma lytic activity in peripheral blood of patients with a good clinical performance status: a clinical phase I study. Br J Cancer, 1998; 77: 1907-1916.

54. Belli F, Arienti F, SuleSuso J, Clemente C, Mascheroni L, Cattelan A, Sanantonio C, Gallino GF, Melani C, Rao S, Colombo MP, Maio M, Cascinelli N, and Parmiani G, Active immunization of metastatic melanoma patients with interleukin-2-transduced allogeneic melanoma cells: Evaluation of efficacy and tolerability. Cancer Immunology Immunotherapy, 1997; 44: 197-203.

55. Pardoll D, Cancer vaccines. Nat Med, 1998; 4: 525-531.

56. Herman JR, Adler HL, Aguilar-Cordova E, Rojas-Martinez A, Woo S, Timme TL, Wheeler TM, Thompson TC, and Scardino PT, In situ gene therapy for adenocarcinoma of the prostate: A phase I clinical trial. Hum Gene Ther, 1999; 10: 1239-1249.

12
Antibody targeted therapy:
delivery of radionuclides, toxins and drugs

A. MURRAY, G. DENTON, M.R. PRICE, and A.C. PERKINS

INTRODUCTION

The concept of using cancer-specific antibodies to kill tumour cells was first suggested by Paul Ehrlich in 1896 when he coined the term "magic bullets". It is probably the apparent simplicity of this concept that makes it so appealing. A 'vehicle' with specificity for a receptor ideally expressed solely on malignant cells serves as a carrier molecule for a cytotoxic agent. Thereby, the agent is delivered to tumour cells and causes specific cell killing while sparing normal cells the cytotoxic effects.

The exquisite specificity of the antibody-antigen interaction is indisputable therefore the antibodies are ideal targeting molecules. After all, this is part of their role in the mammalian immune system. However, it was not until the advent of monoclonal antibody (MAb) technology [1], whereby large amounts of antibody of single and precise specificity are produced, that interest in the field of antibody targeted therapeutics increased dramatically. In the early 1980s there was a general belief that Ehrlich's theory was close to being realised with early publications showing excellent sensitivity and specificity for the *in vivo* detection (immunoscintigraphy) of colon and ovarian cancer and melanoma [2-4]. This raised hopes that antibodies could be used, not only to detect cancer but also to treat it. As we will see, the simple theory of the magic bullet did not take into account the complexities of the human immune system and the initial enthusiasm turned to doubt and disappointment. However research in the field continued, and with the arrival of genetic manipulation we were provided with a means to overcome the problems posed by the use of murine monoclonal antibodies. Antibodies have since moved from the laboratory to clinical trials for the treatment of various malignancies and the first antibody targeted cancer therapy, an anti-CD20 antibody (Rituxin) was approved by the FDA for the treatment of Non-Hodgkin's Lymphoma in 1997 [5].

The field of immunotargeting as a whole consists of numerous diverse strategies, based around the delivery of conventional chemotherapeutic molecules, cytotoxic proteins and therapeutic radionuclides. Such approaches are all common in that they

R.A. Robins and R.C. Rees (eds.), Cancer Immunology, 195–217.

involve some form of an antibody as a targeting agent and a specific receptor on tumour cells (the target). What makes these strategies differ is the nature of the therapeutic payload that the antibody carries and these will be discussed further in this chapter. First, however, it seems appropriate to look at the properties of the molecules on which the success of targeted therapy depends: the receptor (target antigen) and the vector (antibody).

THE BASIC INGREDIENTS OF IMMUNOTARGETING

The target

Antibody targeted therapy exploits the subtle differences between the cancer cell and the normal cell and a variety of cell surface molecules have been used as targets. The only truly tumour-specific antigens are the clonally expressed receptor idiotypes (Ids) on T and B lymphocytes. Unfortunately, the use of anti-Id antibodies to treat lymphoid cancer is limited by the need to create custom-made patient-specific monoclonal antibodies [6]. Instead, tumour-associated rather than tumour specific antigens have been used as targets. These have included differentiation antigens, growth factor receptors, oncofetal antigens, unique carbohydrate antigens or aberrantly expressed normal antigens. One of the first described was carcinoembryonic antigen (CEA) [10] and this antigen is still being used today in the diagnosis and targeted therapy of colorectal cancer (see chapter 5).

Unfortunately, the loss of cellular organisation and control that is a feature of malignancy results in tumour cell antigen expression that is heterogeneous and non-static. This may result in groups of cells within a tumour that have very little or no antigen expression and are thus resistant to antibody targeted therapy. On the other hand, this disregulation of tumour cell function can lead to expression of modified antigens with increased tumour specificity. An example would be that of the MUC1 mucin glycoprotein which is expressed only on the luminal surface of many normal epithelial cells [11]. However, in the malignant state, the polarity of MUC1 expression is lost and the antigen is expressed all over the surface of the cell and thus is exposed to the circulation. In addition, changes in glycosyltransferase and glycosidase patterns within the tumour cell result in truncation of carbohydrate chains covering the molecule. This leads to exposure of cancer-specific epitopes for anti-MUC1 antibodies not usually exposed in the non-malignant state [12].

The target does not, however, necessarily have to be an antigen expressed on the tumour cell itself. The vasculature that supplies the tumour can be the source of useful targets because, unlike the tumour cells, the vascular endothelium is directly accessible to systemic therapeutic agents. In addition, since a capillary may supply a large number of tumour cells, vascular damage can result in widespread tumour cell death [13].

ANTIBODY TARGETED THERAPY

The magic bullet

Some unconjugated antibodies can induce anti-tumour effects by mechanisms that include the activation of effector cells of the immune system (antibody dependant cell-mediated cytotoxicity) or fixation of complement [14]. Others have been shown to have the ability to signal cell cycle arrest or apoptosis [15]. These mechanisms are described in more detail elsewhere.

The main requirement of antibodies used in targeted therapy of cancer is that they must localise to tumour cells, preferably with high affinity. They should also exhibit minimum binding to normal cells. Monoclonal antibodies used as targeting agents in cancer therapy have traditionally been of murine origin. As a consequence the use of these MAbs has been limited by the reaction of the human immune system against the mouse protein which causes a human anti-mouse antibody (HAMA) response. This usually occurs in 1-4 weeks and results in accelerated clearance of subsequently administered MAb conjugates. In addition, the large size (approximately 150 kD) of the antibody limits extravascular tumour penetration [16]. Originally, antibodies were reduced in size by digestion with enzymes such as papain and pepsin to produce Fab and F(ab)$_2$ fragments (Figure 12.1) with retained antigen binding capacity. However such methods produced very low yields.

With the advent of recombinant DNA technology scientists were provided with the tools to redesign antibodies at the genetic level in order to make them smaller and less immunogenic while retaining (and in some cases improving) the tumour specificity and affinity. By isolating the RNA from hybridoma cells, reverse transcribing it into complimentary DNA and then selectively amplifying the sequences encoding the antigen binding domains (Figure 12.1) using Polymerase Chain Reaction (PCR), it is possible to produce large amounts of antibody DNA. This can then be ligated into a suitable vector which is used to transform a host cell such as bacteria or yeast, which expresses and secretes the protein encoded by the recombinant DNA as if it were its own [17].

Figure 1 provides a schematic representation of the types of modification that can be achieved using recombinant DNA technology. In order to reduce the immunogenicity of mouse monoclonal antibodies, chimeric (mouse Fv regions grafted on to human Fc regions) or humanised (mouse hypervariable domains grafted on to human framework and Fc regions) antibodies can be [18, 19]. Chimeric or humanised MAbs have been developed for the treatment of renal cell, ovarian and breast carcinoma, Non-Hodgkin's Lymphoma (NHL), melanoma and neuroblastoma without significant development of HAMA responses [20, 21]. The disadvantage of humanisation is that it can be a laborious process and it is now being superseded by the rapid and direct isolation of human antibodies from phage display libraries. In this approach V_H and V_L domains are PCR-cloned and displayed on the surface of bacteriophage. Antigen specific phage are then selectively recovered by *in vitro* panning against the target antigen [13]. In addition, human antibody genes have been inserted into transgenic mice with endogenous antibody genes deleted. This resulted in mice that could produce human antibodies in response to an antigenic challenge, which could be recovered using standard hybridoma technology [22].

Murine IgG

Antigen Binding Sites (Paratopes)
Comprised of hypervariable domains and framework regions

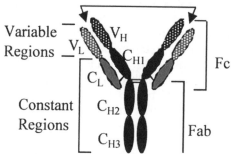

Antibody fragments produced by enzymatic digestion

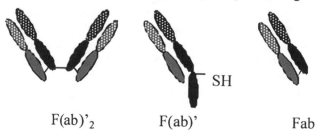

F(ab)'₂   F(ab)'   Fab

Antibody fragments produced by recombinant DNA technology

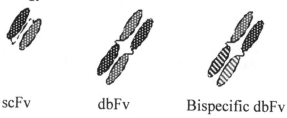

scFv   dbFv   Bispecific dbFv

Figure 12.1. Schematic representation of murine IgG and the structures of the fragments that can be produced by enzymatic digestion of whole antibody and by PCR of antibody encoding mouse genes then expression in host systems such as *E.coli.*

Improved tumour penetration can be achieved using antibody fragments such as Fv heterodimers and single chain Fvs (scFvs), which have a molecular weight of only 25kD [23]. However, one should bear in mind that, after intravenous administration, small size molecules are rapidly cleared from the blood by the kidneys [24]. In addition, these molecules may show decreased avidity due to their monovalency. To overcome these limitations, diabodies (dbFv) have been produced by engineering scFvs with a shortened linker sequence that will allow intermolecular association to produce bivalent antibody fragments [25] that can cross-link cellular receptors more readily. Variations on the dbFv have been produced in the form of double headed antibodies that can bind two different antigens at the same time [26, 27]. These bispecific antibodies have the ability to carry a cytotoxic agent at one paratope while binding to the tumour cell with the other. Bispecific antibodies can also be produced by chemical cross-linking of two MAbs of different specificities or by fusion of two different hybridomas to produce a tetradoma [28], however these constructs are twice the size of a MAb and therefore have poor tumour penetration. The affinity of bispecific antibodies for the cytotoxic agent must be retained *in vivo* and the pharmacokinetics of the loaded antibody must be favourable for good tumour localisation. This approach has shown some success in animals [29].

ACCESSIBILITY OF THE TARGET TUMOUR

In order for targeted therapy to be successful the tumour must be accessible to the immunoconjugate through the chosen route of administration. The systemic route is the classical form of tumour therapy administration. The blood stream has a number of advantages and disadvantages as a route to the tumour site. One of the drawbacks, which has already been discussed, is the reaction of the host immune system to immunoconjugates of murine origin. This results in the formation of HAMA that cause altered biodistribution, increased clearance of subsequent treatments and may even cause serious anaphylactic reactions in the patient. Another problem with systemic administration is the potential toxicity to organs that would normally clear such macromolecules from the circulation such as the kidneys and liver.

Conversely, tumours develop a good blood supply to provide the oxygen and nutrients required for their uncontrolled growth. In addition, tumour vessels are inherently leaky compared with the blood vessels in most normal tissues. This is due to wide inter-endothelial junctions, large numbers of fenestrae and transendothelial channels formed by vesicles as well as discontinuous or absent basement membranes [30, 31]. As a result, capillary permeability of the endothelial barrier in newly vascularised tumours is significantly greater than that of normal tissues [32]. This may lead to increased tumour uptake of immunoconjugates since this is a function of both local blood flow and microvascular permeability. The amount of tissue accumulation of conjugate is proportional to plasma clearance. The enhanced permeability and retention (due to poor lymphatic drainage of the tumour) effect leads to prolonged accumulation and retention of macromolecules in tumour interstitium [33].

One approach to increase the tumour to normal tissue uptake of antibody is to administer the immunoconjugate locally to the site of the tumour. This can be achieved in some cases by injection directly in to the tumour mass. In addition some tumours, such as those in the bladder, grow in body cavities that shield them from the host immune system. Intravesical antibody targeted therapy provides advantages over systemic administration in that no HAMA response is generated [34] and higher doses of therapeutic agent can be given without causing problems of non-target organ toxicity. Of course only a small number of tumour types fulfil the criterion for intravesical therapy and this route of administration will not allow efficient targeting of distant micrometastases.

STRATEGIES FOR TARGETED THERAPY

The type of targeted therapy is often defined by the nature of the therapeutic molecule. Some of the strategies that have been employed for antibody targeted therapy of cancer will now be discussed in more detail.

Radioimmunotherapy (RIT)

Radiotherapy is an established form of cancer therapy whether it is in the form of external beam radiotherapy or systemic administration of cytotoxic radionuclides such as iodine-131 for thyroid cancer and strontium-89 for palliation of bone metastases. The toxic effects of ionising radiation on living cells are well known. External beam radiotherapy causes destruction of the cell nucleus with double or quadruple-strand DNA breaks. However, internal radiation may disrupt the transfer of signals from the cell surface to the nucleus, interfering with signalling at all levels [35].

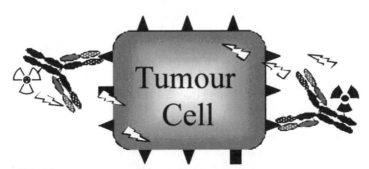

Figure 12.2. Diagrammatic representation of the strategy of radioimmunotherapy (RIT). A therapeutic radionuclide is conjugated to the antibody which carries the radioactivity to the site of the tumour.

Some of the first targeting studies in oncology involved the use of antibodies labelled with gamma emitting radionuclides such as iodine-131, indium-111 and technetium-99m. These were administered to cancer patients and, after a period of time to allow for tumour localisation of the immunoconjugate, an image of the tumour was obtained using a gamma camera. This technique is known as radioimmunoscintigraphy (RIS) and has been used for diagnostic imaging of a wide range of tumours including colorectal, ovarian, breast, lung, prostate and melanoma. It is easy to imagine how it would be straight forward to convert the conjugate from a diagnostic radiopharmaceutical to a therapeutic agent simply by changing the radionuclide to one which emits beta or alpha radiation and increasing the administered dose (Figure 12.2). However, RIT has a number of problems to address when compared to RIS. For imaging, only a proportion of the cancer cells need to be targeted and there is no requirement for tumour penetration, so heterogeneity and tumour size are not an issue. Effective tumour therapy requires that a greater proportion of the cancer cells take up the agent. Clumps of cells with no antigen expression can be a problem. However the penetrating nature of radiation does mean that tumour cells may be killed by antibody localisation on other adjacent or nearby cells (bystander effect), a situation more favourable for effective therapy than conventional chemotherapy which requires the direct action of drug molecules on each tumour cell. In addition, higher residency time of the conjugate on the tumour cell is required for therapeutic efficacy. Nonetheless, a carefully constructed conjugate comprised of an antibody component with good tumour penetration properties (see below) and a radionuclide component with high linear energy transfer (LET) and long physical half-life can overcome these problems.

Choice of Radionuclide

The choice of radionuclide for RIT must take into account the nature and *in vivo* behaviour of the antibody to which it is to be conjugated. Other important factors include the nature of the radiation, the ratio of penetrating (gamma) to non-penetrating (beta and alpha) radiation, the physical half-life ($t_{1/2}$) of the radionuclide and the stability of any daughter nuclides formed. From a practical point of view, the route of production (presence of cold carrier) and the availability may also be important [36]. The properties of some radionuclides commonly used in antibody targeted therapy are given in Table 12.1.

Tumour cell killing is most effectively achieved by radionuclides emitting high LET radiation that deposit the majority of their ionising energy within the targeted tumour. Auger electron and alpha emitting nuclides have powerful cell killing properties but their tumour penetration range is very low and so homogeneous tumour distribution is required. Beta emitters, on the other hand, can yield homogeneous tumour radiation doses even when the radioimmunoconjugate is heterogeneously distributed throughout the tissue. However, high-energy beta-emitters such as yittrium-90 may give rise to a significant radiation dose to the bone marrow.

The gamma radiation associated with many radionuclides can contribute significantly to the whole body radiation dose experienced by radioimmunotherapy patients, but does not contribute significantly to the tumour dose. Highly penetrating gamma radiation (such as that of ^{131}I) can also present a hazard to the patient's carers. However, the advantage of using a therapeutic nuclide that emits gamma radiation is that the presence of the antibody at the site of the tumour (or elsewhere) can be imaged with a gamma camera. This has led to the term radioimmuno-directed therapy (RIDT), which allows calculations of dosimetry to be performed by image analysis and comparison to known standards. An image obtained after intravesicle administration of a copper-67 labelled anti-mucin antibody can be seen in Figure 12.3.

201

Table 12.1. Physical propeties of radionuclides commonly used in RIT. Adapted from Schubiger *et al*, 1996 [36].

Nuclide	Physical Half-Life	Radiation Type (Energy, MeV)	Max Range in Tissue
Iodine-131	8.0 d	β (0.60), γ (0.364)	2.0 mm
Copper-67	2.6 d	β (0.54), γ (0.185)	1.8 mm
Samarium-153	47 h	β (0.80), γ (0.103)	4.4 mm
Silver-111	7.5 d	β (1.05), γ (0.340)	4.8 mm
Rhenium-186	3.8 d	β (1.08), γ (0.131)	5.0 mm
Rhenium-188	17.0 h	β (2.13), γ (0.155)	11.0 mm
Yittrium-90	2.7 d	β (2,28)	12.0 mm
Astatine-211	7.2 h	α (5.90)	65 μm
Bismuth-212	1.0 h	α (7.80), γ (0.720)	70 μm
Iodine-125	60.0 d	Auger, γ (0.027)	10 nm

Ideally, the physical half-life of the therapeutic radionuclide should be similar to the biological half-life of the radioimmunoconjugate at the site of the tumour. A therapeutic dose should be maintained over a long enough period to ensure that all cells are irradiated during the most radio-sensitive M and G_2 phases of the cell cycle [36]. Finally, the route of production of the nuclide may be important. Nuclides produced by bombardment are often contaminated with cold 'parent' element. This can be extremely difficult to remove and can significantly lower the specific activity of the therapeutic nuclide. Generator produced products such as rhenium-188 (resulting from the decay of unstable tungsten-188), have no cold carrier present and therefore relatively high specific activity. Such nuclides also have the advantage of being available on demand simply by eluting the generator with saline [37].

Conjugation Chemistry

Labelling strategies are often based on the utilisation of a multidentate ligand (or chelator) such as DTPA capable of selective chelation of the desired radionuclide [36]. This may be performed as post-labelling in which the chelator is attached to the antibody first then the nuclide is introduced, or pre-labelling (the radionuclide-chelator complex is formed first). Alternatively, a direct approach can be adopted in which the radionuclide is attached directly to the antibody through reaction with suplphydryl

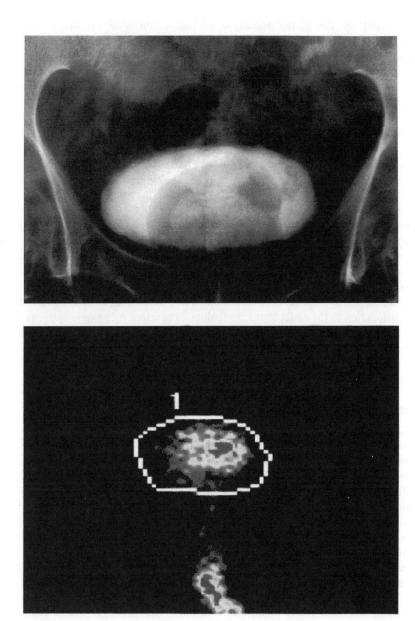

Figure 12.3. Top: Intravenous urogram showing filling defect in the bladder due to a large bladder tumour. Bottom: Anterior gamma camera image of the same patient following instillation and washout of a tracer amount (20MBq) Cu-67-C595 anti-mucin antibody.

groups formed by the partial reduction of inter-chain disulfide bonds within the antibody [38]. Recently, labelling of recombinant antibody fragments with a technetium-99m carbonyl compound at high specific activity has been achieved by linking to an engineered histidine fusion tag [39]. Although not demonstrated, the authors suggest that this labelling method should be applicable to radioimmunotherapeutic approaches with rhenium-188 or rhenium-186.

Immunotoxin therapy (IT)

Immunotoxins consist of potent plant, fungal or bacterial toxins (or toxin subunits) conjugated to a monoclonal antibody. The first immunotoxins were described in the early [40, 41]. The antibody targets a receptor on the tumour cell surface and is internalised by receptor-mediated endocytosis. Some of the internalised immunotoxin is routed via endosomes to the endoplasmic reticulum where the toxin is cleaved from the antibody and translocated to the cytosol. Here the toxin inhibits ribosomal activity leading to blockage of protein synthesis and cell death [17]. Toxins are extremely potent, in fact, only one toxin molecule may be required to kill a cell. In addition, their action is independent of cell cycle stage.

Immunotoxins must be internalised into a non-lysosomal cellular compartment to allow translocation to the endoplasmic reticulum. Therefore membrane antigens such as growth factors which undergo receptor-mediated endocytosis into endosomes or other acidic components make good IT targets [17]. It is important that the target antigen must be present on every tumour cell, since there is no bystander effect.

Characteristics of immunotoxins

Many immunotoxins are comprised of ribosome inactivating proteins (RIPs) derived from plants such as ricin. RIPs are classified into one of two types depending on how many peptide chains they have. Both types block protein synthesis by cleavage of 28s RNA, which inactivates the 60s ribosomal subunit, thus preventing its interaction with elongation factor 2. Type II plant toxins have two chains which are held together by disulphide bonds [42]. The A chain contains the catalytic site and the B chain has galactose binding domains which facilitate cell binding and entry. However, since the B-chain has the ability to bind to all galactose containing glycoproteins and glycolipids, the whole molecule has specificity for any cell. Therefore the B chain must be removed before immunotoxin construction as in the case of ricin A chain immunoconjugates. Type I toxins, on the other hand, only have an A chain and therefore no cell binding domain. Bacterial toxins such as pseudomas exotoxin have a single protein chain with both catalytic and cell binding functions [43]. These toxins inhibit protein synthesis by catalysing the ADP-ribosylation of elongation factor 2 [44]. Toxins derived from plants and bacteria are highly immunogenic and can not be easily humanised.

The chemistry used to link toxins and antibodies must be stable in the circulation and extracellular environment, but must be labile in the cytosol. Many approaches have been based around the formation of disulfide bonds between the two molecules since these can be reduced intracellularly to liberate the toxin. In order to confer resistance to attack by circulating thiols, bulky groups have been placed around the disulfide bonds [45].

Recombinant immunotoxins have also been produced as fusion proteins [46]. These have several advantages over conventionally produced immunotoxins. They can be smaller and so have better tumour penetration properties. Also, they can be engineered to contain sequences that facilitate cell binding and entry or eliminate sequences that induce side effects such as vascular leak syndrome (increased vascular permeability leading to oedema, hypoxia and pulmonary and cardiovascular failure). On the other hand the reduced size of recombinant immunotoxins means that they are more rapidly cleared from the circulation [47].

Applications of Immunotoxins

Clinical trials with the first chemically conjugated immunotoxins began in the late 1980s for treatment of leukaemia and lymphoma in the first instance where dramatic results were [48, 49]. These were closely followed by trials for treatment of solid tumours such as breast [50], colon [51], ovarian [52] and others, however these proved to be less successful [53].

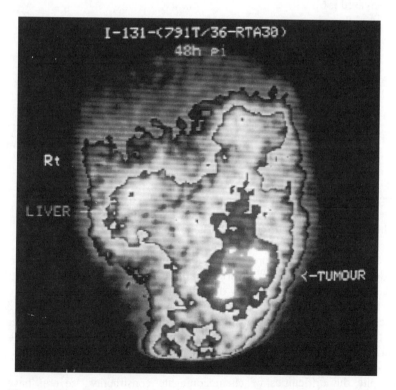

Figure 12.4. Gamma scinitigraphy of the abdomen of a patient with a large recurrent ovarian carcinoma following intraperitoneal injection of a ricin A chain immunoconjugate labelled with iodine-131.

This is probably due to poor penetration of bulky tumours. Figure 12.4 shows a gamma camera image taken 48 hours after intraperitoneal injection of a ricin A chain immunotoxin into a woman with a large recurrent ovarian carcinoma. The immunotoxin was labelled with iodine-131 which allowed its localisation at the site of the tumour to be visualised.

Animal studies would suggest that cocktails of immunotoxins targeting more than one cell surface antigen may have better *in vivo* activity [54]. Combination therapy along with conventional therapeutic regimens has also resulted in improved efficacy in animal models [55].

Chemoconjugate therapy

Conventional anti-cancer drugs can be conjugated to MAbs to produce a chemoconjugate for targeted cytotoxic therapy (Figure 12.5). Chemoconjugate therapy has advantages over conventional chemotherapy in that toxicity to normal cells is reduced, drug uptake into cancer cells is increased and the bioavailability of the toxic agent is increased [56].

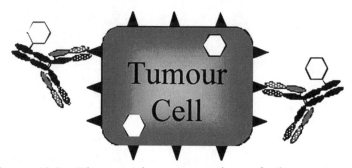

Figure 12.5. Diagrammatic representation of the strategy of chemoconjugate therapy. A cytotoxic drug is conjugated to the antibody which carries the drug to the site of the tumour.

The first chemoconjugate was produced in 1972 by simply mixing chlorambucil with immunoglobulin [57]. Since then, a variety of drugs have been conjugated to antibodies (Table 12.2). This can be achieved by directly linking one to the other, or by coupling indirectly through an intermediate carrier such as human serum albumin [58] or dextran [59]. The second approach has the advantage of allowing more drug molecules to be attached to each antibody. Ideally, the conjugation reaction will not affect the biological activity of either the antibody or the drug. However, in practise, this can be difficult to achieve [60].

Despite the difficulties of chemoconjugate construction, several have been effective *in vitro* and in pre-clinical and clinical trials. Impressive results have been obtained in studies of chemoconjugate therapy in immunosuppressed mice bearing human tumour xenografts [61, 62]. Anti-tumour activity has also been observed in

Phase I clinical trials [60]. Unfortunately chemoconjugate therapy is plagued with the same problems as all types of therapy employing murine monoclonal antibodies – that of normal tissue toxicity and HAMA response. However, studies involving humanised antibodies are underway.

Table 12.2. Examples of cytotoxic drugs that have been conjugated to antibodies for chemoconjugate therapy of a range of types of malignancy.

Mechanisim of Action	Drug	Disease Treated
Antimetabolites	Methotrexate	Lung and colon cancer, T cell lymphoma
	5-Fluorouracil	B cell leukaemia
	5'-Fluoro-2'-deoxyuridine	Colon carcinoma
Alkylating agents	Chlorambucil	Melanoma
	Mitomycin C	Lung cancer
	Cysplatinum	ovarian carcinoma
Anthracyclines	Doxorubicin/ adriamycin	Melanoma, ovararian carcinoma, breast cancer, T & B-cell lymphoma, colon carcinoma
	Daunomycin	Neuroblastoma, soft tissue sarcoma, Hepatoma
Antimitotic agents	Vinca alkaloids	Lung adenocarcinoma

Antibody directed enzyme prodrug therapy (ADEPT)

ADEPT is a two step approach which attempts to increase the concentration of cytotoxic drug at the site of the tumour while decreasing the toxic effect of the drug. In the first step, an antibody that is conjugated to an enzyme with specificity for a cytotoxic prodrug is administered and accumulates at the site of the tumour. Time is allowed for clearance of unbound conjugate from the blood and normal tissues before the second step when a non-toxic, inactive prodrug is administered. This is carried in the circulation until it encounters the immunoconjugate at the tumour site, which converts the prodrug to its active form (Figure 12.6). The interval between the two steps is optimised to produce minimal systemic toxicity by achieving satisfactory accumulation of the conjugate at the tumour with clearance from the circulation and normal tissues [63]. An advantage of ADEPT over other antibody targeted therapeutic approaches is that there is inherent amplification due to the fact that one enzyme molecule may catalyse the conversion of many drug molecules. Lower doses of immunoconjugate may therefore be given to obtain equivalent therapeutic responses and higher concentrations of drug may be achieved at the tumour site compared to administration of drug alone [64]. In addition, as the drug diffuses through the tumour it produces a bystander effect, killing antigen negative cells [65].

The idea of administering an inactive precursor, which is converted to a cytotoxic agent at the tumour site predates the development of monoclonal antibodies. In fact one of the first prodrugs used was nitrogen mustard which can be reduced to its highly toxic aniline and p-phenylenediamine derivatives by an enzyme system present in high amounts in hepatocellular carcinoma known as xanthine oxidase. The derivatives are extremely potent alkylating agents with established anti-tumour activity [66].

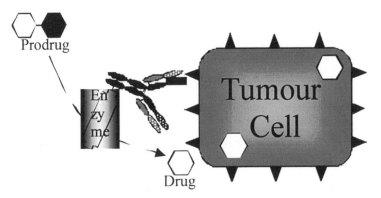

Figure 12.6. Diagrammatic representation of the strategy of ADEPT. An enzyme that catalyses the conversion of an inactive prodrug to a cytotoxic agent is conjugated to a tumour targeting antibody. Following tumour localisation and clearance of unbound immunoconjugate from the circulation, the prodrug is administered and is converted to its active form by the enzyme at the tumour site.

ANTIBODY TARGETED THERAPY

Antibodies for use in ADEPT

High affinity antibodies are required for successful ADEPT since these have slow off-rates with resulting long residency time on the tumour cell. This will allow satisfactory time for clearance of circulating immunoconjugate before the prodrug is administered. Unconjugated antibody fragments provide better tumour penetration than intact IgG, but this potential benefit is hampered by the size of the enzyme used. The rapid blood clearance demonstrated by antibody fragments can be an advantage after tumour localisation, however it also results in lower tumour uptake levels and therefore higher doses of antibody-enzyme conjugate need to be administered. Finally, the covalent linking of the antibody and enzyme should not disrupt the biological activity of either molecule. A wide range of antibodies, targeting antigens such as CEA and β-human chorionic gonadotrophin are now under investigation in *in vivo* and *in vitro* trials of ADEPT [65].

The Enzyme

The function of enzymes used in ADEPT is to catalyse the conversion of the inactive prodrug to its cytotoxic derivative exclusively at the site of the tumour. To achieve this, the enzyme must function and be stable under physiological conditions. Enzymes with pH and temperature optima of 7.0-7.4 and 37°C respectively are best suited although enzymes with characteristics other than these can be used but will work with lower efficiency. In addition, a requirement for co-factors not present in extracellular fluid is not ideal since these would need to be administered together with the prodrug. A high catalytic turnover will allow greater concentrations of active drug at the tumour site, which will produce a steeper diffusion gradient into the cell. Finally, an ideal enzyme for ADEPT would have the ability to activate a panel of cytotoxic drugs.

In order for the therapy to be tumour specific the enzyme must not be widely expressed on normal human tissue. Enzymes of non-mammalian origin such as carboxypeptidase G2 (CPG2), a zinc metalloenzyme originally isolated from Pseudomonas species, have been used [63]. This enzyme is not found in mammalian cells and so activation of the prodrug in the blood and normal tissues is avoided. It catalyses the cleavage of a glutamate moiety from a benzoic acid mustard [67]. This enzyme has been cloned into *E. coli* and so is readily available on a large scale [68]. The main disadvantage however, of non-mammalian enzymes is that they tend to elicit immune responses in the human that can prevent repeated treatment cycles [69]. Antibodies developed against CPG2 in cancer patients have been shown to neutralise the activity of CPG2 at the tumour site as well as clear it from the plasma [70]. The immunosuppresive drug, cyclosporin A, which acts by blocking cytokine synthesis leading to inhibition of T-cell proliferation, has been used successfully to delay the host response to CPG2 in mice and humans, however, the immunosuppresive agent was found to contribute significantly to the side effects experienced by patients [70].

Some non-mammalian enzymes have human analogues and as such, may be less immunogenic. An example would be that of β−glucuronidase which has both human and bacterial forms. The human form is mainly found intracellularly in lysosomes and microsomes and therefore should not cause systemic toxicity after *in vivo* prodrug administration. In addition, the bacterial form has a optimum pH of around 6.8 compared with 5.4 for the human form. The bacterial form is therefore far more efficient under the physiological conditions of the tumour. Epirubicin is excreted in the form epirubicin-glucuronide by patients treated with the drug. This has been isolated from urine and used as a prodrug in conjunction with an antibody-β-glucuronidase conjugate, which cleaves the gluronide to release active epirubicin [71].

Enzymes of mammalian origin such as alkaline phosphatase, which hydrolytically removes phosphate from phosphorylated cytotoxic drug derivatives, are far less immunogenic than bacterial enzymes. However, their ubiquitous nature makes them far from ideal as enzymes for ADEPT.

The Prodrug-Drug System

The main requirement for a prodrug is to be a suitable substrate for the enzyme used under physiological conditions. There should be a large difference in toxicity between the drug and its precursor and the prodrug should not be converted by endogenous enzymes. A very potent drug with a very short half-life offers the optimal combination since the amount of drug diffusing from the tumour and reaching the circulation would be negligible. If the development of host immune responses against the immunoconjugate is a potential problem, the drug should be able to achieve maximum cell killing within a limited number of cycles of treatment with the mode of action being dose-dependent and independent of cell cycle stage [65]. The pharmacological and pharmacokinetic characteristics of the drug should be optimal. The extent of transfer of drug from the circulation to the tumour cell is dependent on the chemical structure of the molecule and the properties of the barrier. Drugs with high lipophilicity may provide better tumour penetration. Drug resistance should also be taken into consideration when the prodrug system is chosen [72].

The design of a non-toxic prodrug, which on activation by an enzyme will be converted, to a highly cytotoxic metabolite requires an in-depth knowledge of the structure-action relationships of both molecules. This is why most ADEPT prodrugs are derived from established anti-cancer agents of which the pharamcological and pharmacokinetic parameters are well known. However there is a group of drugs, the second generation nitrogen mustard compounds such as ZD2767 which have been designed with specific ADEPT requirements in mind [73]. For a comprehensive review of prodrugs developed for ADEPT the reader is referred to the article by Niulescu-Duvaz and Springer [64].

Immunoliposomes

Liposomes have been proposed to be useful carriers for targeted drug delivery systems and are under investigation in several therapeutic fields [74]. They consist of one or more concentric phospholipid bilayers each enclosing an aqueous compartment to form a lipid vesicle of around 40-100 nm in diameter [75] (Figure 12.7). The usual composition is phosphatidylcholine or cholesterol with or without polyethylene glycol (PEG). A large variety of therapeutic agents have been successfully incorporated into liposomes and several types of ligand have been conjugated for targeting purposes such as vitamins [76], glycoproteins [77], peptides [78], and oligonucleotide aptamers [79] as well as antibodies and antibody fragments [80]. When bound to the target cell, delivery of encapsulated drug can take place via four different mechanisms: (1) the drug may be released extracellularly and then taken up by the tumour cell, (2) lipophilic drugs may be transferred from the liposomal membrane to the plasma membrane of tumour cells, (3) the liposomal membrane may fuse with the tumour cell membrane, releasing its contents into the cytosol, (4) cell surface receptor bound immunoliposomes may be taken into the cell by endocytosis and release their contents there (Mastrobattista *et al*, 1999). Under optimal conditions, up to 25,000 liposomes can be taken up by a cell [17].

An advantage of immunoliposomes over other immunoconjugates is that they can accommodate a very wide range of therapeutic agents, regardless of size, solubility etc. and can carry the drug at high concentration. Drug encapsulation also reduces systemic toxicity and increases the biological half-life. The ideal characteristics of immunoliposomes for therapy of cancer are: (1) The blood clearance of the immunoliposome must be low compared with the rate of extravasation to the tumour. (2) Immunoliposome loading and retention of the drug must be efficient. (3) The drug and antibody incorporation must be stable enough to permit liposomal entry into the tumour cell without loss of either agent. (4) The antibody must remain immunoreactive when bound to the liposome [81].

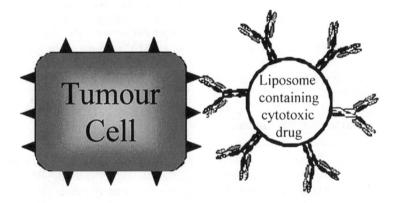

Figure 12.7. Diagrammatic representation of the strategy of immunoliposome therapy. A cytotoxic drug is conjugated to the antibody which carries the drug to the site of the tumour.

Potential Problems of Immunoliposome Therapy

Many *in vitro* experiments have demonstrated high specific binding of immunoliposomes to target cells. However, despite the excellent targeting properties *in vitro*, only a limited number of preclinical studies report successful targeting of immunoliposomes *in vivo* [80]. Accessibility of tumour cells is a critical issue when targeting solid tumours with immunoliposomes. They have great potential for the intracavity treatment of tumours, however when tumour targeting via the systemic route is the only option a number of problems are presented in terms of the transport of the immunoconjugate as well as tumour targeting and treatment.

The circulatory environment exposes liposomes to a number of factors that might compromise their integrity. Adsorption of serum proteins can cause liposome aggregation leading to increased phagocytic clearance rate as well as inducing leakage of their contents [82, 83]. In addition, antibodies reactive against phospholipids have been detected in the human circulation, that have the ability to bind liposomes and activate the complement cascade [84]. Even without aggregation, the immunoliposome provides a tempting target for cells of the mononuclear phagocyte system (MPS) such as macrophages in the liver and spleen [85]. Recently, progress has been made in overcoming these problems by coating the liposome surface with PEG. This is thought to provide a highly hydrated layer around the construct, which stearically inhibits electrostatic and hydrophobic interactions of serum proteins. The result is that these 'stealth' liposomes have longer circulating times and reduced uptake by the MPS [86-88].

Liposomes bearing whole antibodies are prone to Fc-receptor-mediated phagocytosis by cells of the MPS, leading to rapid clearance with the rate of clearance being dependent on antibody density at the liposome surface [89]. However, tumour targeting efficacy is also related to antibody density therefore there is a trade off between highly efficient targeting and low plasma clearance rate. A solution to this problem may be to use antibody fragments with no Fc regions as targeting agents [81]). In addition, liposomes incorporating murine antibodies do not differ from any other type of immunoconjugate in that they induce a HAMA response. In fact, antibodies conjugated to liposomes are more immunogenic than those given in a free form. Surprisingly, however, the production of anti-liposome antibodies has not been documented [90].

In Vivo Immunoliposome Studies

Despite the potential problems of immunoliposome therapy of cancer, research in the field continues. Intracavity tumours are readily accessible to liposomes and intraperitineal administration of liposomes loaded with 5'-palmitoyl-5-fluorouridine targeting the CAR-3 antigen, abundantly expressed on ovarian cancer cells, resulted in a drastic reduction in tumour mass in a nude mouse xenograft model [91]. Haematological malignancies also seem to be readily accessible to intravenously administered immunoliposome preparations. Significant increases in survival have been demonstrated by immunoliposome treatment of human B-cell lymphoma mouse models [92, 93]. However, when treating circulating tumour cells there is a potential risk of agglutination due to the multivalent interaction of immunoliposomes with more than one tumour cell. This can cause occlusion of small capillaries and in extreme cases has led to death of laboratory animals [94]. The abnormal blood vessel structures associated with tumour angiogenesis have been exploited for the extravasation of liposomes following their intravenous administration for the treatment of solid tumours. In order for this approach to be successful the liposomes must be small and exhibit long circulation times. However, studies in experimental animal models of solid tumours such as human breast cancer xenografts give conflicting evidence as to the efficacy of targeted liposome preparations [80]. Nevertheless, doxorubicin encapsulated in PEG-liposomes (Doxil®) has recently been approved for the treatment of AIDS-related

Kaposi's sarcoma in the USA and Europe. This drug is currently in clinical trials for the treatment of breast, ovarian and various other forms of solid tumours [81].

CONCLUSIONS AND FUTURE PERSPECTIVES

Research in the field of antibody targeted therapy has provided a heterogeneous class of anti-tumour agents with remarkable efficacy in the treatment of experimental cancers in animals. Ongoing research is aimed at developing immunoconjugates with increased potency and decreased immunogenicity and toxicity in order to improve their therapeutic index. The most marked successes in humans, however, have so far been observed in the treatment of blood borne malignancies. The disappointing results obtained from trials of systemic targeted therapy of solid tumours may be due to poor tumour penetration properties of the immunoconjugates, heterogeneity of antigen expression and uptake in some normal tissues. It is apparent from ongoing clinical trials that bone marrow toxicity is a major problem to overcome. Success in the treatment of solid tumours will require clinical selection of small cellular deposits that are easily accessible, as well as the use of smaller antibody constructs that exhibit improved tumour penetration. Intracavity administration is certainly one option which may prove to be clinically viable, for example in the therapy of ovarian or bladder cancer

Another significant drawback of the use of murine monoclonal antibodies is the development of HAMA responses and the potential for anaphylactic reactions following subsequent doses of antibody However, there is now a suggestion that such a patient response following an immune challenge may have some therapeutic benefit for the patient. Humanisation has greatly enhanced the utility of antibodies for therapy, but this is being superseded by phage display techniques that facilitate the rapid selection of human antibodies with the desired characteristics of affinity and specificity. While modern fermentation production techniques are resulting in higher antibody yields, the standards required to gain approval by the regulatory bodies are becoming increasingly difficult to attain. Despite this, the future optimisation of the antibody vehicle and the cytotoxic moiety should result in effective cancer treatment.

REFERENCES

1. Kohler, G and Milstein, C. (1975) Continuous cultures of fused cells secreting antibody of predefined specificity. Nature 256, 495-497.
2. Deland, F. and Goldenberg, D.M. (1985) Diagnosis and treatment of neoplasms with radionuclide-labeled antibodies. Semin. Nucl. Med. 15, 2-11.
3. Divigi, C.R. and Larson, S.M. (1989) Radiolabeled monoclonal antibodies in the diagnosis and treatment of malignant melanoma Semin. Nucl. Med. 19, 252-261.
4. Larson, S.M. (1991) Radioimmunology. Imaging and therapy. Cancer 67, 1253-1260.
5. Anderson, D.R., Grillo-Lopez, A., Varns, C., Chambers, K.S. and Hanna, N. (1997) Targeted anticancer therapy using rituximab, a chimeric anti-CD20 antibody (IDECC2B8) in the treatment of non-Hodgkin's B-cell lymphoma. Biochem. Soc. Trans. 25, 705-708
6. Brown, S.L., Miller, R.A. and Levy, R. (1989) Antiidiotypic antibody therapy of B-cell lymphoma. Semin. Oncol. 16, 199-210

7. Waldmann, T.A. (1991) Monoclonal antibodies in diagnosis and therapy. Science 252, (5013), 1657-1662.
8. Dillman, R.O. (1994) Antibodies as cytotoxic therapy. J. clin. Oncol. 12, 1497-1515.
9. Choy, E.H.S., Panayi, G.S. and Kingsley, G.H. (1995) Therapeutic monoclonal antibodies. Br. J. Rheumatol. 34, 707-715.
10. Gold, P. and Freedman, S.O. (1965) Demonstration of tumour specific antigens in human colonic carcinoma by immunological tolerance and absorption techniques. J. Exp. Med. 121, 439-459.
11. Price, M.R., (1988) High molecular weight epithelial mucin as markers in breast cancer. Eur. J. Cancer Clin. Oncol. 24, 1799-1804.
12. Burchell, J. and Taylor-Papadimitriou, J. (1993) Effect of modification of carbohydrate side chains on the reactivity of antibodies with core protein epitopes of the MUC1 gene product. Epith. Cell Biol. 2, 155-162.
13. Carter, P. and Merchant, A.M. (1997) Engineering antibodies for imaging and therapy. Curr. Opin. Biotechnol. 8, 449-454.
14. Dyer, M.J.S., Hale, G., Hayhoe, F.G.J. and Waldmann, H. (1989) Effects of CAMPATH-1 antibodies in vivo in patients with lymphoid malignancies: influence of antibody isotype. Blood 73, 1431-1439.
15. Ghetie, M-A., Podar, E.M., Ilgen, A., Gordon, B.E., Uhr, J.W. and Vitetta, E.S. (1997) Homodimerization of tumor-reactive monoclonal antibodies markedly increases their ability to induce growth arrest or apoptosis of tumor cells. Proc. Natl. Acad. Sci. USA 94, 7509-7514.
16. Moshakis, V., McIlhinney, R.A. and Neville, A.M. (1981) Cellular distribution of monoclonal antibody in human tumours after i.v. administration. Br. J. Cancer 44, 663-669.
17. Farah, R.A., Clinchy, B., Herrera, L. and Vitetta, E.S. (1998) The development of monoclonal antibodies for the therapy of cancer. Critical Rev. Eukaryotic Gene Expression 8, 321-356.
18. Owens, R.J. and Young, R.J. (1994) The genetic engineering of monoclonal antibodies. J. Immunol. Methods 168, 149-165.
19. Rapley, R. (1995) The biotechnology and applications of antibody engineering. Mol. Biotechnol. 3, 139-154.
20. Osterwijk, E., Debruyne, F.M.J. and Schalken, J.A. (1995) The use of monoclonal antibody G250 in the therapy of renal cell carcinoma. Semin. Oncol. 22, 34-41.
21. Adair, J.R. and Bright, S.M. (1995) Progress with humanised antibodies – an update. Exp. Opin. Invest. Drugs 4, 863-870.
22. Green, L.L., Hardy, M.C., Maynard-Currie, C.E., Tsuda, H., Louie, D.M., Mendez, M.J., Abderrahim, H., Noguchi, M., Smith, D.H., Zeng, Y., David, M.E., Sassai, H., Garza, D., Brenner, D.G., Hales, J.F., McGuiness, R.P., Capon, D.J., Klapholz, S. and Jakobovits, A. (1994) Antigen-specific human monoclonal antibodies from mice engineered with human heavy and light chain YACs. Nature Gen. 7, 13-21.
23. Yokota, T., Milenic, D.E., Whitlow, M. and Schlom, J. (1992) Rapid tumour penetration of a single-chain Fv and comparison with other immunoglobulin forms. Cancer Res. 52, 3402-3408.
24. Boucher, Y., Baxter, L.T. and Jain, R.K. (1990) Interstitial pressure gradients in tissue-isolated and subcutaneous tumours: implications for therapy. Cancer Res. 50, 4478-4484.
25. Denton, G., Brady, K., Lo, B.K.C., Murray, A., Graves, C.R.L., Hughes, O.D.M., Tendler, S.J.B., Laughton, C.A. and Price, M.R. (1999) Production and characterisation of an anti-(MUC1 mucin) recombinant diabody. Cancer Immunol. Immunother. 48, 29-38.
26. DeJonge, J., Heirman, C., DeVeerman, M., Van Miervenne, S., Demanet, S., Brissinck, J. and Thielemans, K. (1997) Bispecific antibody treatment of murine B cell lymphoma. Cancer Immunol. Immunother. 45, 162-165.
27. Pluckthun, A. and Pack, P. (1997) New protein engineering approaches to multivalent and bispecific antibody fragments. Immunotechnology 3, 83-105.
28. Staerz, U.D., Kanagawa, O. and Bevan, M.J. (1985) Hybrid antibodies can target sites for attack by T cells. Nature 314, 628-631.
29. Schmidt, M. and Wels, W. (1996) Targeted inhibition of tumour cell growth by a bispecific single-chain toxin containing an antibody domain and TGF alpha. Br. J. Cancer 74, 853-862.
30. Jain, R.K. (1987) Transport of molecules across tumor vasculature. Cancer Metastasis Rev. 6, 559-593.
31. Dvorak, H.F., Nagy, J.A., Dvorak, J.T. and Dvorak, A.M. (1988) Identification and characterisation of the blood vessels of solid tumors that are leaky to circulating macromolecules. Am. J. Pathol. 133, 95-109.
32. Jain, R.K. and Gerlowski, L.E. (1986) Extravascular transport in normal and tumor tissue. Crit. Rev. Oncol. Hematol. 5, 115-170.

33. Maeda, H. (1992) The tumor blood vessel as an ideal target for macromolecular anticancer agents. J. Controlled Release 19, 315-324.
34. Hughes, O.D.M., Bishop, M.C., Perkins, A.C., Wastie, M.L., Denton, G., Price, M.R., Frier, M., Denley, H., Rutherford, R. and Schubiger, P.A. (2000) Targeting of superficial bladder cancer by the intravesical administration of copper-67 labelled anti-MUC1 mucin monoclonal antibody C595. J. Clin. Oncol. 18, 363-370.
35. Britton, K.E. (1997) Towards the goal of cancer specific imaging and therapy. Nucl. Med. Commun. 18, 992-1007.
36. Schubiger, P.A., Alberto, R. and Smith A. (1996) Vehicles, chelators and radionuclides: choosing the building blocks of an effective therapeutic radioimmunoconjugate. Bioconjugate Chem. 7, 165-179.
37. Knapp Jr., F.F., Bleets, A.L., Guhlke, S., Zamora, P.O., Bender, H., Palmedo, H. and Biersack, H-J. (1997). Availability of rhenium-188 from the alumin-based tungsten-188/rhenium-188 generator for preparation of rhenium-188-labeled radiopharmaceuticals for cancer treatment. Anticancer Res., 17, 1783-1796.
38. Griffiths, G.L., Goldenberg, D.M. and Knapp, F.F. (1991). Direct radiolabelling of monoclonal antibodies with generator-produced rhenium-188 for radioimmunotherapy: labeling and animal biodistribution studies. Cancer Res. 51, 4594-4602.
39. Waibel, R., Alberto, R., Willuda, J., Finnern, R., Schibli, R., Stichelberger, A., Egli, A., Abram, U., Mach, J-P., Plückthun, A. and Schubiger, A. (1999) Stable one-step technetium-99m labeling of his-tagged recombinant proteins with a novel Tc(I)-carbonyl complex. Nature Biotechnol. 17, 897-901.
40. Krolick, K.A., Villemez, C., Isakson, P., Uhr, J.W. and Vitetta, E.S. (1980) Selective killing of normal or neoplastic B cells by antibodies coupled to the A chain of ricin. Proc. Natl. Acad. Sci. USA 77, 5419-5423.
41. Raso, V. and Griffin, T. (1980) Hybrid antibodies with dual specificity for the delivery of ricin to immunoglobulin-bearing target cells. Cancer Res. 41, 2073-2078.
42. Barbieri, L., Battelli, M.G. and Stirpe, F. (1993) Ribosome-inactivating proteins from plants. Biochim. Biophys. Acta 1154, 237-282.
43. Brinkmann, U. and Pastan, I. (1994) Immunotoxins against cancer. Biochim. Biophys. Acta Rev. Cancer 1198, 27-45.
44. Middlebrook, J.L. and Dorland, R.B. (1984) Bacterial toxins: cellular mechanisms of action. Microbiol. Rev. 48, 199-221.
45. Thorpe, P.R., Wallace, P.M., Knowles, P.P., Relf, M.G., Brown, A.N.F., Watson, G.J., Knyba, R.E., Wawrzynczak, E.J. and Blakey, D.C. (1987) New coupling agents for the synthesis of immunotoxins containing a hindered disulfide bond with improved stability in vivo. Cancer Res. 47, 5924-5931.
46. Pastan, I., Chaudhary, V. and FitzGerald, D.J. (1992) Recombinant toxins as novel therapeutic agents. Annu. Rev. Biochem. 61, 331-3544.
47. Benhar, I., Reiter, Y., Pai, L.H. and Pastan, I. (1995) Administration of disulphide-stabilised Fv-immunotoxins B1 (dsFv)-Pe38 and B3 (dsFv)-PE38 by continuous infusion increases their efficacy in curing large tumour xenografts in nude mice. Int. J. Cancer, 62, 351-355.
48. Hertler, A.A., Schlossman, D.M. and Borowitz, M.J. (1988) A phase I study of T101-ricin A chain immunotoxin in refractory chronic lymphocytic leukemia. J Biol. Response Modifiers 7, 97-113.
49. LeMaistre, C.F., Rosen, S., Frankel, A., Kornfeld, S., Saria, E., Meneghetti, C., Drajesk, J., Fishwild, D., Scannon, P. and Byers, V. (1991) Phase I trial of H65-RTA immunoconjugate in patients with cutaneous T-cell lymphoma. Blood 78, 1173-1182.
50. Weiner, L.M., O'Dwyer, J., Kitson, J., Comis, R.L., Frankel, A.E., Bauer, R.J., Konrad, M.S. and Groves, E.S. (1989) Phase I evaluation of an anti-breast carcinoma monoclonal antibody 260F9-recombinant ricin A chain immuno-conjugate. Cancer Res. 49, 4062-4067.
51. Byers, V.S., Rodvien, R., Grant, K., Durrant, L.G., Hudson, K.H., Baldwin, R.W. and Scannon, P.J. (1989) Phase I study of monoclonal antibody-ricin A chain immunotoxin XomaZyme-791 in patients with metastatic colon cancer. Cancer Res. 49, 6153-6160.
52. Pai, L.H., Bookman, M.A., Ozols, R.F., Young, R.C., Smith, J.W., Longo, D.L., Gould, B., Frankel, A., McClay, E.F., Howell, S., Reed, E., Willingham, M.C., FitzGerald, D.J. and Pastan, I. (1991) Clinical evaluation of intraperitoneal Pseudomonas exotoxin immunoconjugate OVB3-PE in patients with ovarian cancer. J. Clin. Oncol. 9, 2095-2103.
53. Ghetie, M-A. and Vitteta, E.S. (1994) Immunotoxins in the therapy of cancer: from bench to the clinic. Pharmacol. Ther. 63, 209-234.

54. Flavell, D.J., Boehm, D.M., Emery, L., Noss, A., Ramsay, A. and Flavell, S.U. (1995) Therapy of human B-cell lymphoma bearing SCID mice is more effective with anti-CD19-saporin and anti-CD38-saporin immunotoxins used in combination than with either toxin used alone. Int. J. Cancer 62, 337-344.

55. Ghetie, M-A., Tucker, K., Richardson, J., Uhr, J.W. and Vitteta, E.S. (1994) Eradication of minimal disease in severe combined immunodeficient mice with disseminated Daudi lymphoma using chemotherapy and an immunotoxin cocktail. Blood 84, 702-707.

56. Dillman, R.O., Johnson, D.E., Shawler, D.L. and Koziol, J.A. (1988) Superiority of an acid-labile daunorubicin-monoclonal antibody immunoconjugate compared to free drug. Cancer Res. 48, 6097-6102.

57. Ghose, T., Norvell, S.T., Guclu, A., Cameron, D., Bodurtha, A. and MacDonald, A.S. (1972) Immunotherapy of cancer with chlorambucil-carrying antibody. Br. Med. J. 3, 495-499.

58. Garnett, M.C., Embleton, M.J., Jacobs, E. and Baldwin, R.W. (1983) Preparation and properties of a drug-carrier-antibody conjugate showing selective antibody-directed cytotoxicity in vitro. Int. J. Cancer 31, 661-670.

59. Bernstein, A., Hurwitz, E., Maron, R., Arnon, R., Seal, M. and Wilchek, M. (1978) Higher anti-tumour efficacy of daunomycin when linked to dextran: in vivo and in vitro studies. J. Natl. Cancer Inst. 60, 379-384.

60. Pietersz, G.A. and Krauer, K. (1994) Antibody targeted drugs for the therapy of cancer. J. Drug Targeting 2, 183-215.

61. Trail, P.A., Willner, D., Lasch, S.J., Henderson, A.J., Hofstead, S., Casazza, A.M., Firestone, R.A., Hellstrom, I. and Hellstrom, K.E. (1993) Cure of xenografted human carcinomas by BR96-doxorubicin immunoconjugates. Science 261, 212-215.

62. Lui, C.N., Tadayoni, B.M., Bourret, L.A., Mattocks, K.M., Derr, S.M., Widdison, W.C., Kedsrsha, N.L., Ariniello, P.D., Goldmacher, V.S., Lambert, J.M., Blättler, W.A. and Chari, R.V. (1996) Eradication of large colon tumor xenografts by targeted delivery of maytansinoids. Proc. Natl. Acad. Sci. USA 93, 8618-8623.

63. Bagshawe, K.D. (1987) Antibody directed enzymes revive anti-cancer prodrugs concept. Br. J. Cancer 56, 531-532.

64. Niculescu-Duvas, I. and Springer, C.J. (1997) Antibody-directed enzyme prodrug therapy (ADEPT): a review. Adv. Drug Delivery Rev. 26, 151-172.

65. Syrigos, K.N. and Epenetos, A.A. (1999) Antibody directed enzyme prodrug therapy (ADEPT): A review of the experimental and clinical considerations. Anticancer Res. 19, 605-614.

66. Connors, T.A., Foster, A.B., Gelsenan, A.M., Jarman, M. and Tisdale, M.J. (1972) Chemical trapping of a reactive metabolite. The metabolism of the AZO-mustard 2'-carboxy-4-di-(2-chloroethyl)amino-2-methylazobenzene. Biochem. Pharmacol. 21, 1309-1316.

67. Springer, C.J., Bagshawe, K.D., Sharma, S.K., Searle, F., Boden, J.A., Antoniw, P., Burke, P.J., Rogers, G.T., Sherwood, R.F. and Melton, R.G. (1991) Ablation of human choriocarcinoma xenografts in nude mice by antibody directed enzyme prodrug therapy (ADEPT) with three novel compounds. Eur. J. Cancer 27, 1361-1366.

68. Minton, N.P., Atkinson, T., Bruton, C.J. and Sherwood, R.F. (1984) The complete nucleotide sequence for caoboxypeptidase G2. Gene 31, 31-38.

69. Senter, P.D., Wallace, P.M., Svensson, H.P., Vrudhula, V.M., Kerr, D.E., Hellström, I. and Hellström, K.E. (1993) Generation of cytotoxic agents by targeted enzymes. Bioconjugate Chem. 4, 3-9.

70. Sharma, S.K. (1996) Immune responses in ADEPT. Adv. Drug Delvery. Rev. 22, 369-376.

71. Haisma, H.J., van Muijen, M., Pinedo, H.M. and Boven, E. (1994) Comparison of two anthracycline-based prodrugs for activation by a monoclonal antibody-beta-glucuronidase conjugate in the specific treatment of cancer. Cell Biophys. 24-25, 185-192.

72. Baldini, N. (1997) Multidrug resistance - a complex phenomenon. Nature Med. 3, 378-380.

73. Springer, C.J., Dowell, R.L., Burke, P.J., Hadley, E., Davies, D.H., Blakey, D.C., Melton, R.G. and Niculescu-Duvaz, I. (1995) Optimization of alkylating agent prodrugs derived from phenol and aniline mustards: a new clinical candidate prodrug (ZD2767) for ADEPT. J. Med. Chem. 38, 5051-5065.

74. Lasic, D. (1993) Application of liposomes in pharmacology and medicine, in: D. Lasic (ed) Liposomes From Physics to Applications, Elsevier, Amsterdam pp. 262-471.

75. Gregoriadis, G. (1995) Engineering liposomes for drug delivery: progress and problems. Trends Biotechnol, 13, 527-537.

76. Lee, R.J. and Low, P.S. (1997) Folate-targeted liposomes for drug delivery. J. Liposome Res. 7, 455-466.

77. Kikuchi, A., Sugaya, S., Ueda, H., Tanaka, K., Aramaki, Y., Hara, T., Arima, H., Tsuchiya, S. and Fuwa, T. (1996) Efficient gene transfer to EGF receptor overexpressing cancer cells by means of EGF-labeled cationic liposomes. Biochem. Biophys. Res. Commun. 227, 666-671.

78. Oku, N., Tokudome, Y., Koike, C., Nishikawa, N., Mori, H., Saiki, I. and Okada, S. (1996) Liposomal Arg-Gly-Asp analogs effectively inhibit metastatic B16 melanoma colonization in murine lungs. Life Sci. 58, 2263-2270.

79. Willis, M.C., Collins, B., Zhang, T., Green, L.S., Sebesta, D.P., Bell, C., Kellogg, E., Gill, S.C., Magallanez, A., Knauer, S., Bendele, R.A., Gill, P.S. and Janjic, N. (1998) liposome-anchored vascular endothelial growth factor aptamers. Bioconjugate. Chem. 9, 573-582.

80. Mastrobattista, E., Koning, G.A. and Storm, G. (1999) Immunoliposomes for targeted delivery of antitumor drugs. Adv. Drug Delivery Rev. 40, 103-127.

81. Maruyama, K., Ishida, O., Takizawa, T. and Moribe, K. (1999) Possibility of active targeting of tumor cells with liposomes. Adv. Drug Delivery Rev. 40, 89-102.

82. Jones, M.N. and Nicholas, A.R. (1991) The effect of blood serum on the size and stability of phospholipid liposomes. Biochim. Biophys. Acta 1065, 145-152.

83. Hernandez-Caselles, T., Villalain, J. and Gomes-Fernandez, J.C. (1993) Influence of liposome charge and composition on their interaction with human blood serum proteins. Mol. Cell Biochem. 120, 119-126.

84. Szebeni, J., Wassef, N.M., Rudolph, A.S. and Alving, C.R. (1996) Complement activation in serum by liposome-encapsulated hemoglobin: the role of natural anti-phospholipid antibodies. Biochim. Biophys. Acta 1285, 127-130.

85. Derksen, J.T., Morselt, H.W. and Sherphof, G.L. (1988) Uptake and processing of immunoglobulin-coated liposomes by sub-populations of rat liver macrophages. Biochim. Biophys. Acta 971, 127-136.

86. Alving, C.R. and Wassef, N.M. (1992) Complement-dependent phagocytosis of liposomes: suppression by 'stealth' liposomes. J. Liposome Res. 2, 383-395.

87. Chonn, A. and Cullis, P.R. (1992) Ganglioside Gm, and hydrophylic polymers increase liposome circulation times by inhibiting the association of blood proteins. J. Liposome Res. 2, 397-410.

88. Storm, G., Belliot, S.O., Daemen, T. and Lasic, D.D. (1995) Surface modification of nanoparticles to oppose uptake by the mononuclear phagocyte system. Adv. Drug Delivery Rev. 17, 31-48.

89. Aragnol, D. and Leserman, L.D. (1986) Immune clearance of liposomes inhibited by an anti-Fc receptor antibody in vivo. Proc. Natl. Acad. Sci. USA 83, 2699-2703.

90. Harding, J.A., Engbers, C.M., Newman, M.S., Goldstein, N.I. and Zalipsky, S. (1997) Immunogenicity and pharmokinetic attributes of poly(ethylene glycol)-grafted immunoliposomes. Biochim. Biophys. Acta 1327, 181-192.

91. Crosasso, P., Brusa, P., Dosio, F., Arpicco, S., Pacchioni, D., Schuber, F. and Cattel, L. (1997) Antitumoral activity of liposomes and immunoliposomes containing 5-fluorouridine prodrugs. J. Pharm. Sci. 86, 832-839.

92. Lopes de Menezes, D.E., Pilarski, L.M. and Allen, T.M. (1998) In vitro and in vivo targeting of immunoliposomal doxorubicin to B-cell lymphoma. Cancer Res. 58, 3320-3330.

93. Tseng, Y.L., Hong, R.L., Tao, M.H. and Chang, F.H. (1999) Sterically stabilised anti-idiotype immunoliposomes improve the therapeutic efficacy of doxorubicin in a murine B-cell lymphoma model. Int. J. Cancer 80, 723-730.

94. Bankert, R.B., Yokota, S., Ghosh, S.K., Mayhew, E. and Jou, Y.H. (1989) Immunospecific targeting of cytosine arabinonucleoside containing liposomes to the idiotype on the surface of a B-cell tumor in vitro and in vivo. Cancer Res. 49, 301-308.

217

13
ESCAPE MECHANISMS IN TUMOUR IMMUNITY

GRAHAM PAWELEC

INTRODUCTION

There is now much evidence that tumours can be immunogenic, ie. that they frequently do express antigens in a form recognizable by the host immune system. This has been shown not only in experimental animals but also for spontaneously arising human tumours. Tumour progression may therefore require the evolution of variants which can "escape" the immune response. Mechanisms for the escape of tumours from immune responses (endogenous or therapeutic) include:

- downregulation of immune responses by the tumour and / or associated T cells and their products
- altered expression of MHC and/or tumour antigens by tumour cells
- altered expression of adhesion or accessory molecules by tumour and / or dendritic cells
- usurpation of the immune response to the advantage of the tumour ("immunostimulation")

The purpose of this chapter is to consider the current status of knowledge concerning these different tumour escape strategies, focussing on clinical studies wherever possible. Animal models will only be considered to illustrate points of potential importance to studies in humans where data in the latter are scarce or absent. This area is very fast-moving and for this reason, predominantly literature from the last 5 years will be reviewed. Some of the overall concepts have been recently discussed in a "Symposium-in-Writing" published in October 1999 (see ref.[1]). Weight will be given to those studies that not only contribute to defining the nature of the event associated with tumour escape, but point to possible ways for preventing this occurence.

R.A. Robins and R.C. Rees (eds.), Cancer Immunology, 219–247.

DOWNREGULATION OF IMMUNE RESPONSES BY THE TUMOUR AND / OR ASSOCIATED T CELLS AND THEIR PRODUCTS

Downregulation of immune responses by cytokines

There is a large body of data clearly indicating that cytokines secreted by the tumour and/or tumour-associated immune cells can have deleterious as well as stimulatory effects on the immune response. Potentially suppressive cytokines such as IL-10 and TGF-ß have received much attention. Earlier studies concentrated on characterising cytokine secretion from tumour cell lines. These data will not be extensively reviewed here; rather, in situ cytokine expression and clinical relevance of cytokine profiles will be discussed.

High levels of TGF-ß have been found in serum of cancer patients in correlation to the degree of tumour progression, and shown to decrease after resection[2]. In patients with disseminated melanoma, TGF-ß levels in plasma are higher than in patients with local melanoma[3]. Colorectal cancers in patients responding to immunotherapy were found not to express TGF-ß mRNA, whereas non-responders did; the expression of IL-1, IL-6, IL-8, IL-10 and TNF-alpha was variable between responders and non-responders, underlining the paramount importance of TGF-ß expression[4]. Consistent with these data, addition of TGF-ß-neutralising antibodies to autologous lymphocyte/tumour cell cocultures increased the frequency of cultures showing positive responses[5].

IL-6 levels in the serum of cancer sufferers are also commonly elevated[6] as is IL-10 (see below). In lung cancer patients, levels of serum IL-6 are greater even than in patients with chronic obstructive pulmonary disease and acute infection; thus it is unlikely that the increases in IL-6 simply reflect a systemic inflammatory response[7]. In melanoma, patients responding to therapy showed a serum IL-6 level only twice that of controls, whereas in nonresponders this factor was 11-fold, suggesting a strong correlation between IL-6 level and clinical status[8]. In breast cancer, patients with more metastases and patients refractory to therapy had higher levels of IL-6 in their serum; they also had poorer survival such that multivariate analysis showed that IL-6 and disease-free interval were the major prognostic factors[9].

Elevated serum IL-10 concentrations have also been frequently reported in patients with various solid tumours, including melanoma[10] and pancreatic carcinoma[11], as well as haematological malignancies. In non-Hodgkin's lymphoma and Hodgkin's disease the IL-10 titer represented a prognostic factor[12] but in diffuse large cell lymphoma this was apparently not the case[13,14]. Quite the reverse, in B-CLL, the presence of IL-10 mRNA was associated with non-progression[15]. Pisa et al.[16] found large amounts of IL-10 but no IL-2 locally in ovarian tumours. Berghella et al. noted increased serum IL-10 and decreased IL-2 during progression from adenoma to colorectal carcinoma[17]. Kim et al.[18] described secretion of IL-10 by BCC and SCC cells and showed that intra-lesional treatment with IFN-α induced tumour regression, associated with downregulation of IL-10 mRNA. We have shown that CML cells spontaneously secrete large amounts of IL-10 ex vivo and that IFN-α acts to decrease this while increasing IL-1ß secretion without altering TNF-α[19]. Other reports implicating IL-10 as a prognostic marker in various cancers continue to appear. For example, a recent study of nasopharyngeal carcinoma documented that 5 year survival of the IL-10-negative patient group (negative by immunohistochenmistry locally in the tumour) was nearly 90% of patients compared to only 15% in the IL-10-positive group[20]. In gastrointestinal carcinoma, De Vita et al. showed that pre-chemotherapy levels of IL-10 were increased, and that pretreatment levels represented a prognostic criterion for response to therapy[21]. Nakagomi et al.[22] found IL-10 mRNA in freshly isolated renal carcinoma cells (RCC), but not in RCC cell lines, patients´ PBMC or normal kidney tissue. They did not detect IL-2, 3 or 4 mRNA in any tissue. RCC cells may also induce IL-10 as well as PGE2 production by monocytes, which can have downregulatory effects on immune responses[23]. Yamamura et al.[24] found IL-4, IL-5 and IL-10 locally in basal cell carcinoma lesions, but IL-2, IFN-γ and TNF-ß in benign skin lesions. Young et al.[25] noted that freshly excised human head and neck cancers released PGE2, IL-10 and TGF-ß which was associated with a reduced level of CD8 but not CD4 cells in the TIL. Despite equivalent numbers of CD4 cells, it is likely that their function was compromized, because they expressed less CD25 and secreted less IL-2 and IFN-gamma. These patterns were more extreme in metastatic compared to primary cancers. Rabinowich[26] noted that in ovarian carcinoma, both tumour cells and TIL expressed elevated IL-10 mRNA and protein levels. In breast tumours, IL-10 mRNA but not IL-2 and IL-4 mRNA was commonly found[27]. IL-10 mRNA is found in both melanoma and normal melanocytes, but unlike the former, the latter did not secrete IL-10 protein[28]. Huang et al.[29] reported that both NSCLC lines and freshly isolated tumour cells secreted IL-10, and that exposure of the cells to IL-4 or TNF-α augmented IL-10 secretion. Hishii et al.[30] reported that human glioma cells secreted IL-10 which downregulated HLA-DR expression on monocytes and inhibited IFN-γ and TNF-α effects. Non-small cell lung cancer commonly contained large amounts of IL-10, TGF-ß and IL-6 mRNA but little IL-2[31].

There may well be various other cytokines which tumours secrete and which influence the immune response. One candidate not extensively examined so far, for example, is monocyte chemo-attractant protein-1, MCP-1, which, when secreted by a tumour in a mouse model, blocks the generation of tumour-reactive T cells[32]. Melanoma cells may secrete IL-15, which enhances expression of downregulatory NKIR on T cells (see below) as well as possibly depressing the level of expression of MHC class I molecules on the tumour cells[33]. In human primary melanoma, mRNA for GM-CSF, IL-2 and IL-15 was higher in spontaneously regressing lesions than in progression, whereas TNF-α expression was similar in both[34]. Moretti et al. further showed that nevi and thin primary melanomas expressed few cytokines except TNF-α, TGF-ß and IL-8, whereas these and others (including IL-6 and IL-6R), but not IL-2, were upregulated in thick melanomas[35]. Consistent with this, another study found high levels of IL-8 mRNA in necrotic areas of melanoma metastases, but not in primary lesions or non-necrotic metastases; high level expression was associated with induction by anoxia[36].

CANCER IMMUNOLOGY

The Th1 / Th2 Paradigm in Tumour Escape

Cytokines such as IL-10 are characteristic of Th2 cells involved primarily in humoural immunity and anti-inflammatory activity, whereas Th1 cells and cytokines mediate DTH. The diversion of the immune response towards Th2 and humoural immunity, for which B cells are required, associated with disabling the Th1 and DTH response, may be critical for tumour tolerance[37]. B cells may inhibit IFN-γ production by a mechanism involving downregulation of CD40-ligand-induced IL-12 production by APC[38], perhaps by competition binding of T cell CD40L. It has been suggested that antibodies may be generated which can mask the epitopes recognized by CTL and thereby block tumour cell lysis[39]. T cell lines and clones derived from TIL commonly possess the characteristics of Th2 cells (secretion of IL-3, IL-4, IL-6, IL-10, GM-CSF but not IL-2, IFN-gamma, TNF-alpha or TNF-beta, and mediating cytotoxicity only in 18 h assays[40]). Th2 cells are thought not to be efficient anti-cancer effectors. In a mouse lymphoma model, the presence of tumour-specific CTL could be demonstrated in both susceptible and resistant hosts, but in the susceptible hosts the helper response was dominated by Th2-phenotype cells and in the resistant hosts the dominant response was Th1-phenotype[41]. This is a striking finding because although the tumour was immunogenic and even stimulated CTL responses, the presence of Th2 responses was overiding and was still associated with fatal outcome[41]. In humans, there is a prevalence of IL-10 production in certain CD4+ melanoma-specific T cell clones[42]. CD4 T cell clones generated in the presence of IL-10 had little proliferative capacity and secreted large amounts of IL-10 but not IL-2; moreover, they suppressed the response of other CD4 cells to antigen and showed suppressive activity in vivo[43]. Moreover, IL-10 and TGF-ß may be synergistic in inducing or maintaining T cell suppression[44] and in diverting T cell responses from Th1 to Th2 phenotypes[11]. It may therefore be possible clinically to influence the course of disease by giving cytokines which can facilitate Th1-type responses. For example, in Sezary syndrome, tumour-specific CTL can be revealed by in vitro treatment with IFN-γ or IL-12[45]. In a comparison of spontaneously regressing with non-regressing melanomas, Lowes et al. found elevated levels of mRNA for Th1 cytokines IL-2, TNF-ß and IFN-γ in the former compared to the latter, although they found no differences in Th 2 cytokines IL-10, IL 13, or pro-inflammatory cytokines IL-1, IL-6, IL-8, TNF-α or the factors GM-CSF and TGF-ß[46].

In some models, successful immunotherapy of established tumour is associated with a change in the balance of T cell subsets from Th2 to Th1 phenotype (eg.[47]). Other models are consistent with these results in showing even a pathogenic role of Th2 cells[48]. Tumour-derived TGF-ß can induce over-production of IL-10, stimulating suppression of anti-tumour responses; conversely, in vivo administration of anti-TGF-ß resulted in prevention of Th2 dominance, reversed immunosuppression and reconstituted a Th1 response[49]. However, it may be some aspects of the Th1 and Th2 cell function which are important in this context, rather than always a clear Th1/Th 2 dichotomy; thus, Handel-Fernandez reported that it is the downregulation of IL-12 production, rather than a shift from Th1 to Th2 phenotype *per se*, which causes impaired IFN-gamma production in mammary tumour-bearing mice[50]. IL-12 may indeed by a critical cytokine, since for example, in the murine C26 colon carcinoma model, it is the graded amount of IL-12 locally available at the tumour site that determines the nature and quantity of the T cell infiltrate and thus clinical outcome[51]. In colon cancer patients, a preferential accumulation of Th2 cells has been reported, which might contribute to suppression and blockade of Th1 effectors[52].

The presumption that Th1 predominance indicates host-mediated tumour rejection, but that Th2 predominance inhibits this process may not apply universally, of course. In some models, Th2 cells together with CD8 cells can mediate tumour rejection[53]. The "classical" Th2 cytokine IL-4 can enhance rather than inhibit immunogenicity and induce efficient tumour rejection in certain models[54]. In certain murine models, IL-4-transduced tumour vaccines trigger type 2 polarization in both CD4 and CD8 cells; the CD8 cells are instrumental in rejecting the tumours, in an IL-4-dependent fashion involving other CD8 cells and probably also NK cells[55]. In humans, the expression of TNF-alpha and IL-4 was found to be more common in TIL from primary than metastatic colon carcinomas and that expression of either was associated with better overall 5 year survival. In contrast, IL-10 and TGF-ß were expressed by colon carcinoma cells and TIL, but there was no correlation with survival for these cytokines[56]. IL-4 is also effective in reversing the decline of CTL activity observed during in vivo progression of a murine B cell lymphoma[57]. There is even evidence that IL-10 can also enhance tumour rejection[58], elicit cytotoxic immune memory due to the combined action of NK cells, CD8$^+$ T cells and neutrophils[59], and in conjunction with CD80-CD28 co-stimulation can prime tumour reactive CTL[60]. This is consistent with the ability of IL-10 to prevent T cell apoptosis[61,62] and enhance the proliferation of CD4[63] and CD8[64] cells under certain circumstances. Kirkin et al. defined four groups of melanoma-specific CTL directed against differentiation antigens or "progression" antigens and found that treatment of tumour cells in vitro with IL-10 could upregulate CTL responses against the former but not the latter[65]. In addition, IL-10 has been shown to exert anti-angiogenic and anti-metastatic effects in certain murine models[66], so that it is remains difficult to dissect out the contradictory activities of this cytokine in tumour immunology.

Downregulation of immune responses by shed molecules other than cytokines

Sera of cancer patients commonly contain immunosuppressive proteins, many of which may be acute phase reactants with non-specific inhibitory properties. Reactivity to non-tumour antigens may be depressed in cancer patients and contribute to their increased susceptibility to infection. In stage IV melanoma, for example, only 36% of HLA-A2+ patients reacted to influenza matrix peptide, compared to 75% of normal A2+ controls[67]. The tumour cells themselves may be the source of immune system-specific factors which can mediate suppressive effects, eg. Altomonte et al.[68] reported that melanoma cells express large amounts of CD58 (LFA-3), that the patients´ serum contained soluble CD58, and that this inhibited melanoma cell lysis which was to a great extent dependent on CD58-CD2 interactions. Becker et al. described secretion of soluble CD54 (ICAM 1) from melanoma cell lines at levels able to block conjugate formation between melanoma-specific TIL clones and tumour cells[69]. More recently, increased levels of sICAM-1 in the plasma of cancer patients has been reported to correlate with disease progression[70,71], but there was no correlation with sICAM-1 shedding by tumours and their level of ICAM-1 expression at the cell surface[72]. However, in glioblastoma, there appears to be no increase in circulating soluble ICAM-1 or VCAM-1 levels[73].

Breast cancer cells synthesize isoferritin-associated p43 molecules which have been reported to inhibit lymphocyte stimulation in breast cancer patients T cells´ but not in normal T cells[74]. Molecules commonly over-expressed in tumour cells, such as MUC-1, may also be immunosuppressive for T cells in soluble form[75,76], although there may be some doubt whether the MUC molecule itself is always the responsible entity[77]. In any event, elevated serum levels of MUC-1 are associated with poor survival and poor anti-cancer responses in patients on immunotherapy[78]. Recent data also suggest that in extra-hepatic bile duct carcinoma, higher MUC-1 levels correlated with a higher degree of liver metastasis and poorer patient survival[79]. Another candidate suppressive substance is soluble Annexin II, which is over-expressed in several tumours, and which may inhibit T cell proliferation[80].

Tumours may also be non-specifically suppressive, eg. by secreting adenosine as a result of their hypoxic metabolism. Adenosine directly suppresses tumouricidal lymphocyte function[81]. This group more recently confirmed that both murine tumours grown in syngeneic hosts and human tumours grown in nude mice produced sufficient levels of adenosine to mediate immunosuppressive effects[82]. A different mechanism recently described is the secretion of a decoy receptor found eg. in about half of primary lung and colon cancers[83]. This soluble decoy receptor binds to fas-ligand and inhibits apoptosis by blocking fas/fas-ligand interactions (see 2.4). Tumour gangliosides may be shed in large amounts and can be highly immunosuppressive, thereby contributing to escape[84]. One mechanism of action of suppressive gangliosides is paralysis of NF-kappa-B transcription factor activity, which occurs without prevention of NF-kappa-B inhibitor degradation[85]. This is somewhat different from the mechanism of action of IL-10 (see 2.1) where inhibitor degradation is also blocked by the cytokine[86].

Alterations in signal transducing molecules

The phenomenon first described in mice bearing slowly growing colon carcinoma which showed an altered pattern of protein tyrosinase phosphorylation, a reduction of the protein tyrosine kinases (PTKs) p56^{lck} and p59^{fyn} and decreased expression of CD3 zeta chain[87] has subsequently been confirmed and extended to a variety of human tumours, including renal, colorectal, ovarian, liver, gastric, oral, prostate, pancreatic and cervical carcinomas, glioblastomas and melanomas[88-95]. Alterations in other molecules involved in the activation of lymphocyte functions have also been described. Abnormalities in NF-κB sequence motif-specific binding activity were found in patients with renal cell carcinoma (RCC)[96]. Unlike activated T cells from normal individuals, RCC T cells, post stimulation, had little or no detectable NF-κB component RelA (p65) in nuclear extracts. Also in RCC patients, failure to degrade the I-κBα constitutive inhibitor of NF-κB may contribute to lack of response[97]. Taken together, these observations argue that several distinct signal transducing pathways can be impaired in cancer patient T and NK cells.

Of particular interest is the repeatedly documented correlation between these alterations and the disease stage in many different cancers[88,91,92,95,98-101]. Gunji et al.[99] found structurally abnormal TCR/CD3 complexes on PBL from colon carcinoma patients as well as patients with several other types of malignancies, and described a correlation between decreased zeta chain levels and cancer stage. Abnormal association between zeta chains and other CD3 components was associated with the first stage of immunosuppression followed by the total disappearance of zeta from the cell surface in more advanced stages. In oral carcinomas, higher levels of zeta expressed by TIL were associated with survival, and, together with stage and lymph node status, prognostically highly significant[95]. In patients with colorectal carcinoma, T cells in PBL from patients with lymph node involvement, or with distant metastatic spread had significantly less zeta chain than patients with localized disease as measured with a flow cytometric method[100]. In agreement with these findings, immunohistochemical studies have recently demonstrated that compared with normal gut mucosa, the number of TCR-zeta-expressing lymphocytes was decreased in colorectal tumours, being lowest in more advanced tumours[101]. In contrast, cells which expressed Granzyme B which has an important role in exocytosis-mediated cytotoxic processes, were more frequent in less advanced tumours than in normal mucosa, but disappeared from advanced stage tumours. In PBL from patients with cervical cancer, a marked decrease in the expression of signal-transducing CD3 zeta chain has been found[91]. In the same study, PBL isolated from patients with cervical intraepithelial neoplasia (CIN) to a lesser but significant extent, expressed reduced CD3 zeta levels as compared to those from healthy donors, raising the possibility that alterations in signal transducing molecules may already occur at relatively early stages in some types of cancer. In the same study, CD3 zeta chain expression significantly correlated with the ability of the PBL to produce TNF in response to anti-CD3 stimulation. There was a significant decrease in IFN-γ production but IL-10 was unaffected, leading to the suggestion that downregulation of the zeta chain occured only in Th1 not Th2 cells[102]. Given the findings on the linkage of caspase activation and zeta downregulation (see following), these findings are consistent with the resistance of Th2 cells to activation-induced cell death, and the susceptibility of Th1 cells to this type of apoptosis[103].

It must be noted, however, that these TCR alterations are not specific to the cancer-bearing host. Thus, the alterations in signal-transduction in T cells from PBL and synovial fluid of patients with rheumatoid arthritis, which are known to have poor mitogenic T cell responses, are also associated with decreased CD3 zeta expression[104,105]. T cells from many patients with SLE lack CD3 zeta[106], and T lymphocytes from leprosy patients present alterations in nuclear transcription factors and in CD3 zeta chain expression[107]. Perhaps analogous to the tumour situation, chronic inflammatory processes might involve the same mechanism. Indeed, one report examined lymphocytes from non-malignant inflammatory secondary lymphoid tissues and concluded that they showed similar functional defects to TIL, indicating lack of tumour specificity in these phenomena[108].

Nonetheless, cell-surface losses of zeta chains, or abnormal association between zeta chains and other CD3 components, might explain the observed gradual decline of cell-mediated responses in patients and experimental animals with growing tumours (and other conditions). In this respect, however, it must be borne in mind that under certain conditions, extinction of zeta-signalling may not necessarily inhibit T cell responses[109], and decreased levels of CD3 zeta chain in cancer patients may not correlate with their proliferative or cytotoxic capacity[110]. Conversely, it has been reported that T cells from PBMC in early breast cancer patients do not show zeta chain deficiencies but are nonetheless functionally compromized[102]. However, others have reported that peripheral blood T cells from breast cancer patients do contain low zeta[111]; the reason for this discrepancy is unclear, but may relate to the latter data applying to later-stage disease. In that report, the T cells also possessed increased levels of the MKP-1 phosphatase, which may contribute to further downregulation of responsiveness[111]. Nonetheless, flow-cytometric analysis of zeta levels on PBL and biopsy material might provide an easy-to-perform method for monitoring the immune status of cancer patients. CD3 zeta levels might also be prognostic indicators. Zea et al.[92] demonstrated that melanoma patients with low TCR zeta levels had significantly shorter overall survival than patients with normal TCR zeta levels. TCR zeta-deficient patients also tended to have faster growing tumours.

Inconsistencies in reports of CD3 ζ downregulation have appeared in mouse and humans. In experimental mouse tumour models the generality of the phenomenon of alterations in signal transducing molecules has been questioned. Levey & Srivastava[112] reported that even in mice with very large serially transplanted tumours they were unable to detect alterations in CD3 zeta, lck, fyn or ZAP. A rapidly growing transplantable tumour is, however, a poor model for slowly progressing human tumours. Slowly progressing primary tumours induced by chemical carcinogens in mice may be more appropriate model to study the immune dysfunction in patients. In human, Camardi et al.[113] using flow cytometric and Western blot analysis studied the expression of ζ chain in CD3+ PBLs and TILs from RCCs, as well as in PBLs from normal healthy donors. In contrast to earlier findings in patients with RCC[89], these authors found similarly high levels of zeta expression in all three groups. Although the authors did observe a small but significant decrease in CD3 zeta expression in 3 of the TILs as compared to the PBLs of the same patients, they concluded that this could not explain the anergic state of TIL. The reason for the absence of consistent ζ alterations in RCC patients in this study may be methodological. Proteolytic degradation of mouse splenocyte zeta and p56[lck] by granulocyte-associated cathepsin G, which occurred during sample processing, is another concern[114]. This would have to be a specific proteinase effect, since despite this, these investigators maintained that the decreased activity of nuclear c-rel and NF-κB factors cited above was not caused by granulocyte contamination. More recent work from this group has shown that the alterations in NF-κB family proteins, specifically the translocation of p65 to the nucleus, precedes the decrease in zeta chain[115]. As levels of zeta chain remained reduced in human PBL even in the presence of additional protease inhibitors of cathepsin G activity[114], this potential in vitro artefact may be less of a concern in human PBL. Also, T cells analysed by flow cytometry are much less prone to in vitro degradation of zeta as compared to those studied by biochemical methods with solubilized cells. Nonetheless, Deakin et al., using peripheral blood T cells from colon cancer patients to detect zeta chain by flow cytometry, Western blotting and immunohistochemistry, could find no evidence for its downregulation[116]. Therefore, there is still no general consensus on this topic.

Not only tumour cells themselves and their products, but tumour-infiltrating macrophages may be to induce alterations in signal transducing molecules. Aoe et al.[117] described decreased CD3ζ expression even on freshly isolated normal T cells cocultured with tumour-derived macrophages. Kono et al.[118] showed that macrophages isolated from metastatic lymph nodes of melanoma patients were able to down-regulate CD3-zeta levels in autologous PBL. Again, this was not tumour-specific, because LPS-stimulated monocytes from normal PBMC did the same. Because treatment with catalase prevented this, and H_2O_2 duplicated it, it was concluded that reactive oxygen metabolites produced by activated monocytes were responsible for zeta chain downregulation[118]. Otsuji et al.[119] also found that oxidative stress caused by tumour-derived macrophages suppressed zeta chain expression. This could be prevented by treating the macrophages with an anti-oxident, as duplicated by treatment of responders with H_2O_2, similar to the phenomenon in cancer patients discussed above. The final mechanism of action of this oxidative stress-induced CD3 zeta loss may be via activation of components of the apoptotic pathway. Thus, oxidative stress triggers many cellular responses including pro-apoptotic factors such as p53; indeed, in a model system, loss of CD3 zeta chain may be directly mediated by one of the enzymes intimately involved in the apoptotic pathway, caspase-3[120]. Moreover, the induction of apoptosis in T cells by fas-ligand-bearing ovarian carcinoma cells is accompanied by zeta downregulation and inhibitors of fas or apoptosis prevent this[121]. These observations therefore suggest that chronic inflammatory conditions in advanced cancer and in certain infectious and autoimmune conditions will alter the redox potential of macrophages, causing them to exert an immunosuppressive effect on the host immune system via secretion of factors such as H_2O_2. These factors will rapidly shut off the effector functions of CTL and NK cells. Research aimed at developing drugs which can counteract suppression of anti-tumour activity and which should be given in combination with immunotherapy should provide new and promising avenues for the treatment of cancer.

Downregulation of immune responses by apoptosis induction

The most radical way for a tumour to induce non-responsiveness would be to kill the attacking T cells. Some examples of this have been forthcoming. Perhaps the most extreme but unsurprising example is the finding that secreted protein from tumours may be presented in the thymus and cause tolerance induction by clonal deletion, just like any normal protein would[122].

Peripheral T cell clonal deletion may also be an option open to tumours. Many tumours have now been shown to express fas-ligand, which, upon interaction with CD95 (fas) expressed by activated T cells may under approproiate conditions trigger apoptosis of the latter. Niehans et al.[123] found fas-ligand on 16 of 16 lung carcinoma cell lines and 23 of 28 resected fresh tumours. Melanoma cells commonly express fas-ligand, and induce apoptosis of fas+ susceptible T cells[124], although these findings have been challenged on the basis of PCR and functional assays, with disparities put down to technical differences[125]. There may be variation in tumour stage, within lesions or after selection to help account for these discrepancies. Thus, Shiraki et al.[126] found that while only 2 of 7 primary human colonic adenocarcinomas expressed fas-ligand, 4/4 hepatic metastatic tumours were fas-ligand positive. A whole variety of tumours including astrocytoma, ovarian carcinoma, pancreatic adenocarcinoma and head and neck squamous carcinoma, hepatocellular carcinoma may also express fas-ligand[121,127,131]. In many reports, the fas-ligand expressed was shown to be functional, ie. its ligation of fas resulted in apoptosis of the target cell.

In esophageal cancer, upregulation of fas-ligand and downregulation of fas was found to be an early indicator of progression[132]; in this cancer, fas-ligand was found to be functional in triggering apoptosis of the TIL[133]. Longitudinal studies in melanoma reveal that fas-ligand expression by primary tumour was weak and rare whereas in metastases, including those of these primary tumours, fas-ligand expression was stronger and commoner[134].

On the other hand, although ligand or antibody interaction with CD95 on T cells commonly results in their apoptosis, this is not always the case. CD8+ (and CD4+) melanoma-specific CTL may resist apoptosis induced by fas-ligand+ tumour or other cells[135]. Moreover, under certain circumstances, fas-mediated costimulation rather than destruction may result[136]. This possibly helps to explain some instances where the expression of fas-ligand results in enhanced destruction rather than protection of the fas-ligand-bearing cells. However, it must be said that this mechanism has not yet been observed; a case reported where transfected fas-ligand resulted in enhanced destruction was in fact due to neutrophil activity, and was T and B cell-independent[137]. Moroever, because T cells are also fas-ligand positive, the fas/fas-ligand interaction can be a double-edged sword and result in the killing of fas+ tumour cells by fas-ligand-positive T cells[138]. Here again, tumour escape mechanisms may come into play; thus, fas+ tumour cells may develop resistance to fas-mediated killing[128], possibly by over-expressing the anti-apoptotic protein cFLIP[139,140]. Loss of fas function in tumours may thus contribute to progression and metastasis[141]. One mechanism for this may be the over-expression of a fas decoy receptor, mentioned above[83]. It has also been observed that fas/fas-ligand interactions between tumour-specific T cells can result in downregulated responses, even where the tumour itself appears to be fas-ligand-negative[142]. On the other hand, it has also been demonstrated that maximal proliferation of CD8 cells may even require stimulation via the fas-ligand that they express[143]. Therefore, the weight of evidence currently suggest that fas/fas-ligand interactions commonly but not necessarily result in effects detrimental to the T cell anti-tumour response.

Moreover, fas/fas-ligand-interactions may not be the only tumour cell / T cell interactions which trigger apoptosis. MUC-1, a well-known tumour antigen expressed on pancreatic and gynecological cancer, was also reported to induce apoptosis in T cells[144]. However, Agrawal et al. were subsequently unable to find evidence for MUC-1-induced apoptosis, although they were able to show that soluble MUC-1 indeed inhibited T cell proliferation, but in a way more akin to anergy [76]. It seems that these results concerning the inability of MUC-1 to induce apoptosis have been confirmed by the laboratory which originally reported that apoptosis was inducible by MUC-1[145]. Nonetheless, it does seem clear that MUC-1 can downregulate T cell responses[146]. However, there is an increasing appreciation that immunoregulatory pathways may involve MUC-1 in the normal functioining of the immune system as well as in tumour-bearing hosts[147].

Downregulation of immune responses by anergy induction

However, perhaps equally or more effective may be the ability of tumours to induce non-responsiveness in the T cells without destroying them and thereby possibly triggering compensatory responses on the part of the host. Even powerful antigen-presenting cells such as DC can be subverted by tumour products, eg. IL-10, as discussed above, to anergise rather than activate anti-tumour cells[148]. Anergy-induction is antigen-specific and is an early event associated with tumour progression[149]. Anergic cells remain present and can continue to perform several functions; thus, anergy is a state of partial nonresponsiveness. It can be induced by stimulating T cells via the TCR in the absence of costimulation[150], or by partial agonist ligands (PALs)[151] or by preventing proliferation of responding cells by neutralising the autocrine IL-2 pathway[152,153]. Of great potential interest is a report that documents the existence of naturally ocurring peptide sequences from endogenous as well as foreign proteins which can act as partial agonists for the melanoma antigen MART1/Melan A (27-35) and which could anergise anti-tumour T cells by cross-presentation[154]. This may parallel the type of "original antigenic sin" recorded for CTL whereby confrontation of the immune system with rechallenge by a variant antigen still results only in a response to the original, now irrelevant, variant[155]. Also dangerously for immunotherapy, under certain circumstances, anergy can be induced by vaccination with immunogenic peptides representing tumour antigens[156]. However, the presence of IL-2 can prevent anergy at least when it is induced via the first two pathways. T cell proliferation *per se* seems not to be critical; rather it is the triggering of proliferation by the IL-2R common gamma chain which prevents anergy[157]. T helper cells stimulated to release IL-2 may therefore help to prevent anergy induction in CD8 CTL. CD8 cells are not just ineffective in the absence of CD4 products, they may be actively tolerized[158]; this may be one part of the explanation of the requirement for CD4 cells for optimal CD8 anti-tumour function. Vaccination of mice with tumour peptides in the absence of any "help" may itself also result in the induction of anergy, with the result that the immunized mice could no longer reject tumours that even non-immunized mice could [159].

Particularly since non-hematopoeitic cells rarely express CD80/86-family costimulatory molecules, anergy induction by MHC^+ tumours could be very important. A survey of 6 primary melanomas and 19 lines, for example, revealed that although about half expressed CD80 mRNA, cell surface expression of the protein was very low or absent in the majority[160]. In a transgenic model of tumourigenesis, Antonia et al. [161] found that once tumour-specific T cells had been lost, tumours emerging in the animals did express CD80 (whereas they were usually CD80-negative). In progressing compared to spontaneously regressing melanoma in humans, 5/5 regressors expressed both CD80 and 86 on the tumour cells themselves[162]. Here, the TIL expressed CD28 but not CTLA-4, and were present in areas with histological signs of tumour rejection. Since CTLA-4 transmits negative signals to the T cells, its absence may be important for the anti-tumour response. The paramount importance of negative signalling by CTL-4 can be demonstrated in some mouse models and further studies may reveal critical contributions in human tumour stimulation also. Thus, Leach et al.[163] reported that blockade of CTLA-4 with antibody in vivo could by itself enhance antitumour immunity. In adoptive transfer immunotherapy models, CD8+ tumour-specific T cells otherwise rendered anergic and ineffective may be maintained in an active state via a mechanism involving CD4+ cells by CTLA-4-blockade[164]. Furthermore, there may be further downregulatory co-receptors and their ligands, the existence of which is only now being learned, and these could also be dysregulated in cancer[165]. The in vivo relevance of these mechanisms in a clinical context has recently become susceptible to analysis by employing technology to identify tumour antigen-specific T cells in patients. Thus, the use of soluble tetramer/peptide complexes between HLA-A2 and common melanoma antigens such as tyrosinase (368-376) allow the direct demonstration of clonally-expanded antigen-specific CD8 cells in melanoma patients. These effector cells were demonstrated to be anergic, being unable to lyse target cells or secrete cytokines on activation[166].

ALTERED EXPRESSION OF MHC AND/OR TUMOUR ANTIGENS BY TUMOUR CELLS

HLA-loss phenotypes

As reviewed a number of times recently (eg. see ref.[167]), loss of HLA antigens from tumour cells is common and clinically important[168,169]. Poor prognosis has been documented in association with HLA loss[170] and there may be a higher frequency of selective loss of HLA class I specificities in metastases compared to primary lesions[171]. Single HLA alleles, groups of alleles or even total loss of HLA expression is not uncommon. For example, in breast cancer, total class I loss was found in >50% of patients, with a further 35% showing selective losses; only 12% of tumours retained a full HLA-class I complement[172]. Therefore, downregulation of MHC antigen may provide a powerful strategy for the avoidance of T cell immunity by tumours.

Causes of HLA loss

A common reason for decreased class I expression is the loss of peptide transporter gene expression. This has been shown for TAP-1 and -2 in several tumours[173-178]. In the absence of TAP, antigenic peptides derived from the tumour cannot be presented. TAP defects may be corrected by treatment with with IFN-γ [173-176]. For example, transfection of IFN-γ genes into HLA-deficient small cell lung cancer cells resulted in HLA upregulation and subsequent recognition of the tumour by MAGE-3-specific CTL [179]. This may represent a general finding[180]. The clinical relevance of TAP for tumour development has recently been demonstrated in a mouse model, where TAP-positive cells were unable to generate tumours in normal mice, but did so in nude mice[181]. Clinical consequences of such phenomena have also been implicated in man. Maeurer et al.[182] reported a melanoma patient whose tumour was resected in 1987, at which time expression of MART-1 was recorded. The patient subsequently relapsed and tumour was tested again in 1993. At this time, expression of MART-1 had been lost, concomittant with downregulation of TAP-1. Co-transfection of both TAP and MART was required for re-expression, demonstrating that two selection events must have occured in the tumour, not just loss of peptide transporter.

Other mechanisms of HLA loss may include additional pathways involved in antigen processing and peptide presentation. In the murine B16 melanoma, transfection of hsp65 resulted in increased class I expression and CTL lysis[183]. Therefore, loss of class I because of altered expression of molecular chaperones involved in peptide loading might also be a general mechanism of MHC downregulation and tumour escape. Mutations resulting in splicing defects in HLA pre-mRNA may also contribute to the allele-specific loss commonly observed[184]. And, of course, mutation causing loss of ß2m represents a relatively common mechanism accounting for global HLA loss[185] and has also been observed in patients vaccinated with tumour antigen peptides[186]. Such mutations may themselves reflect particularly severe genetic instability, the so-called "mutator phenotype". Thus, a survey of HLA expression in colorectal adenocarcinoma lines showed that 4/37 failed to express ß2m. Only these four lines had mutator phenotypes; the others, which were non-mutators, had retained HLA expression[187].

Altered HLA / tumour antigen expression under immunological selection, and its consequences

Where levels of MHC class I expression are too low to trigger an immune response, they may still be high enough to act as restriction elements for presensitized cells[188]. Therefore, despite natural progression of tumour, adoptive immunotherapy with in vitro sensitized cells might still be effective. Tumours lacking MHC class I expression and therefore capable of escaping CTL responses might become susceptible to immunotherapy based on NK cells. In fact, it may only be necessary for tumours to decrease their level of HLA expression to become susceptible to NK lysis[189]. In melanoma patients under immunotherapy, tumour variants no longer expressing MHC class I were indeed found to be susceptible to lysis by autologous NK cells[190]. The molecular basis for the increased NK susceptibility as a result of loss of MHC class I expression came with the characterization of NK inhibitory receptors that impede the lytic activity upon interaction with the correct HLA haplotype[191], while failing to do so when interacting with HLA loss variants which as a consequence are lysed. However, a proportion of CTL can also express these NKIR[192], and one might therefore expect these more efficiently to kill tumours which have lost expression of particular class I

231

alleles (other than than tumour antigen restriction element of course). This type of CTL expressing a KIR has actually been reported. In one patient, a melanoma line was established at surgery and found to express at least five different antigens restricted by HLA-A28, B13, B44 and Cw3 and recognized by autologous CTL derived from the PBMC. Five years later the patient developed metastases from which another tumour line was derived. This line could not be killed by any of the previous CTL, because it now expressed only HLA-24. New CTL were isolated recognizing a different antigen presented by A24. This was the first demonstration for tumour escape by evolution of HLA loss variants under selective pressure of CTL in vivo[193]. The new antigen presented by HLA-A24 has now been cloned and designated FRAME[194]. Interestingly, the FRAME-specific HLA-A24-restricted CTL failed to lyse the original melanoma cells from this patient (despite their being FRAME+ and A24+). The reason for this was found to be the recognition of HLA-Cw7 on the tumour cells by NK inhibitory receptors (NKIR) on the CTL, illustrating another mechanism for tumour escape, namely, that HLA class I molecules on the tumours can deliver negative signals to CTL via NKIR[194], who demonstrated that CTL derived from a melanoma patient expressed an NK inhibitory receptor that inhibits its lytic activity upon interaction with HLA-Cw7 molecules. As a consequence, these CTL were able to kill a melanoma line isolated late during disease progression, but not a tumour line isolated earlier, as this tumour expressed HLA-Cw7. The authors proposed that such CTL, active against tumour cells showing partial HLA loss, may constitute an intermediate line of anti-tumour defense between the CTL, which recognize highly specific tumour antigens, and the NK cells, which recognize HLA loss variants[195]. This may indeed be a general phenomenon in melanoma patients[196]. The expression of NKIR may be upregulated by cytokines such as IL-15[197] which can be produced by melanoma cells[33], as well as TGF-ß, commonly produced by tumours[198]. However, inhibitory interactions may also be blocked by antibodies against the NKIR[199], holding out hope for therapeutic intervention. Antibody blockade should also be effective against tumours upregulating non-classical HLA molecules forming ligands for NKIR. Thus, for example, melanoma biopsies were found to express more HLA-G than normal skin; and melanoma lines expressing HLA-G were resistant to NK-lysis[200]. HLA-G may also mediate inhibition of antigen-specific lysis by CTL; this can also be blocked by specific antibody[201].

Robbins et al. reported that HLA-A24-restricted tyrosinase-specific TIL could mediate regression of tumour in the patient. Two years later, relapse occurred and an A24-restricted TIL was isolated that failed to recognize tyrosinase. This may be an example of changed antigen expression on the tumour, which remained HLA-A24+, although it also remained tyrosinase+ as well[202]. Thus, the mechanism of escape here is not clear, but might be due to the tumour no longer expressing the same tyrosinase-derived peptide because of the development of antigen processing variants. In melanoma, antigens commonly targeted in immunotherapy are expressed in a heterogeneous manner in different tumour deposits and within the same deposits; many lesions may have lost expression of these antigens altogether, for example gp100 and MART-1/Melan-A[203]. Another study revealed that MART-1/Melan-A-positivity decreased with clinical stage, being 100% at stage I but only 75% by stage IV[204]. There are increasingly examples where peptide vaccination results in the eventual appearance of metastases lacking the corresponding antigen[205]. Using immunotherapy directed against a single tumour antigen would then be unlikely to target all of the tumour cells even at the beginning of treatment. Thus, CTL precursors specific for MAGE-3 peptide 271-279 have been found in a proportion of melanoma patients, but cells sensitized to synthetic peptide were unable to lyse native tumour cells. In contrast, CTL generated against another MAGE-3 peptide, 168-176, did lyse native tumour cells. It was suggested that the expression of 271-279 by the tumours was too low to allow CTL recognition, despite the existence of antigen-specific precursors in the patients[206]. Along these lines, MAGE-1-specific CTL lysing some but not all MAGE-1+ melanoma cell lines have been reported. PCR-analysis indicated that lines expressing too little MAGE-1 mRNA were not lysed, and that a certain threshold amount of message correlated with lysability[207].

More direct, but still circumstantial, evidence for antigen loss under selective pressure in vivo comes from studies where patients are immunized with defined tumour antigens. Jäger et al.[208] have reported results after vaccination of melanoma patients with Melan A / MART-1 peptide or tyrosinase peptide. Regression of metastases with persistent antigen expression was noted, but those metastases which progressed were found not to express the relevant antigen, although (or presumably because) the patient possessed CTL specific for that antigen. These results suggest that CTL responses to melanocyte differentiation antigens can be boosted in melanoma patients by peptide vaccination and that these CTL may mediate regression of antigen-positive tumours and select for antigen-loss variants in vivo[208]. The same group also reported that in unvaccinated patients repeated biopsies of metastatic lesions showed gradual loss of Melan A/MART-1 expression in 4/5 and tyrosinase expression in 2/5 in association with tumour progression[209]. However, three other patients showed progression without loss of melanoma antigen, and their tumours were shown to have lost HLA instead. Thus, in some cases at least, there may be independent loss of either MHC or tumour antigen under immunoselective pressure[209].

ALTERED EXPRESSION OF ADHESION OR ACCESSORY MOLECULES BY TUMOUR AND / OR DENDRITIC CELLS

Dendritic cells

Anti-tumour responses are commonly triggered by presentation of tumour antigen to T cells by host dendritic cells (DC). If these are compromized in their function, tumour immunity will be severely affected. Chaux et al.[210] reported that DC in the infiltrates of human colorectal carcinomas were strongly MHC class II+ but essentially failed to express the important costimulatory molecules CD80 or CD86, whereas DC in inflammatory infiltrates such as in Crohn's disease lesions were all CD80/86+. In hepatocellular carcinoma, DC in the tumour microenvironment produce more nitric oxide and TNF-α but stimulate lymphocytes less well than DC from liver cirrhosis patients or normal controls[211]. In sunlight-induced basal cell carcinoma, only 5 - 10% of tumour-associated DC expressed costimulatory ligands CD80 and CD86, compared to 38 - 73% of DC from non-tumourous dermatoses, although they expressed high levels of HLA-DR[212]. Presentation of tumour antigen by HLA-DR in the absence of sufficient costimulation might induce anergy in the responding tumour-specific T cells (see 2.5). In rare patients presenting simultaneously with progressing and regressing melanoma metastases, DC showed markedly different characteristics in the two types of lesion. DC from progressing lesions had depressed CD86 expression and secreted IL-10 and induced anergy in autologous CD4+ cells, whereas DC from regressing lesions secreted IFN-γ and IL-12 and did not induce anergy[213]. In breast cacinoma, all samples analysed (32 of 32) showed the presence of immature DCs in the tumour bed, which was attributed to the presence of high local levels of MIP-3α, whereas mature DCs were only present in 20 of 32 cases and were restricted to the peritumoural areas[214]. IL-10 itself may be the factor having an inhibitory effect on the function of DC, inhibiting their differentiation from circulating precursors (P. Allavena, cited in[215]), the accumulation of DC within tumours[216], antigen presentation function and IL-12 production capacity[217]. Moreover, DC exposed to IL-10 may induce anergy in peptide-specific anti-tumour CTL instead of activating them[148]. IL-10-pretreated DC also tend to prime IL-4-secreting T cells, perhaps by default due to the downregulation of IL-12 production[218].

Tumour cells

Where tumour cells themselves do in fact express CD80, it has been observed that progressive variants may arise which have decreased levels of CD80; in contrast, altered levels of CD86 or MHC class class I expression did not correlate with tumourigenicity in this model[219]. Although generally thought to be required only for sensitization and not for effector function, costimulatory molecules such as CD80 may indeed also be required for efficient effector function, at least in some models[220]. In human primary gastric carcinoma, expression of both CD80 and CD86 seems quite common; however, metastases rarely expressed CD80, while CD86 remained high, in agreement with the mouse data above[221]. Indeed, high expression of CD86 may be deleterious, as there is some evidence for selective stimulation of Th2 cells and increased IL-4 production on CD86-costimulation. In one mouse model, this results in suppression of anti-tumour immunity[222].

Melanoma cells may also express other important costimulatory molecules, such as CD40; Von Leoprechting et al. reported that advanced stages were CD40-negative whereas primary tumours and even metastases were CD40+[223]. Moreover, CD40 ligation of melanoma cells enhanced their susceptibility to lysis by MelanA/MART-1-specific CTL, so loss of CD40 expression would prevent this and contribute to escape[223].

Effector cells, once generated, must interact with their target cells, initially via antigen non-specific adhesive mechanisms. Tumour cells of different histologies frequently show relatively decreased levels of important adhesion molecules, such as ICAM-1[224], which may have functional consequences. For example, Pandolfi et al.[225]showed that the degree of TIL kill of autologous melanoma cells correlated with level of expression of adhesion molecules (especially ICAM-1 and LFA-3) - low expression resulted in low kill. Low expression of LFA-3 also results in low level cytokine secretion by CTL interacting with melanoma cells[226]. Anichini et al.[227] further demonstrated that upregulation of ICAM-1 expression by cytokines or gene transfer enhanced the lysability of melanoma cells by CTL clones (but not LAK cells). Anichini et al. also showed[228] that melanoma clones derived from the same metastatic lesion could differ in the amount of intergrins VLA-2 -5 and -6 (CDw49b, e and f) that they expressed, where high expressors were more susceptible to lysis by CTL.

USURPATION OF THE IMMUNE RESPONSE TO THE ADVANTAGE OF THE TUMOUR ("IMMUNOSTIMULATION")

Cytokines produced by T cells reacting to the tumour may well encourage tumour growth. Receptors for IL-10 have been found on melanoma cells and it has been reported that IL-10 may function as a growth stimulating factor for melanoma as well as reducing cell surface expression of HLA and adhesion molecules[229]. In this case, melanoma cells may also produce the IL-10 themselves, making it an autocrine growth factor; but as alluded to above, infiltrating T cells may provide a rich source of IL-10 as well. A further remarkable example of immunostimulation was reported recently where mucosa-associated B cell lymphomas develop secondary to H. pylori infection in the stomach; their growth was shown to depend on the presence of H. pylori-specific CD4+ T cells[230]. Similarly, but without direct evidence, it has been suggested that the pathogenesis of hepatocellular carcinoma is dependent upon the immune response to HBV[231]. Novel and unsuspected mechanisms continue to be discovered, as illustrated by the recent finding that a T cell and monocyte-proinflammatory cytokine identified as macrophage migration inhibitory factor (MIF) inhibits the tumour suppressor activity of p53[232].

Mechanisms other than cytokine production may also be involved in immunostimulation of the tumour. An intriguing report from Hersey´s group showed that many melanoma cells express CD40, which was on occasion upregulatable by IFN-gamma. While CD40 may engage CD154 on activated T cells and possibly deliver costimulatory signals, it is well known that on B cells CD40 itself delivers stimulatory signals required for target cell activation. According to Thomas et al.[233] the same may be true in melanoma, where ligating CD40 with mAb resulted in enhanced cell division. Thus, anti-melanoma cells expressing CD154 (CD40-ligand) may interact with melanoma cells and directly stimulate them via CD40.

Another aspect of immunostimulation of tumour growth is represented by the finding that TIL can also secrete angiogenic factors contributing to vascularisation of the tumours (basic fibroblast growth factor) and factors directly stimulating tumour cells (heparin-binding epidermal growth factor-like GF)[234]. TIL may also secrete other factors which indirectly assist the growth of tumour, eg. vascular endothelial growth factor, which enhances angiogenesis[235]. In this study, in situ hybridisation showed that T cells infiltrating bladder and prostate cancer expressed VEGF mRNA and protein, and that isolated T cells could secrete bioactive VEGF.

CONCLUDING REMARKS

Tumour escape from the immune response represents the last hurdle to successful immunotherapy of cancer[1]. Despite an intense and continuing effort, the problem of how immunogenic tumours evade the host immune response is still not completely resolved. This rapidly progressing area of research offers tremendous therapeutic potential by defining mechanisms of tumour escape from immunotherapy and developing interventions for preventing this. However, a major challenge for the future remains the identification of small numbers of variant tumour cells in the patient, in order to determine their mechanism of escape and prepare a therapeutic approach tailor-made to circumvent this. Here, also, immunological methods of tumour cell identification and localisation will play an increasingly important part in individual treatment strategies.

ACKNOWLEDGEMENTS

The author is currently supported by the Deutsche Forschungsgemeinschaft (Pa 361/5-2), the Mildred Scheel Foundation (10-1173-Pa3), the VERUM Foundation, the Dieter Schlag Foundation, the fortüne program of the University of Tübingen Medical Faculty and the European Commission (BMHI-CT-98-3058; QLK6-CT-1999-02031).

REFERENCES

1. Pawelec G. Tumour escape from the immune response: the last hurdle for successful immunotherapy of cancer? Cancer Immunol Immunother 1999;48(7):343-5.
2. Tsushima H, Kawata S, Tamura S, et al. High levels of transforming growth factor beta 1 in patients with colorectal cancer: Association with disease progression. Gastroenterology 1996;110(2):375-82.
3. Krasagakis K, Tholke D, Farthmann B, Eberle J, Mansmann U, Orfanos CE. Elevated plasma levels of transforming growth factor (TGF)-beta 1 and TGF-beta 2 in patients with disseminated malignant melanoma. Br J Cancer 1998;77(9):1492-4.
4. Doran T, Stuhlmiller H, Kim JA, Martin EW, Triozzi PL. Oncogene and cytokine expression of human colorectal tumors responding to immunotherapy. J Immunother 1997;20(5):372-6.
5. Vanky F, Nagy N, Hising C, Sjovall K, Larson B, Klein E. Human ex vivo carcinoma cells produce transforming growth factor beta and thereby can inhibit lymphocyte functions in vitro. Cancer Immunol Immunother 1997;43(6):317-23.
6. Mantovani G, Maccio A, Esu S, et al. Lack of correlation between defective cell-mediated immunity and levels of secreted or circulating cytokines in a study of 90 cancer patients - Clinical study. Int J Oncol 1994;5(6):1211-7.
7. Dowlati A, Levitan N, Remick SC. Evaluation of interleukin-6 in bronchoalveolar lavage fluid and serum of patients with lung cancer. J Lab Clin Med 1999;134(4):405-9.

8. Mouawad R, Khayat D, Merle S, Antoine EC, GilDelgado M, Soubrane C. Is there any relationship between interleukin-6/ interleukin-6 receptor modulation and endogenous interleukin-6 release in metastatic malignant melanoma patients treated by biochemotherapy? Melanoma Res 1999;9(2):181-8.

9. Zhang GJ, Adachi I. Serum interleukin-6 levels correlate to tumor progression and prognosis in metastatic breast carcinoma. Anticancer Res 1999;19(2B):1427-32.

10. Fortis C, Foppoli M, Gianotti L, et al. Increased interleukin-10 serum levels in patients with solid tumours. Cancer Lett 1996;104(1):1-5.

11. Bellone G, Turletti A, Artusio E, et al. Tumor-associated transforming growth factor-beta and interleukin-10 contribute to a systemic Th2 immune phenotype in pancreatic carcinoma patients. Amer J Pathol 1999;155(2):537-47.

12. Philip T, Negrier S, Lasset C, et al. Patients with Metastatic Renal Carcinoma Candidate for Immunotherapy with Cytokines - Analysis of a Single Institution Study on 181 Patients. Br J Cancer 1993;68(5):1036-42.

13. Sarris AH, Kliche KO, Pethambaram P, et al. Interleukin-10 levels are often elevated in serum of adults with Hodgkin's disease and are associated with inferior failure-free survival. Ann Oncol 1999;10(4):433-40.

14. Cortes JE, Talpaz M, Cabanillas F, Seymour JF, Kurzrock R. Serum levels of interleukin-10 in patients with diffuse large cell lymphoma: Lack of correlation with prognosis. Blood 1995;85(9):2516-20.

15. Sjoberg J, Aguilarsanteleises M, Sjogren AM, et al. Interleukin-10 mRNA expression in B-cell chronic lymphocytic leukaemia inversely correlates with progression of disease. Br J Haematol 1996;92(2):393-400.

16. Pisa P, Halapi E, Pisa EK, et al. Selective Expression of Interleukin-10, Interferon-gamma, and Granulocyte Macrophage Colony-Stimulating Factor in Ovarian Cancer Biopsies. Proc Natl Acad Sci USA 1992;89:7708-12.

17. Berghella AM, Pellegrini P, Delbeato T, Adorno D, Casciani CU. IL-10 and sIL-2R serum levels as possible peripheral blood prognostic markers in the passage from adenoma to colorectal cancer. Cancer Biother Radiopharm 1997;12(4):265-72.

18. Kim J, Modlin RL, Moy RL, et al. IL-10 production in cutaneous basal and squamous cell carcinomas - A mechanism for evading the local T cell immune response. J Immunol 1995;155(4):2240-7.

19. Pawelec G, Schlotz E, Rehbein A. IFN-alpha regulates IL-10 production by CML cells in vitro. Cancer Immunol Immunother 1999;48(8):430-4.

20. Fijieda S, Lee K, Sunaga H, et al. Staining of interleukin-10 predicts clinical outcome in patients with nasopharyngeal carcinoma. Cancer 1999;85(7):1439-45.

21. DeVita F, Orditura M, Galizia G, et al. Serum interleukin-10 levels in patients with advanced gastrointestinal malignancies. Cancer 1999;86(10):1936-43.

22. Nakagomi H, Pisa P, Pisa EK, et al. Lack of interleukin-2 (IL-2) expression and selective expression of IL-10 mRNA in human renal cell carcinoma. Int J Cancer 1995;63(3):366-71.

23. MenetrierCaux C, Bain C, Favrot MC, Duc A, Blay JY. Renal cell carcinoma induces interleukin 10 and prostaglandin E-2 production by monocytes. Brit J Cancer 1999;79(1):119-30.

24. Yamamura M, Modlin RL, Ohmen JD, Moy RL. Local Expression of Antiinflammatory Cytokines in Cancer. J Clin Invest 1993;91:1005-10.

25. Young MRI, Wright MA, Lozano Y, Matthews JP, Benefield J, Prechel MM. Mechanisms of immune suppression in patients with head and neck cancer: Influence on the immune infiltrate of the cancer. Int J Cancer 1996;67(3):333-8.

26. Rabinowich H, Suminami Y, Reichert TE, et al. Expression of cytokine genes or proteins and signaling molecules in lymphocytes associated with human ovarian carcinoma. Int J Cancer 1996;68(3):276-84.

27. Venetsanakos E, Beckman I, Bradley J, Skinner JM. High incidence of interleukin 10 mRNA but not interleukin 2 mRNA detected in human breast tumours. Br J Cancer 1997;75(12):1826-30.

28. Krugerkrasagakes S, Krasagakis K, Garbe C, et al. Expression of interleukin 10 in human melanoma. Br J Cancer 1994;70(6):1182-5.

29. Huang M, Wang JY, Lee P, et al. Human non-small cell lung cancer cells express a type 2 cytokine pattern. Cancer Res 1995;55(17):3847-53.

CANCER IMMUNOLOGY

30. Hishii M, Nitta T, Ishida H, et al. Human glioma-derived interleukin-10 inhibits antitumor immune responses in vitro. Neurosurgery 1995;37(6):1160-6.
31. AsselinPaturel C, Echchakir H, Carayol G, et al. Quantitative analysis of Th1, Th2 and TGF-beta 1 cytokine expression in tumor, TIL and PBL of non-small cell lung cancer patients. Int J Cancer 1998;77(1):7-12.
32. Peng LM, Shu SY, Krauss JC. Monocyte chemoattractant protein inhibits the generation of tumor-reactive T cells. Cancer Res 1997;57(21):4849-54.
33. Barzegar C, Meazza R, Pereno R, et al. IL-15 is produced by a subset of human melanomas, and is involved in the regulation of markers of melanoma progression through juxtacrine loops. Oncogene 1998;16(19):2503-12.
34. Wagner SN, Schultewolter T, Wagner C, et al. Immune response against human primary malignant melanoma: A distinct cytokine mRNA profile associated with spontaneous regression. Lab Invest 1998;78(5):541-50.
35. Moretti S, Pinzi C, Spallanzani A, et al. Immunohistochemical evidence of cytokine networks during progression of human melanocytic lesions. Int J Cancer 1999;84(2):160-8.
36. Kunz M, Hartmann A, Flory E, et al. Anoxia-induced up-regulation of interleukin-8 in human malignant melanoma - A potential mechanism for high tumor aggressiveness. Amer J Pathol 1999;155(3):753-63.
37. Qin ZH, Richter G, Schuler T, Ibe S, Cao XT, Blankenstein T. B cells inhibit induction of T cell-dependent tumor immunity. Nature Med 1998;4(5):627-30.
38. Wijesuriya R, Maruo S, Zou JP, et al. B cell-mediated down-regulation of IFN-gamma and IL-12 production induced during antitumor immune responses in the tumor-bearing state. Int Immunol 1998;10(8):1057-65.
39. Manson LA. Does Antibody-Dependent Epitope Masking Permit Progressive Tumour Growth in the Face of Cell-Mediated Cytotoxicity? Immunol Today 1991;12:352-5.
40. Kharkevitch DD, Seito D, Balch GC, Maeda T, Balch CM, Itoh K. Characterization of autologous tumor-specific T-helper 2 cells in tumor-infiltrating lymphocytes from a patient with metastatic melanoma. Int J Cancer 1994;58(3):317-23.
41. Lee PP, Zeng DF, McCaulay AE, et al. T helper 2-dominant antilymphoma immune response is associated with fatal outcome. Blood 1997;90(4):1611-7.
42. Brady MS, Eckels DD, Lee F, Ree SY, Lee JS. Cytokine production by CD4+T-cells responding to antigen presentation by melanoma cells. Melanoma Res 1999;9(2):173-80.
43. Groux H, Ogarra A, Bigler M, et al. A CD4(+) T-cell subset inhibits antigen-specific T-cell responses and prevents colitis. Nature 1997;389(6652):737-42.
44. Zeller JC, PanoskaltsisMortari A, Murphy WJ, et al. Induction of CD4(+) T cell alloantigen-specific hyporesponsiveness by IL-10 and TGF-beta(1). J Immunol 1999;163(7):3684-91.
45. Seo N, Tokura Y, Matsumoto K, Furukawa F, Takigawa M. Tumour-specific cytotoxic T lymphocyte activity in Th2-type Sezary syndrome: its enhancement by interferon-gamma (IFN-gamma) and IL-12 and fluctuations in association with disease activity. Clin Exp Immunol 1998;112(3):403-9.
46. Lowes MA, Bishop GA, Crotty K, Barnetson RS, Halliday GM. T helper 1 cytokine mRNA is increased in spontaneously regressing primary melanomas. J Invest Dermatol 1997;108(6):914-9.
47. Gabrilovich DI, Nadaf S, Corak J, Berzofsky JA, Carbone DP. Dendritic cells in antitumor immune responses .2. Dendritic cells grown from bone marrow precursors, but not mature DC from tumor-bearing mice, are effective antigen carriers in the therapy of established tumors. Cell Immunol 1996;170(1):111-9.
48. Yashiro Y, Tai XG, Toyooka K, et al. A fundamental difference in the capacity to induce proliferation of naive T cells between CD28 and other co-stimulatory molecules. Eur J Immunol 1998;28(3):926-35.
49. Maeda H, Shiraishi A. TGF-beta contributes to the shift toward Th2-type responses through direct and IL-10-mediated pathways in tumor-bearing mice. J Immunol 1996;156(1):73-8.
50. Handelfernandez ME, Cheng XF, Herbert LM, Lopez DM. Down-regulation of IL-12, not a shift from a T helper-1 to a T helper-2 phenotype, is responsible for impaired IFN-gamma production in mammary tumor-bearing mice. J Immunol 1997;158(1):280-6.
51. Colombo MP, Vagliani M, Spreafico F, et al. Amount of interleukin 12 available at the tumor site is critical for tumor regression. Cancer Res 1996;56(11):2531-4.

52. Pellegrini P, Berghella AM, Delbeato T, Cicia S, Adorno D, Casciani CU. Disregulation in TH1 and TH2 subsets of CD4+ T cells in peripheral blood of colorectal cancer patients and involvement in cancer establishment and progression. Cancer Immunol Immunother 1996;42(1):1-8.

53. Nishimura T, Iwakabe K, Sekimoto M, et al. Distinct role of antigen-specific T helper type 1 (Th1) and Th2 cells in tumor eradication in vivo. J Exp Med 1999;190(5):617-27.

54. Golumbek PT, Lazenby AJ, Levitsky HI, et al. Treatment of Established Renal Cancer by Tumor Cells Engineered to Secrete Interleukin-4. Science 1991;254:713-6.

55. Rodolfo M, Zilocchi C, Accornero P, Cappetti B, Arioli I, Colombo MP. IL-4-transduced tumor cell vaccine induces immunoregulatory type 2 CD8 T lymphocytes that cure lung metastases upon adoptive transfer. J Immunol 1999;163(4):1923-8.

56. Barth RJ, Camp BJ, Martuscello TA, Dain BJ, Memoli VA. The cytokine microenvironment of human colon carcinoma -Lymphocyte expression of tumor necrosis factor-alpha and interleukin-4 predicts improved survival. Cancer 1996;78(6):1168-78.

57. Santra S, Ghosh SK. Interleukin-4 is effective in restoring cytotoxic T cell activity that declines during in vivo progression of a murine B lymphoma. Cancer Immunol Immunother 1997;44(5):291-300.

58. Richter G, Krugerkrasagakes S, Hein G, et al. Interleukin-10 Transfected into Chinese Hamster Ovary Cells Prevents Tumor Growth and Macrophage Infiltration. Cancer Res 1993;53(18):4134-7.

59. Giovarelli M, Musiani P, Modesti A, et al. Local release of IL-10 by transfected mouse mammary adenocarcinoma cells does not suppress but enhances antitumor reaction and elicits a strong cytotoxic lymphocyte and antibody-dependent immune memory. J Immunol 1995;155(6):3112-23.

60. Yang GC, Hellstrom KE, Mizuno MT, Chen LP. In vitro priming of tumor-reactive cytolytic T lymphocytes by combining IL-10 with B7-CD28 costimulation. J Immunol 1995;155(8):3897-903.

61. Taga K, Cherney B, Tosato G. IL-10 Inhibits Apoptotic Cell Death in Human T-Cells Starved of IL-2. Int Immunol 1993;5(12):1599-608.

62. Pawelec G, Hambrecht A, Rehbein A, Adibzadeh M. Interleukin 10 protects activated human T lymphocytes against growth factor withdrawal-induced cell death but only anti-fas antibody can prevent activation-induced cell death. Cytokine 1996;8(12):877-81.

63. Pawelec G, Pohla H, Scholtz E, et al. Interleukin 10 is a human T cell growth factor in vitro. Cytokine 1995;7(4):355-63.

64. Vanbergen CAM, Smit WM, Vansluijters DA, Rijnbeek M, Willemze R, Falkenburg JHF. Interleukin-10, interleukin-12, and tumor necrosis factor-alpha differentially influence the proliferation of human CD8(+) and CD4(+) T-cell clones. Ann Hematol 1996;72(4):245-52.

65. Kirkin AF, Straten PT, Zeuthen J. Differential modulation by interferon gamma of the sensitivity of human melanoma cells to cytolytic T cell clones that recognize differentiation or progression antigens. Cancer Immunol Immunother 1996;42(4):203-12.

66. Huang SY, Ullrich SE, BarEli M. Regulation of tumor growth and metastasis by interleukin-10: The melanoma experience. J Interferon Cytokine Res 1999;19(7):697-703.

67. Scheibenbogen C, Lee KH, Stevanovic S, et al. Analysis of the T cell response to tumor and viral peptide antigens by an IFN gamma-elispot assay. Int J Cancer 1997;71(6):932-6.

68. Altomonte M, Gloghini A, Bertola G, et al. Differential Expression of Cell Adhesion Molecules CD54/CD11a and CD58/CD2 by Human Melanoma Cells and Functional Role in Their Interaction with Cytotoxic Cells. Cancer Res 1993;53(14):3343-8.

69. Becker JC, Termeer C, Schmidt RE, Brocker EB. Soluble Intercellular Adhesion Molecule-1 Inhibits MHC-Restricted Specific T-Cell Tumor Interaction. J Immunol 1993;151(12):7224-32.

70. Grothey A, Heistermann P, Philippou S, Voigtmann R. Serum levels of soluble intercellular adhesion molecule-1 (ICAM-1, CD54) in patients with non-small-cell lung cancer: correlation with histological expression of ICAM-1 and tumour stage. Br J Cancer 1998;77(5):801-7.

71. SanchezRovira P, Jimenez E, Carracedo J, Barneto IC, Ramirez R, Aranda E. Serum levels of intercellular adhesion molecule 1 (ICAM-1) in patients with colorectal cancer: Inhibitory effect on cytotoxicity. Eur J Cancer 1998;34(3):394-8.

72. Fonsatti E, Lamaj E, Coral S, et al. In vitro analysis of the melanoma endothelium interaction increasing the release of soluble intercellular adhesion molecule 1 by endothelial cells. Cancer Immunol Immunother 1999;48(2-3):132-8.

73. Salmaggi A, Eoli M, Frigerio S, Ciusani E, Silvani A, Boiardi A. Circulating intercellular adhesion molecule-1 (ICAM-1), vascular cell adhesion molecule-1 (VCAM-1) and plasma thrombomodulin levels in glioblastoma patients. Cancer Lett 1999;146(2):169-72.

74. Rosen HR, Ausch C, Reiner G, et al. Downregulation of lymphocyte mitogenesis by breast cancer-associated p43. Cancer Lett 1994;82(1):105-11.

75. Chan AK, Lockhart DC, vonBernstorff W, et al. Soluble MUC1 secreted by human epithelial cancer cells mediates immune suppression by blocking T-cell activation. Int J Cancer 1999;82(5):721-6.

76. Agrawal B, Krantz MJ, Reddish MA, Longenecker BM. Cancer-associated MUC1 mucin inhibits human T-cell proliferation, which is reversible by IL-2. Nature Med 1998;4(1):43-9.

77. Paul S, Bizouarne N, Paul A, et al. Lack of evidence for an immunosuppressive role for MUC1. Cancer Immunol Immunother 1999;48(1):22-8.

78. Maclean GD, Reddish MA, Longenecker BM. Prognostic significance of preimmunotherapy serum CA27.29 (MUC-1) mucin level after active specific immunotherapy of metastatic adenocarcinoma patients. J Immunother 1997;20(1):70-8.

79. Takao S, Uchikura K, Yonezawa S, Shinchi H, Aikou T. Mucin core protein expression in extrahepatic bile duct carcinoma is associated with metastases to the liver and poor prognosis. Cancer 1999;86(10):1966-75.

80. Aarli A, Kristoffersen EK, Jensen TS, Ulvestad E, Matre R. Suppressive effect on lymphoproliferation in vitro by soluble annexin II released from isolated placental membranes. Am J Reprod Immunol 1997;38(5):313-9.

81. Hoskin DW, Reynolds T, Blay J. Adenosine as a possible inhibitor of killer T-cell activation in the microenvironment of solid tumors. Int J Cancer 1994;59(6):854-5.

82. Blay J, White TD, Hoskin DW. The extracellular fluid of solid carcinomas contains immunosuppressive concentrations of adenosine. Cancer Res 1997;57(13):2602-5.

83. Pitti RM, Marsters SA, Lawrence DA, et al. Genomic amplification of a decoy receptor for Fas ligand in lung and colon cancer. Nature 1998;396(6712):699-703.

84. McKallip R, Li RX, Ladisch S. Tumor gangliosides inhibit the tumor-specific immune response. J Immunol 1999;163(7):3718-26.

85. Uzzo RG, Rayman P, Kolenko V, et al. Renal cell carcinoma-derived gangliosides suppress nuclear factor-kappa B activation in T cells. J Clin Invest 1999;104(6):769-76.

86. Schottelius AJG, Mayo MW, Sartor RB, Badwin AS. Interleukin-10 signaling blocks inhibitor of kappa B kinase activity and nuclear factor kappa B DNA binding. J Biol Chem 1999;274(45):31868-74.

87. Mizoguchi H, Oshea JJ, Longo DL, Loeffler CM, McVicar DW, Ochoa AC. Alterations in Signal Transduction Molecules in Lymphocytes-T from Tumor-Bearing Mice. Science 1992;258:1795-8.

88. Lai P, Rabinowich H, Crowley-Nowick PA, Bell MC, Mantovani G, Whiteside TL. Alterations in expression and function of signal-transducing proteins in tumor-associated T and natural killer cells in patients with ovarian carcinoma. Clinical Cancer Research 1996;2:161-73.

89. Finke JH, Zea AH, Stanley J, et al. Loss of T-Cell Receptor zeta-Chain and p56(lck) in T-Cells Infiltrating Human Renal Cell Carcinoma. Cancer Res 1993;53(23):5613-6.

90. Nakagomi H, Petersson M, Magnusson I, et al. Decreased Expression of the Signal-Transducing zeta-Chains in Tumor-Infiltrating T-Cells and NK Cells of Patients with Colorectal Carcinoma. Cancer Res 1993;53(23):5610-2.

91. Kono K, Ressing ME, Brandt RM, et al. Decreased expression of signal-transducing zeta chain on peripheral T cells and NK cells in patients with cervical cancer. Clinical Cancer Research 1996;2:1825.

92. Zea AH, Curti BD, Londo DL, et al. Alterations in T cell receptor and signal-transduction molecules in melanoma patients. Clinical Cancer Research 1995;1:1327-35.

93. Morford LA, Elliott LH, Carlson SL, Brooks WH, Roszman TL. T cell receptor-mediated signaling is defective in T cells obtained from patients with primary intracranial tumors. J Immunol 1997;159(9):4415-25.

94. Healy CG, Simons JW, Carducci MA, et al. Impaired expression and function of signal-transducing zeta chains in peripheral T cells and natural killer cells in patients with prostate cancer. Cytometry 1998;32(2):109-19.

95. Reichert TE, Day R, Wagner EM, Whiteside TL. Absent or low expression of the zeta chain in T cells at the tumor site correlates with poor survival in patients with oral carcinoma. Cancer Res 1998;58(23):5344-7.

96. Li X, Liu J, Park J-K, et al. T cells from renal carcinoma patients show an abnormal pattern of kappa B-specific DNA-binding activity: a preliminary analysis. Cancer Res 1994;54:5424-9.

97. Ling WJ, Rayman P, Uzzo R, et al. Impaired activation of NF Kappa B in T cells from a subset of renal cell carcinoma patients is mediated by inhibition of phosphorylation and degradation of the inhibitor, I Kappa B alpha. Blood 1998;92(4):1334-41.

98. Rossi E, Matutes E, Morilla R, Owusuankomah K, Heffernan AM, Catovsky D. Zeta chain and CD28 are poorly expressed on T lymphocytes from chronic lymphocytic leukemia. Leukemia 1996;10(3):494-7.

99. Gunji Y, Hori S, Aoe T, et al. High frequency of cancer patients with abnormal assembly of the T cell receptor-CD3 complex in peripheral blood T lymphocytes. Jpn J Cancer Res 1994;85:1189-92.

100. Matsuda M, Petersson M, Lenkei R, et al. Alterations in the signal-transducing molecules of T cells and NK cells in colorectal tumor-infiltrating, gut mucosal and peripheral lymphocytes: Correlation with the stage of the disease. Int J Cancer 1995;61(6):765-72.

101. Mulder WM, Bloemena E, Stukart MJ, Kummer JA, Wagstaff J, Scheper RJ. T cell receptor zeta and granzyme B expression in mononuclear cell infiltrates in normal colon mucosa and colon carcinoma. Gut 1997;40:113.

102. Nieland JD, Loviscek K, Kono K, et al. PBLs of early breast carcinoma patients with a high nuclear grade tumor unlike PBLs of cervical carcinoma patients do not show a decreased TCR zeta expression but are functionally impaired. J Immunother 1998;21(4):317-22.

103. Varadhachary AS, Perdow SN, Hu CG, Ramanarayanan M, Salgame P. Differential ability of T cell subsets to undergo activation-induced cell death. Proc Natl Acad Sci USA 1997;94(11):5778-83.

104. Maurice MM, Lankester AC, Bezemer AC, et al. Defective TCR-mediated signaling in synovial T cells in rheumatoid arthritis. J Immunol 1997;159(6):2973-8.

105. Matsuda M, Ulfgren AK, Lenkei R, et al. Decreased expression of signal-transducing CD3 zeta chains in T cells from the joints and peripheral blood of rheumatoid arthritis patients. Scand J Immunol 1998;47(3):254-62.

106. Liossis SNC, Ding XZ, Dennis GJ, Tsokos GC. Altered pattern of TCR/CD3-mediated protein-tyrosyl phosphorylation in T cells from patients with systemic lupus erythematosus - Deficient expression of the T cell receptor zeta chain. J Clin Invest 1998;101(7):1448-57.

107. Zea AH, Ochoa MT, Ghosh P, et al. Changes in signal transduction molecules in patients with lepromatous leprosy. Infect Immun 1997;(in press).

108. Agrawal S, Marquet J, DelfauLarue MH, et al. CD3 hyporesponsiveness and in vitro apoptosis are features of T cells from both malignant and nonmalignant secondary lymphoid organs. J Clin Invest 1998;102(9):1715-23.

109. Ardouin L, Boyer C, Gillet A, et al. Crippling of CD3-zeta ITAMs does not impair T cell receptor signaling. Immunity 1999;10(4):409-20.

110. Choi SH, Chung EJ, Whang DY, Lee SS, Jang YS, Kim CW. Alteration of signal-transducing molecules in tumor-infiltrating lymphocytes and peripheral blood T lymphocytes from human colorectal carcinoma patients. Cancer Immunol Immunother 1998;45(6):299-305.

111. Kurt RA, Urba WJ, Smith JW, Schoof DD. Peripheral T lymphocytes from women with breast cancer exhibit abnormal protein expression of several signaling molecules. Int J Cancer 1998;78(1):16-20.

112. Levey DL, Srivastava PK. T cells from late tumor-bearing mice express normal levels of p56(lck), p59(fyn), ZAP-70, and CD3 zeta despite suppressed cytolytic activity. J Exp Med 1995;182(4):1029-36.

113. Cardi G, Heaney JA, Schned AR, Phillips DM, Branda MT, Ernstoff MS. T-cell receptor xi-chain expression on tumor-infiltrating lymphocytes from renal cell carcinoma. Cancer Res 1997;57(16):3517-9.

114. Franco JL, Ghosh P, Wiltrout RH, et al. Partial degradation of T-cell signal transduction molecules by contaminating granulocytes during protein extraction of splenic T cells from tumor-bearing mice. Cancer Res 1995;55(17):3840-6.

115. Correa MR, Ochoa AC, Ghosh P, Mizoguchi H, Harvey L, Longo DL. Sequential development of structural and functional alterations in T cells from tumor-bearing mice. J Immunol 1997;158(11):5292-6.

116. Deakin AM, Singh K, Crowe JS, et al. A lack of evidence for down-modulation of CD3 zeta expression in colorectal carcinoma and pregnancy using multiple detection. Clin Exp Immunol 1999;118(2):197-204.

117. Aoe T, Okamoto Y, Saito T. Activated macrophages induce structural abnormalities of the T cell receptor-CD3 complex. J Exp Med 1995;181(5):1881-6.

118. Kono K, Salazaronfray F, Petersson M, et al. Hydrogen peroxide secreted by tumor-derived macrophages down-modulates signal-transducing zeta molecules and inhibits tumor-specific T cell- and natural killer cell-mediated cytotoxicity. Eur J Immunol 1996;26(6):1308-13.

119. Otsuji M, Kimura Y, Aoe T, Okamoto Y, Saito T. Oxidative stress by tumor-derived macrophages suppresses the expression of CD3 zeta chain of T-cell receptor complex and antigen-specific T-cell responses. Proc Natl Acad Sci USA 1996;93(23):13119-24.

120. Gastman BR, Johnson DE, Whiteside TL, Rabinowich H. Caspase-mediated degradation of T-cell receptor zeta-chain. Cancer Res 1999;59(7):1422-7.

121. Rabinowich H, Reichert TE, Kashii Y, Gastman BR, Bell MC, Whiteside TL. Lymphocyte apoptosis induced by Fas ligand-expressing ovarian carcinoma cells - Implications for altered expression of T cell receptor in tumor-associated lymphocytes. J Clin Invest 1998;101(11):2579-88.

122. Lauritzsen GF, Hofgaard PO, Schenck K, Bogen B. Clonal deletion of thymocytes as a tumor escape mechanism. Int J Cancer 1998;78(2):216-22.

123. Niehans GA, Brunner T, Frizelle SP, et al. Human lung carcinomas express Fas ligand. Cancer Res 1997;57(6):1007-12.

124. Hahne M, Rimoldi D, Schroter M, et al. Melanoma cell expression of Fas(Apo-1/CD95) ligand: Implications for tumor immune escape. Science 1996;274(5291):1363-6.

125. Chappell DB, Restifo NP. T cell-tumor cell: a fatal interaction? Cancer Immunol Immunother 1998;47(2):65-71.

126. Shiraki K, Tsuji N, Shioda T, Isselbacher KJ, Takahashi H. Expression of Fas ligand in liver metastases of human colonic adenocarcinomas. Proc Natl Acad Sci USA 1997;94(12):6420-5.

127. Walker PR, Saas P, Dietrich PY. Role of Fas ligand (CD95L) in immune escape: The tumor cell strikes back - Commentary. J Immunol 1997;158(10):4521-4.

128. Ungefroren H, Voss M, Jansen M, et al. Human pancreatic adenocarcinomas express Fas and Fas ligand yet are resistant to Fas-mediated apoptosis. Cancer Res 1998;58(8):1741-9.

129. Gastman BR, Atarashi Y, Reichert TE, et al. Fas ligand is expressed on human squamous cell carcinomas of the head and neck, and it promotes apoptosis of T lymphocytes. Cancer Res 1999;59(20):5356-64.

130. Kume T, Oshima K, Yamashita Y, Shirakusa T, Kikichi M. Relationship between Fas-ligand expression on carcinoma cell and cytotoxic T-lymphocyte response in lymphoepithelioma-like cancer of the stomach. Int J Cancer 1999;84(4):339-43.

131. Nagao M, Nakajima Y, Hisanaga M, et al. The alteration of Fas receptor and ligand system in hepatocellular carcinomas: How do hepatoma cells escape from the host immune surveillance in vivo? Hepatology 1999;30(2):413-21.

132. Gratas C, Tohma Y, Barnas C, Taniere P, Hainaut P, Ohgaki H. Up-regulation of Fas (APO-1/CD95) ligand and down-regulation of Fas expression in human esophageal cancer. Cancer Res 1998;58(10):2057-62.

133. Bennett MW, OConnell J, OSullivan GC, et al. The Fas counterattack in vivo: Apoptotic depletion of tumor-infiltrating lymphocytes associated with Fas ligand expression by human esophageal carcinoma. J Immunol 1998;160(11):5669-75.

134. Terheyden P, Siedel C, Merkel A, Kampgen E, Brocker EB, Becker JC. Predominant expression of Fas (CD95) ligand in metastatic melanoma revealed by longitudinal analysis. J Invest Dermatol 1999;112(6):899-902.

135. Rivoltini L, Radrizzani M, Accornero P, et al. Human melanoma-reactive CD4(+) and CD8(+) CTL clones resist Fas ligand-induced apoptosis and use Fas/Fas ligand-independent mechanisms for tumor killing. J Immunol 1998;161(3):1220-30.

136. Alderson MR, Armitage RJ, Maraskovsky E, et al. Fas Transduces Activation Signals in Normal Human T-Lymphocytes. J Exp Med 1993;178(6):2231-5.

137. Kang SM, Schneider DB, Lin ZH, et al. Fas ligand expression in islets of Langerhans does not confer immune privilege and instead targets them for rapid destruction. Nature Med 1997;3(7):738-43.

138. Tsutsui T, Mu J, Ogawa M, et al. Administration of IL-12 induces a CD3(+)CD4(-)CD8(-)B220(+) lymphoid population capable of eliciting cytolysis against Fas-positive tumor cells. J Immunol 1997;159(6):2599-605.

139. Medema JP, deJong J, vanHall T, Melief CJM, Offringa R. Immune escape of tumors in vivo by expression of cellular FLICE-inhibitory protein. J Exp Med 1999;190(7):1033-8.

140. Djerbi M, Screpanti V, Catrina AI, Bogen B, Biberfeld P, Grandien A. The inhibitor of death receptor signaling, FLICE-inhibitory protein defines a new class of tumor progression factors. J Exp Med 1999;190(7):1025-31.

141. OwenSchaub LB, vanGolen KL, Hill LL, Price JE. Fas and fas ligand interactions suppress melanoma lung metastasis. J Exp Med 1998;188(9):1717-23.

142. Zaks TZ, Chappell DB, Rosenberg SA, Restifo NP. Fas-mediated suicide of tumor-reactive T cells following activation by specific tumor: Selective rescue by caspase inhibition. J Immunol 1999;162(6):3273-9.

143. Suzuki I, Fink PJ. Maximal proliferation of cytotoxic T lymphocytes requires reverse signaling through Fas ligand. J Exp Med 1998;187(1):123-8.

144. Gimmi CD, Morrison BW, Mainprice BA, et al. Breast cancer-associated antigen, DF3/MUC1, induces apoptosis of activated human T cells. Nature Med 1996;2(12):1367-70.

145. Boussiotis V, Freeman GJ, Gribben JG, Hayes DF, Nadler LM. No evidence for MUC 1-induced apoptosis. Nature Med 1998;4:1093.

146. Agrawal B, Gendler SJ, Longenecker BM. The biological role of mucins in cellular interactions and immune regulation: prospects for cancer immunotherapy. Mol Med Today 1998;4(9):397-403.

147. Agrawal B, Krantz MJ, Parker J, Longenecker BM. Expression of MUC1 mucin on activated human T cells: Implications for a role of MUC1 in normal immune regulation. Cancer Res 1998;58(18):4079-81.

148. Steinbrink K, Jonuleit H, Muller G, Schuler G, Knop J, Enk AH. Interleukin-10-treated human dendritic cells induce a melanoma-antigen-specific anergy in CD8(+) T cells resulting in a failure to lyse tumor cells. Blood 1999;93(5):1634-42.

149. StaveleyOCarroll K, Sotomayor E, Montgomery J, et al. Induction of antigen-specific T cell anergy: An early event in the course of tumor progression. Proc Natl Acad Sci USA 1998;95(3):1178-83.

150. Gimmi CD, Freeman GJ, Gribben JG, Gray G, Nadler LM. Human T-Cell Clonal Anergy Is Induced by Antigen Presentation in the Absence of B7 Costimulation. Proc Natl Acad Sci USA 1993;90(14):6586-90.

151. Sloanlancaster J, Evavold BD, Allen PM. Induction of T-Cell Anergy by Altered T-Cell-Receptor Ligand on Live Antigen-Presenting Cells. Nature 1993;363(6425):156-9.

152. Desilva DR, Urdahl KB, Jenkins MK. Clonal Anergy Is Induced Invitro by T-Cell Receptor Occupancy in the Absence of Proliferation. J Immunol 1991;147:3261-7.

153. Jenkins MK. The Role of Cell Division in the Induction of Clonal Anergy. Immunol Today 1992;13:69-73.

154. Loftus DJ, Squarcina P, Nielsen MB, et al. Peptides derived from self-proteins as partial agonists and antagonists of human CD8(+) T-cell clones reactive to melanoma/melanocyte epitope MART1(27-35). Cancer Res 1998;58(11):2433-9.

155. Klenerman P, Zinkernagel RM. Original antigenic sin impairs cytotoxic T lymphocyte responses to viruses bearing variant epitopes. Nature 1998;394(6692):482-5.

156. Toes REM, Offringa R, Blom RJJ, Melief CJM, Kast WM. Peptide vaccination can lead to enhanced tumor growth through specific T-cell tolerance induction. Proc Natl Acad Sci USA 1996;93(15):7855-60.

157. Boussiotis VA, Barber DL, Nakarai T, et al. Prevention of T cell anergy by signaling through the gamma(c) chain of the IL-2 receptor. Science 1994;266(5187):1039-42.

158. Antoniou A, McCormick D, Scott D, et al. T cell tolerance and activation to a transgene-encoded tumor antigen. Eur J Immunol 1996;26(5):1094-102.

159. Toes REM, Blom RJJ, Offringa R, Kast WM, Melief CJM. Enhanced tumor outgrowth after peptide vaccination -Functional deletion of tumor-specific CTL induced by peptide vaccination can lead to the inability to reject tumors. J Immunol 1996;156(10):3911-8.

160. Hersey P, Si ZY, Smith MJ, Thomas WD. Expression of the co-stimulatory molecule B7 on melanoma cells. Int J Cancer 1994;58(4):527-32.

161. Antonia SJ, Munozantonia T, Soldevila G, Miller J, Flavell RA. B7-1 expression by a non-antigen presenting cell-derived tumor. Cancer Res 1995;55(11):2253-6.

162. Denfeld RW, Dietrich A, Wuttig C, et al. In situ expression of B7 and CD28 receptor families in human malignant melanoma: Relevance for T-cell-mediated anti-tumor immunity. Int J Cancer 1995;62(3):259-65.

163. Leach DR, Krummel MF, Allison JP. Enhancement of antitumor immunity by CTLA-4 blockade. Science 1996;271(5256):1734-6.

164. Shrikant P, Khoruts A, Mescher MF. CTLA-4 blockade reverses CD8(+) T cell tolerance to tumor by a CD4(+) T cell-and IL-2-dependent mechanism. Immunity 1999;11(4):483-93.

165. Hutloff A, Dittrich AM, Beier KC, et al. ICOS is an inducible T-cell co-stimulator structurally and functionally related to CD28. Nature 1999;397(6716):263-6.

166. Lee PP, Yee C, Savage PA, et al. Characterization of circulating T cells specific for tumor-associated antigens in melanoma patients. Nature Med 1999;5(6):677-85.

167. Garrido F, Ruizcabello F, Cabrera T, et al. Implications for immunosurveillance of altered HLA class I phenotypes in human tumours. Immunol Today 1997;18(2):89-95.

168. Goepel JR, Rees RC, Rogers K, Stoddard CJ, Thomas WEG, Shepherd L. Loss of Monomorphic and Polymorphic HLA Antigens in Metastatic Breast and Colon Carcinoma. Br J Cancer 1991;64:880-3.

169. Kageshita T, Hirai S, Ono T, Hicklin DJ, Ferrone S. Down-regulation of HLA class I antigen-processing molecules in malignant melanoma - Association with disease progression. Amer J Pathol 1999;154(3):745-54.

170. Amiot L, Onno M, Lamy T, et al. Loss of HLA molecules in B lymphomas is associated with an aggressive clinical course. Br J Haematol 1998;100(4):655-63.

171. Geertsen RC, Hofbauer GFL, Yue FY, Manolio S, Burg G, Dummer R. Higher frequency of selective losses of HLA-A and -B allospecificities in metastasis than in primary melanoma lesions. J Invest Dermatol 1998;111(3):497-502.

172. Cabrera T, Fernandez MA, Sierra A, et al. High frequency of altered HLA class I phenotypes in invasive breast carcinomas. Hum Immunol 1996;50(2):127-34.

173. Restifo NP, Esquivel F, Kawakami Y, et al. Identification of Human Cancers Deficient in Antigen Processing. J Exp Med 1993;177:265-72.

174. Cromme FV, Airey J, Heemels MT, et al. Loss of Transporter Protein, Encoded by the Tap-1 Gene, Is Highly Correlated with Loss of HLA Expression in Cervical Carcinomas. J Exp Med 1994;179(1):335-40.

175. Korkolopoulou P, Kaklamanis L, Pezzella F, Harris AL, Gatter KC. Loss of antigen-presenting molecules (MHC class I and TAP-1) in lung cancer. Br J Cancer 1996;73(2):148-53.

176. Sanda MG, Restifo NP, Walsh JC, et al. Molecular characterization of defective antigen processing in human prostate cancer. J Nat Cancer Inst 1995;87(4):280-5.

177. Chen HL, Gabrilovich D, Tampe R, Girgis KR, Nadaf S, Carbone DP. A functionally defective allele of TAP1 results in loss of MHC class I antigen presentation in a human lung cancer. Nat Genet 1996;13(2):210-3.

178. Seliger B, Hohne A, Jung D, et al. Expression and function of the peptide transporters in escape variants of human renal cell carcinomas. Exp Hematol 1997;25(7):608-14.

179. Traversari C, Meazza R, Coppolecchia M, et al. IFN-gamma gene transfer restores HLA-class I expression and MAGE-3 antigen presentation to CTL in HLA-deficient small cell lung cancer. Gene Therapy 1997;4(10):1029-35.

180. Johnsen A, France J, Sy MS, Harding CV. Down-regulation of the transporter for antigen presentation, proteasome subunits, and class I major histocompatibility complex in tumor cell lines. Cancer Res 1998;58(16):3660-7.

181. Johnsen AK, Templeton DJ, Sy MS, Harding CV. Deficiency of transporter for antigen presentation (TAP) in tumor cells allows evasion of immune surveillance and increases tumorigenesis. J Immunol 1999;163(8):4224-31.

182. Maeurer MJ, Gollin SM, Martin D, et al. Tumor escape from immune recognition - Lethal recurrent melanoma in a patient associated with downregulation of the peptide transporter protein TAP-1 and loss of expression of the immunodominant MART-1/Melan-A antigen. J Clin Invest 1996;98(7):1633-41.

183. Wells AD, Rai SK, Salvato MS, Band H, Malkovsky M. Restoration of MHC class I surface expression and endogenous antigen presentation by a molecular chaperone. Scand J Immunol 1997;45(6):605-12.

184. Wang ZG, Marincola FM, Rivoltini L, Parmiani G, Ferrone S. Selective histocompatibility leukocyte antigen (HLA)-A2 loss caused by aberrant pre-mRNA splicing in 624MEL28 melanoma cells. J Exp Med 1999;190(2):205-15.

185. Hicklin DJ, Wang ZG, Arienti F, Rivoltini L, Parmiani G, Ferrone S. beta 2-microglobulin mutations, HLA class I antigen loss, and tumor progression in melanoma. J Clin Invest 1998;101(12):2720-9.

186. Benitez R, Godelaine D, LopezNevot MA, et al. Mutations of the beta(2)-microglobulin gene result in a lack of HLA class I molecules on melanoma cells of two patients immunized with MAGE peptides. Tissue Antigen 1998;52(6):520-9.

187. Branch P, Bicknell DC, Rowan A, Bodmer WF, Karran P. Immune surveillance in colorectal carcinoma. Nat Genet 1995;9(3):231-2.

188. Koeppen H, Acena M, Drolet A, Rowley DA, Schreiber H. Tumors with Reduced Expression of a Cytotoxic T Lymphocyte Recognized Antigen Lack Immunogenicity But Retain Sensitivity to Lysis by Cytotoxic T Lymphocytes. Eur J Immunol 1993;23(11):2770-6.

189. Pende D, Accame L, Pareti L, et al. The susceptibility to natural killer cell-mediated lysis of HLA class I-positive melanomas reflects the expression of insufficient amounts of different HLA class I alleles. Eur J Immunol 1998;28(8):2384-94.

190. Suzue K, Zhou XZ, Eisen HN, Young RA. Heat shock fusion proteins as vehicles for antigen delivery into the major histocompatibility complex class I presentation pathway. Proc Natl Acad Sci USA 1997;94(24):13146-51.

191. Moretta A, Bottino C, Vitale M, et al. Receptors for HLA class-I molecules in human natural killer cells. Annu Rev Immunol; 14619-648.

192. Lanier LL, Phillips JH. Inhibitory MHC class I receptors on NK cells and T cells. Immunol Today 1996;17(2):86-91.

193. Lehmann F, Marchand M, Hainaut P, et al. Differences in the antigens recognized by cytolytic T cells on two successive metastases of a melanoma patient are consistent with immune selection. Eur J Immunol 1995;25(2):340-7.

194. Ikeda H, Lethé B, Lehmann F, et al. Characterization of an antigen that is recognized on a melanoma showing partial HLA loss by CTL expressing an NK inhibitory receptor. Immunity 1997;6:199-208.

195. Ikeda H, Lethe B, Lehmann F, et al. Characterization of an antigen that is recognized on a melanoma showing partial HLA loss by CTL expressing an NK inhibitory receptor. Immunity 1997;6(2):199-208.

196. Speiser DE, Pittet MJ, Valmori D, et al. In vivo expression of natural killer cell inhibitory receptors by human melanoma-specific cytolytic T lymphocytes. J Exp Med 1999;190(6):775-82.

197. Mingari MC, Ponte M, Bertone S, et al. HLA class I-specific inhibitory receptors in human T lymphocytes: Interleukin 15-induced expression of CD94/NKG2A in superantigen- or alloantigen-activated CD8(+) T cells. Proc Natl Acad Sci USA 1998;95(3):1172-7.

198. Guerra N, Benlhassan K, Carayol G, et al. Effect of tumor growth factor-beta on NK receptor expression by allostimulated CD8(+) T lymphocytes. Eur Cytokine Netw 1999;10(3):357-63.

199. Noppen C, Schaefer C, Zajac P, et al. C-type lectin-like receptors in peptide-specific HLA class I-restricted cytotoxic T lymphocytes: differential expression and modulation of effector functions in clones sharing identical TCR structure and epitope specificity. Eur J Immunol 1998;28(4):1134-42.

200. Paul P, RouasFreiss N, KhalilDaher I, et al. HLA-G expression in melanoma: A way for tumor cells to escape from immunosurveillance. Proc Natl Acad Sci USA 1998;95(8):4510-5.

201. LeGal FA, Riteau B, Sedlik C, et al. HLA-G-mediated inhibition of antigen-specific cytotoxic T lymphocytes. Int Immunol 1999;11(8):1351-6.

202. Robbins PF, Elgamil M, Li YF, et al. Cloning of a new gene encoding an antigen recognized by melanoma-specific HLA-A24-restricted tumor-infiltrating lymphocytes. J Immunol 1995;154(11):5944-50.

203. Cormier JN, Abati A, Fetsch P, et al. Comparative analysis of the in vivo expression of tyrosinase, MART-1/Melan-A, and gp100 in metastatic melanoma lesions: Implications for immunotherapy. J Immunother 1998;21(1):27-31.

204. Hofbauer GFL, Kamarashev J, Geertsen R, Boni R, Dummer R. Melan A/MART-1 immunoreactivity in formalin-fixed paraffin-embedded primary and metastatic melanoma: frequency and distribution. Melanoma Res 1998;8(4):337-43.

205. Lee KH, Panelli MC, Kim CJ, et al. Functional dissociation between local and systemic immune response during anti-melanoma peptide vaccination. J Immunol 1998;161(8):4183-94.

206. Valmori D, Lienard D, Waanders G, Rimoldi D, Cerottini JC, Romero P. Analysis of MAGE-3-specific cytolytic T lymphocytes in human leukocyte antigen-A2 melanoma patients. Cancer Res 1997;57(4):735-41.

207. Lethe B, Vanderbruggen P, Brasseur F, Boon T. MAGE-1 expression threshold for the lysis of melanoma cell lines by a specific cytotoxic T lymphocyte. Melanoma Res 1997;7:S83-8.

208. Jager E, Ringhoffer M, Karbach J, Arand M, Oesch F, Knuth A. Inverse relationship of melanocyte differentiation antigen expression in melanoma tissues and CD8(+) cytotoxic-T-cell responses: Evidence for immunoselection of antigen-loss variants in vivo. Int J Cancer 1996;66(4):470-6.

209. Jager E, Ringhoffer M, Altmannsberger M, et al. Immunoselection in vivo: Independent loss of MHC class I and melanocyte differentiation antigen expression in metastatic melanoma. Int J Cancer 1997;71(2):142-7.

210. Chaux P, Moutet M, Faivre J, Martin F, Martin M. Inflammatory cells infiltrating human colorectal carcinomas express HLA class II but not B7-1 and B7-2 costimulatory molecules of the T-cell activation. Lab Invest 1996;74(5):975-83.

211. Ninomiya T, Akbar F, Masumoto T, Horiike N, Onji M. Dendritic cells with immature phenotype and defective function in the peripheral blood from patients with hepatocellular carcinoma. J Hepatol 1999;31(2):323-31.

212. Nestle FO, Burg G, Fah J, Wronesmith T, Nickoloff BJ. Human sunlight-induced basal-cell-carcinoma-associated dendritic cells are deficient in T cell co-stimulatory molecules and are impaired as antigen-presenting cells. Am J Pathol 1997;150(2):641-51.

213. Enk AH, Jonuleit H, Saloga J, Knop J. Dendritic cells as mediators of tumor-induced tolerance in metastatic melanoma. Int J Cancer 1997;73(3):309-16.

214. Bell D, Chomarat P, Broyles D, et al. In breast carcinoma tissue, immature dendritic cells reside within the tumor, whereas mature dendritic cells are located in peritumoral areas. J Exp Med 1999;190(10):1417-25.

215. Girolomoni G, Ricciardicastagnoli P. Dendritic cells hold promise for immunotherapy. Immunol Today 1997;18(3):102-4.

216. Qin ZH, Noffz G, Mohaupt M, Blankenstein T. Interleukin-10 prevents dendritic cell accumulation and vaccination with granulocyte-macrophage colony-stimulating factor gene-modified tumor cells. J Immunol 1997;159(2):770-6.

217. Sharma S, Stolina M, Lin Y, et al. T cell-derived IL-10 promotes lung cancer growth by suppressing both T cell and APC function. J Immunol 1999;163(9):5020-8.

218. Liu LM, Rich BE, Inobe J, Chen WJ, Weiner HL. Induction of T(h)2 cell differentiation in the primary immune response: dendritic cells isolated from adherent cell culture treated with IL-10 prime naive CD4(+) T cells to secrete IL-4. Int Immunol 1998;10(8):1017-26.

219. Thomas GR, Chen Z, Oechsli MN, Hendler FJ, VanWaes C. Decreased expression of CD80 is a marker for increased tumorigenicity In a new murine model of oral squamous-cell carcinoma. Int J Cancer 1999;82(3):377-84.

220. Zheng P, Sarma S, Guo Y, Liu Y. Two mechanisms for tumor evasion of preexisting cytotoxic T-cell responses: Lessons from recurrent tumors. Cancer Res 1999;59(14):3461-7.

221. Koyama S, Maruyama T, Adachi S, Nozue M. Expression of costimulatory molecules, B7-1 and B7-2 on human gastric carcinoma. J Cancer Res Clin Oncol 1998;124(7):383-8.

222. Stremmel C, Greenfield EA, Howard E, Freeman GJ, Kuchroo VK. B7-2 expressed on EL4 lymphoma suppresses antitumor immunity by an interleukin 4-dependent mechanism. J Exp Med 1999;189(6):919-30.

223. vonLeoprechting A, vanderBruggen P, Pahl HL, Aruffo A, Simon JC. Stimulation of CD40 on immunogenic human malignant melanomas augments their cytotoxic T lymphocyte-mediated lysis and induces apoptosis. Cancer Res 1999;59(6):1287-94.

224. Vora AR, Rodgers S, Parker AJ, Start R, Rees RC, Murray AK. An immunohistochemical study of altered immunomodulatory molecule expression in head and neck squamous cell carcinoma. Br J Cancer 1997;76(7):836-44.

225. Pandolfi F, Trentin L, Boyle LA, et al. Expression of Cell Adhesion Molecules in Human Melanoma Cell Lines and Their Role in Cytotoxicity Mediated by Tumor-Infiltrating Lymphocytes. Cancer 1992;69:1165-73.

226. LeGuiner S, LeDrean E, Labarriere N, et al. LFA-3 co-stimulates cytokine secretion by cytotoxic T lymphocytes by providing a TCR-independent activation signal. Eur J Immunol 1998;28(4):1322-31.

227. Anichini A, Mortarini R, Alberti S, Mantovani A, Parmiani G. T-Cell-Receptor Engagement and Tumor ICAM-1 Up-Regulation Are Required to by-Pass Low Susceptibility of Melanoma Cells to Autologous CTL-Mediated Lysis. Int J Cancer 1993;53:994-1001.

228. Anichini A, Mortarini R, Parmiani G. beta(1)-Integrins on Melanoma Clones Regulate the Interaction with Autologous Cytolytic T-Cell Clones. J Immunother 1992;12:183-6.

229. Yue FY, Dummer R, Geertsen R, et al. Interleukin-10 is a growth factor for human melanoma cells and down-regulates HLA class-1, HLA class-II and ICAM-1 molecules. Int J Cancer 1997;71(4):630-7.

230. Koulis A, Diss T, Isaacson PG, Dogan A. Characterization of tumor-infiltrating T lymphocytes in B-cell lymphomas of mucosa-associated lymphoid tissue. Am J Pathol 1997;151(5):1353-60.

231. Nakamoto Y, Guidotti LG, Kuhlen CV, Fowler P, Chisari FV. Immune pathogenesis of hepatocellular carcinoma. J Exp Med 1998;188(2):341-50.

232. Hudson JD, Shoaibi MA, Maestro R, Carnero A, Hannon GJ, Beach DH. A proinflammatory cytokine inhibits p53 tumor suppressor activity. J Exp Med 1999;190(10):1375-82.

233. Thomas WD, Smith MJ, Si Z, Hersey P. Expression of the co-stimulatory molecule CD40 on melanoma cells. Int J Cancer 1996;68(6):795-801.

234. Peoples GE, Blotnick S, Takahashi K, Freeman MR, Klagsbrun M, Eberlein TJ. T lymphocytes that infiltrate tumors and atherosclerotic plaques produce heparin-binding epidermal growth factor-like growth factor and basic fibroblast growth factor: A potential pathologic role. Proc Natl Acad Sci USA 1995;92(14):6547-51.

235. Freeman MR, Schneck FX, Gagnon ML, et al. Peripheral blood T lymphocytes and lymphocytes infiltrating human cancers express vascular endothelial growth factor: A potential role for T cells in angiogenesis. Cancer Res 1995;55(18):4140-5.

Index

INDEX

Immunology and Medicine Series

Kluwer Academic Publishers – Dordrecht / Boston / London